FROM
SILENCE
TO
VOICE

What Nurses
Know and Must
Communicate
to the Public

FROM SILENCE TO VOICE

What Nurses Know and Must Communicate to the Public

Bernice Buresh and Suzanne Gordon

Foreword by Patricia Benner, RN, PhD, FAAN
Afterword by Mary Ellen Jeans, RN, PhD

ILR PRESS
an imprint of
Cornell University Press
Ithaca and London

First published 2000 by Canadian Nurses Association
First printing, ILR Press/Cornell Paperbacks, 2003

Some of the material in this book originally appeared in other forms in the
American Journal of Nursing, Revolution, The Nation, and *Kango: The Japanese
Journal of Nursing.* For further information, visit the *From Silence to Voice*
website at www.silencetovoice.com.

Edited by Wendy McPeake
Designed by Aerographics
Printed in the United States of America

Librarians: A CIP catalog record for this book is available from the Library
of Congress.

Cornell University Press strives to use environmentally responsible suppliers
and materials to the fullest extent possible in the publishing of its books.
Such materials include vegetable-based, low-VOC inks and acid-free papers
that are recycled, totally chlorine-free, or partly composed of nonwood fibers.
For further information, visit our website at www.cornellpress.cornell.edu.

Paperback printing   10 9 8 7 6 5 4 3 2 1

For Peggy O'Malley, RN

And In Memory of Nancy Buresh

CONTENTS

FOREWORD

In *From Silence to Voice*, Bernice Buresh and Suzanne Gordon, two well-known feminist journalists, have given nurses:

- A gift of clearly stated respect for the worth of nursing work.
- A manifesto calling on nurses to apply their courage and develop their skills to speak out forcefully and effectively to the public and in the media.
- A practical step-by-step guide providing inspiring, confident approaches to increasing nurses' visibility and voice in media and policy arenas.

I came to this text with full appreciation for the power that nurses acquire when they articulate the skill and knowledge that is embedded in their practice. For many years, part of my work has been to help nurses construct clinical narratives that are self-informing both professionally and personally. We have found that discerning and describing the knowledge, competence and skill that goes into day-to-day nursing work allows nurses themselves to comprehend their work in a more empowering way. It increases nurses' mastery and appreciation of their own work, and, by extension, nurses' ability to better care for patients. The articulation of nursing work can not only spur hospital management, politicians and policy makers to value and reward nursing, it contributes to nurses valuing themselves and each other.

Buresh and Gordon teach nurses how to give voice and presence to their knowledge in the public media in a vivid and dynamic way. Spending time with this work can be a transformative experience. Reading this book gave me an expanded vision and renewed enthusiasm for improving health care by making nursing practice visible to the public and the media. The authors convincingly explain why nurses must take the risk to be heard and to be visible. They show why it is essential for nurses to bridge the communication gap between the profession and the greater public. Nothing less than living in a safer and healthier society is at stake.

Without the authors' passionate vision for the worth of nursing work, this particular book could not have been written. They do not trivialize nursing by dressing it up in others' power suits. They oppose the sham of false advertising that sells nursing as the latest hot commodity in a fickle marketplace. Rather they direct the reader to the real societal worth of nurses' knowledgeable care of the vulnerable, the sick and the injured. They point to both the wisdom of the heart and mind in nursing practice. They are sure, as they put it, that: "Nurses can articulate their thoughts, find the right words to describe their work, do so in a confident way that doesn't sound boastful or self-aggrandizing, believe in their own knowledge and ability to acquire more, answer tough questions, and tolerate making the occasional mistake. In doing so, nurses will reveal what it really means to be 'just a nurse.'"

The authors write this vivid text with the experience of having covered marginalized groups, and after working with nurses for more than a decade. Bernice Buresh, through her teaching and research, has raised consciousness about the problem of nursing silence in the media. Her astute monitoring of media has demonstrated a sustained absence of nursing knowledge in the coverage of health care.

Both authors practice what they preach and the book is full of their experiential learning. I offer my own anecdote. Shortly after *The Primacy of Caring: Stress and Coping in Health and Illness* was published in 1989, my co-author, Judith Wrubel, and I were surprised to read a review of it in the *Washington Post*. It was written by Suzanne Gordon who clearly understood the worth of caregiving work and insisted that this book should not be lost to the public in the nursing publishing ghetto. We immediately called Gordon and thanked her (a strategy recommended in *From Silence to Voice*). She said she had learned that the journalists who covered health care at the *Post* did not have nurses among their expert sources. She suggested the names of nurses that they could contact. Several years later, Buresh and Gordon developed a directory of nursing sources for journalists.

Since then I have observed Suzanne Gordon's unswerving commitment to increasing public awareness of nursing, as exemplified by her influential 1997 book, *Life Support: Three Nurses on the Frontlines*. As a team, Buresh and Gordon are powerful voices for nursing and teach us how nursing can be heard by the public and in the mass media.

From Silence to Voice is a practical guide. From it nurses can learn how to get their stories, insights, research, and expert opinions to the public and into the media. The authors give away many insider secrets on how the media— print, the Internet, radio, and television—work, how they are interrelated, and, most importantly, how to influence them and the political debate about the future of our health care systems. I commend this book to every nurse and believe that it should be a required text for all nursing students.

Patricia Benner, RN, PhD, FAAN
Professor of Nursing
University of California, San Francisco

ACKNOWLEDGEMENTS

It was not until Suzanne Gordon and I were engaged in writing this book that I understood how central the theme, From Silence to Voice, has been to my life and work. To be sure, the struggle for voice is not limited to women. Anyone involved in the three areas that have occupied my professional life—journalism, education and writing—is grappling with external and internal restraints on free expression. Still, we must not overlook the cultural constraints that have stilled the authentic voices, and writing hands, of so many women.

Women artists and writers began to explore these constraints in earnest in the 1970s. I joined my first women's writers' group then and have since belonged to others. While these groups often focused on practical matters (how to approach an editor or agent with a particular project, for example), they were nothing if not vehicles for women to make the transition from silence to voice in their own art. I wish, now, to thank members of those groups who contributed so much to my understanding of these issues. I am particularly grateful to Janet H. Murray, Diana Korzenik, and Katherine Butler Jones for their interest in and thoughtful suggestions for this book. I would like to thank them also and the following writers—Ann Banks, Celia Gilbert, Phyllis Karas, Gail Mazur, Carolyn Toll Oppenheim, Harriet Reisen, Caryl Rivers, Janet Robertson, Trudy Rubin, and Barbara Sirota—for fundamental support that has been sustaining over the years.

The genesis of this book occurred in a setting dedicated to fostering democratic discourse and political participation—the Joan Shorenstein Center on the Press, Politics and Public Policy at Harvard University's John F. Kennedy School of Government. I was a fellow there in 1989 and was exploring a question that I had found intriguing while covering political movements and in my previous teaching at Boston University. It was: Why are women so underrepresented as "newsmakers" and as expert sources in the media?

The canonical answer was that women would appear in the news when more of them achieved "newsworthy" positions. But that answer raised more questions. Why were certain positions worthy of coverage and others not? What of the professions where women already were in the majority, like health care (as nurses as opposed to doctors), education (as teachers as opposed to professors) and social and caregiving work (as care providers as opposed to policy makers)? Why weren't the activities of these women also worthy of our journalistic attention? These sorts of questions led to my professional association with Suzanne Gordon and to our exploration of who in our society gets to be seen and heard. I am immensely grateful to Marvin Kalb of the Shorenstein Center for providing a launching site for this inquiry, and to Nancy Palmer for her many kindnesses. I would especially like to thank Lawrence K. Grossman for extending his expertise and encouragement for all of these years.

A considerable amount of the writing, editing and thinking that I have done in connection with this book took place in the Writers' Room of Boston, a place that provides the silence for writers to hear their own voices. My heartfelt thanks go to all of the writers who have contributed to the special nature of the Writers' Room. In particular, I would like to thank Ivan Gold, Nancy Kassell and Donald E. Cecich, with whom I have had the pleasure of working closely, for all they have done to make the Writers' Room possible. There are two other people I want to mention for contributing to "voice" in other ways: Elinor M. Siner and Barry Kesselman. I am grateful to Barbara C. Wallace and M. Monteen Lucas for sharing their knowledge about nursing.

The first nurse I ever knew was my aunt Theresa H. Reineck whose work was a source of family pride. Now there are other nurses in the family, my niece, Cathy Buresh, and my cousin Beth Halusan. My mother, Erna H. Byrne, has followed the progress of this book every inch of the way. I am grateful to her and to my brother Theodore F. Buresh and my sister Gail Schank for their support. My greatest thanks go to Irwin Oppenheim, my husband, and to Josh Buresh-Oppenheim, my son, for being never-ending sources of love, strength and sanctuary.

Finally, it may seem peculiar to acknowledge the co-author of a co-authored book. But Suzanne Gordon has been a valued friend and colleague, and, by thinking up the title, *From Silence to Voice*, has crystallized for me, for other women and for caregivers, the passage we must continue to make.

Bernice Buresh
Cambridge, Massachusetts
April 2000

For over a decade, Bernice Buresh and I have been holding a vibrant conversation that has informed this book. Our ability to not only agree, but to disagree—even fight over words, phrases and ideas—has helped me to clarify my ideas about nurses' and women's issues. I am deeply grateful to nursing for bringing me together with this true colleague and dear friend.

I also want to thank my oldest friend, Isabel Marcus, for the intellectual companionship that has been so important to this and to other work.

Claire Fagin and Joan Lynaugh have been my tireless guides into the world of nursing. They have graciously responded to an endless stream of phone calls beginning with the white lie, "Do you have a minute?" when I knew it would be more like an hour. In my work and discussions with Ellen Baer I have come to better grasp the complexity of the tapestry of nursing care. I also want to thank Patricia Benner and Christine Tanner for their extraordinary ability to describe what nurses know and do, and their willingness to share their insights with this non-nurse. There have been countless exchanges with Victoria Palmer Erbs, Elizabeth Grady, Trish Gibbons, and Ptlene Minick for which I am grateful. Kathleen Dracup not only taught me about nursing, she allowed me to be her "nurse" when she needed care. That experience enriched my understanding of how difficult it is to think like a nurse.

Charlene Harrington, Alan Sager, Deborah Socolar, and Timothy McCall have been navigators through the health policy issues that are so critical to this book. I owe a tremendous debt of thanks to Joyce Clifford, Kathy Horvath, Mitchell Rabkin, and Antony Swartz-Lloyd for giving a journalist unrestricted access to the Beth Israel Hospital when I was writing *Life Support: Three Nurses on the Front Lines*. But my largest debt is to Jean Chaisson, Nancy Rumplik and Ellen Kitchen for sharing their lives and work with me for over three years.

I cannot thank Laurie Gottlieb enough for the opportunity to teach nurses at the McGill School of Nursing, and Genevieve E. Chandler for numerous opportunities to share her ideas and meet with her students at the University of Massachusetts School of Nursing at Amherst. I also want to thank Sioban Nelson, Shinya Sato, Masako Hayano, Yumiko Katsuhara, Tom Keighley, Linda Thomas, and Inger Holter for helping to give this book an international scope so that nurses can mount a global challenge to the mistaken idea that caregivers must be silent and invisible.

Suzanne Gordon
Arlington, Massachusetts
April 2000

We are enormously grateful to Maureen Farrington, Ondina Love and Serge Duguay at the Canadian Nurses Association for their work in making this book a reality, and to our editor, Wendy McPeake, for making it a pleasurable experience as well.

We would also like to thank Judith Shindul Rothschild, Karen Daley, Barry Adams, Sandy Eaton, Ann Eldridge, Michael Malone, Paul Lehman, Beth Blacksin, Echo Heron, and Diana J. Mason for their strong voices on behalf of nursing.

The work of Julie Sochalski, Linda H. Aiken and Barbara Norrish has been invaluable in contributing to knowledge about nursing. In Canada, Kathleen Connors, Debra McPherson, Judith Shamian, Carole Presseault, Mary Ellen Jeans, Pat and Hugh Armstrong, and Jackie Larkin have helped us understand what a publicly funded universal health care system can offer to both caregivers and those they care for.

We are very grateful to the following for responding so generously to our many requests in the midst of their demanding schedules: Chuck Idelson at the California Nurses Association, Anne Schott at the New York State Nurses Association, David Schildmeier at the Massachusetts Nurses Association, Joan Meehan Hurwitz at the American Nurses Association, Dan Mezibov at the American Association of Colleges of Nursing, Art Moses at the British Columbia Nurses Union, Vera Chernecki at the Manitoba Nurses' Union, Jamie Cohen at the Service Employees International Union, and Rick Brooks, Linda McDonald, and the nurses at the United Nurses & Allied Professionals in Rhode Island.

BB and SG

INTRODUCTION

When we began working on the relationship between nursing and public communication more than a decade ago, we were convinced that the key to increasing the public visibility of the nursing profession lay in reversing the media's indifference to nursing. We believed that once we documented the lack of coverage of nursing and understood why journalists seemed to ignore nursing, it would be possible for nurses and nursing organizations to master communication recipes and construct a plan to make themselves more visible.

Our assumption was based on years of experience covering marginalized groups that had succeeded in getting national attention. We have been journalists and writers all of our professional lives. Although our careers differ, between the two of us we have covered most of the political and social movements in the United States from the 1960s to the end of the 20th century. We have known and written about participants in the civil rights, women's, anti-war, gay rights, labor, and community organizing movements, to name a few. We have also covered mainstream elective politics. Throughout this period, marginalized and subjugated groups won important legal and social victories by bringing their agendas to the forefront of public attention.

Although the issues confronting nursing in terms of its public visibility are not identical to those of other groups, we felt then, and still do, that much can be learned from the experiences of others. Over the years, however, we learned that we had initially underestimated the complexity of cultural imperatives in the relationship between nursing and the external public world. We once thought that nursing could become significantly more visible by using more or less standard public relations techniques—and even wrote a first draft of a book for nurses just on public relations and communications skills. Now we believe that the subject must be approached differently. We believe that a paramount obstacle is the reluctance of nurses to use communication skills. Hence our metaphors have changed. We started out thinking in terms of the "invisibility" and "visibility" of nursing. Now we see the operative terms as "silence" and "voice." That is why we call this book *From Silence to Voice*.

Our inquiry into nursing and public communication began in 1990 when we served as consultants on journalism to a national public relations campaign in the US known as Nurses of America (NOA). NOA's goal was to rectify the nursing shortage by attracting high-quality candidates into the field. The Pew Charitable Trusts contributed almost a million dollars to this project which was administered by a council consisting of major nursing organizations.

Nurses of America sponsored activities designed to analyze public attitudes toward nurses and to project a positive image of contemporary nursing. The project undertook studies, monitored the media, distributed press materials, media-trained nurses so that they would be more skilled in talking to reporters and appearing on television, and conducted "media events" to stimulate coverage of nursing. We describe these activities in more detail in this book.

We were particularly interested in press coverage of nursing. We wanted to know whether and to what degree journalists used nurses and nursing organizations as sources of information on health and health care. We devised a study to examine the representation of nurses in the health coverage of three major newspapers.[1] This is an important line of inquiry because today a profession's public status and legitimacy is linked to having its expertise acknowledged in the journalistic media.

We were quite sure that nursing—the largest health care profession by far—would be shown to be vastly under-represented in news coverage. But we didn't expect nursing to be virtually missing from health reportage. This is what the study—Who Counts in News Coverage of Health Care?—documented.

According to our findings, practically everyone had more of a public voice on health and health care than nurses. When we analyzed the sources of 908 direct quotations by "occupation," we found that physicians were by far the most frequently quoted occupational group. They accounted for nearly one-third of the quotations. But nurses were not a close second, third, or even fourth. After physicians, 11 other groups were quoted more frequently than nurses. These included sources from government, business, nonprofit groups, education, public relations, and medical organizations, as well as patients, family members, and an assortment of professional and nonprofessional health workers. Nurses were at the bottom of the list accounting for only 10 (1.1 percent) of the quotations. No matter how we analyzed public visibility, nurses were either in or tied for last place.

This was a disturbing discovery and one with far-reaching implications. If there was little trace of nursing in the serious coverage of health and health care, then how could anyone, including those in a position to supply nursing with needed resources, understand and recognize its value? When medicine is consistently depicted as the center of the health care universe, then physicians will get credit for every contribution to health care, even in those instances when credit should go to nursing or another profession.

Concerned about what might be a systematic journalistic bias against nursing, we were determined to acquaint our fellow journalists, particularly those who specialize in health and medical reporting, with this serious omission in their reporting. Armed with the study, we and small groups of nurses met with journalists to discuss the fact that they seemed to be ignoring nurses as sources of health care information and nursing issues as news. We made sure our study was widely circulated. It was distributed to journalists at conferences and was reported on in the journalism trade press.

Many journalists acknowledged they knew nothing about nursing. To help them get a better grasp of the field, we prepared a media packet that presented basic information on nursing as well as materials on newsworthy nursing projects and biographies of nurses. These materials linked nursing with contemporary health care issues, suggested potential stories, and gave reporters the names of expert nurses to talk to.

Later on, with the support of major nursing organizations, we created a nursing source directory for journalists so that they would have the names of nurses, instead of just physicians, to call for information on health care.[2] This project was suggested by the Ms. Foundation for Communication and Education, Inc., which provided a grant to develop the directory.

In general, reporters and editors welcomed this material. Some readily acknowledged that they had not paid much attention to nursing. Many said they were interested in doing stories that included nurses. When groups of nurses provided them with materials on current health care issues, many in fact did do stories in which nurses were primary spokespersons. In most cases, when nurses sought a meeting with editorial boards to discuss health coverage, they received a positive response and engaged in serious discussions about how coverage could be improved.

At this point, the approaches to increasing the visibility of nursing seemed straightforward enough. The news media constituted the major conduit. Nurses had to work on educating journalists about nursing so that they would be more receptive to covering the profession. Nurses and nursing organizations had to be much more active in presenting journalists with newsworthy material. All this could be accomplished if more nurses developed public communication skills. Indeed, we would write a public communications book for nurses that would help them develop these skills.

We anticipated that the Nurses of America project would provide the foundation for an ongoing communication program carried out cooperatively by the nursing organizations involved, and there was some discussion of such a plan. We also expected nurses who had been media trained to take an active role in media outreach. We wrote articles about nursing ourselves and thought that more journalists would routinely cover nursing.

As nursing came under siege in the health care upheaval that began in the mid-1990s, some courageous nurses did speak up. But this was still not enough. Indeed, journalists complained that when they sought out nursing sources, they were frustrated in their attempts to find nurses who would do even the basics of communication—return their phone calls or answer simple questions about their work.

These complaints were echoed by public relations specialists in nursing organizations and nursing schools who were trying to increase coverage. They might interest a journalist in a story idea and then be unable to find nurses willing to talk to reporters, even about non-controversial subjects or to describe positive examples of nursing practice.

Ten years later journalists are still saying that information about nursing does not come to them routinely. While doctors who conduct medical research are usually willing to explore the implications of their work, nurses, they say, often shut down when asked to express an informed opinion. Nurses, many reporters tell us, seem terrified of expressing strong opinions and seem overly concerned that they might offend someone. In fact, nurses don't reach out to journalists and don't make journalists' work easier, or even possible, by providing necessary information and by returning telephone calls to journalists trying to reach a nurse before deadline.

This has also been our experience in writing about nursing and in speaking with nurses. Despite what nurses, nursing institutions and nursing organizations say about wanting nursing to gain more recognition from the public, we have found great reluctance on the part of individual nurses and nursing organizations to do what is necessary to create such recognition. Indeed, nurses often seem as hesitant to tell their friends and relatives about their work as they are to tell the *New York Times* or the *Globe and Mail*.

Public communication skills are important to nurses. That's why half of this book is devoted to them. But the willingness of nurses to use these skills is even more important. Over the last decade we have come to believe that there is a profound ambivalence in nursing about whether it is even advisable to be more visible, more vocal, and to have a larger role on the public stage.

Therefore, the first chapter of this book, "Ending the Silence," envisions the benefits to nurses and to health care if the public knew and understood the importance of nursing.

In chapter two we take a serious look at the systematic, although often unacknowledged, conditioning that goes on within nursing to inhibit the public communication that would make nursing known. We introduce the concept of a "voice of agency"—a concept that could make it possible for nurses to move comfortably from silence to voice.

Taking the private voice public, as Genevieve E. Chandler[3] describes it, is an incremental process that begins in the workplace, in the home, and in the community. Even nurses who never have contact with the news media are public communicators through the way they present themselves. Therefore, chapter three concentrates on self-presentation and first impressions. In chapter four, "Tell the World What You Do," we define "the world" as being the people nurses know and work with every day as well as the mass media or larger public, and the "what you know" as being the intellectual and experiential knowledge of nurses. While it is critically important for nurses to communicate through the mass media, we also believe there are many other "publics" nurses must educate. The techniques a nurse uses in talking with a patient, a family member, a neighbor, or a friend about her work are vitally important, and they are transferable. A nurse who can talk comfortably about nursing with family or friends can also talk effectively on the radio or television or to a reporter. So we start the communication process by describing how to communicate with the people nurses encounter in every day life. This chapter also examines fears and internal obstacles nurses have told us they confront. Many of these inhibitions can be understood and managed by exploring their sources and by testing them in the real world.

Because the mass media are so powerful in shaping people's views of reality, and because they reflect the visibility of a profession, the second half of this book concentrates on mass communication and the media. It is clear that the media have too often neglected nursing or even promoted unfortunate stereotypes of the profession. But a careful examination reveals that when nurses have engaged in outreach and exerted pressure, the results have been very promising.

In section II readers will learn how to write a news release—the basic tool for communicating with the media; how to assemble other press materials; and how to develop media strategies to achieve specific goals. We also show how nursing groups have organized special events and media campaigns to publicize their programs and further their goals.

This section devotes a chapter to publicizing nursing research, one of the most promising ways of acquainting the public with nursing expertise in health care. But communicating the knowledge that goes into nursing is not the exclusive province of nurses who are scholars, researchers or organizational leaders. Every nurse, as we explain in chapter nine, can learn how to write letters to the editor and newspaper op-ed essays. We demonstrate the elements of these forms so that every nurse can present her or his experience, insights, innovations, and policy proposals.

The elements of communication are similar whether they are used in print, on the Internet, or on radio and television. All communication depends on organizing messages to get across the most important points. We devote a chapter specifically to communication techniques for radio and television because they are the most popular media in our society.

Sometimes nurses berate themselves because they feel they don't have good public communication skills. They assume that knowledge in this field is instinctual, when, in fact, it is learned. Most nurses went to school to learn how to take care of patients, not how to speak about nursing on television.

Effective public communication depends on writing and speaking skills. These skills are learned, practiced and constantly refined. Successful communicators in every field become effective through instruction and practice. So can nurses. But nurses don't have to be expert in every aspect of public communication. They can call upon the assistance of public relations specialists whose work we describe in chapter seven.

We'd like to explain our choice of certain language in *From Silence to Voice*. Most of the time, for expediency, we use "we" in recounting situations involving one or the other or both of us. We refer to ourselves as Gordon or Buresh when it is necessary for clarity.

Although we talk a great deal about women's culture and its influence on nursing, our intention is not to exclude men who are nurses. Our purpose is to explore the legacy of women's socialization and gender stereotypes to nursing. Men in nursing are affected by these influences as well as women. Because the vast majority of nurses are women, the feminine pronoun is given preference.

Throughout this book we avoid the use of the word "consumer" or "customer" to describe the people nurses care for. This is a deliberate choice. The word consumer, as defined by the dictionary, has two meanings. One meaning is someone who consumes, spends, wastes or destroys. The second meaning, "a person who uses goods and services to satisfy his needs," pertains to economics. The first definition is negative, and the second is an extremely narrow, marketplace definition of human beings in relationship to sickness and health. We feel it seriously miscasts the relationship between caregivers and the people who seek their care and services.

Even though we understand the term's appeal in countering paternalistic language, replacing "patient" with a market term like "consumer" (or "customer") puts clinicians on very shaky ground. For the clinician, the moral injunction to do no harm can too easily be hijacked by the market ethic of *caveat emptor*, "Let the buyer beware." From the public communication perspective, talking about nurses in relation to consumers shifts attention from the hospital, home, clinic, or hospice to the shopping mall. It suggests that human beings can choose health the way they choose a new dress and can, therefore, exercise control when they are the least able to. We prefer to use the words "human being," "individual," "people," "patient," and "family."

We recognize that the problem of silence in nursing is an international one. In fact, this book itself is representative of an international approach to increasing the visibility of nursing. Written by American journalists, it is being published by a Canadian nursing organization. We hope this book will further the conversation about this topic among nurses throughout the world.

Like everyone else in journalism, and much of the public, we started out knowing nothing about nursing. No doubt, we accepted many of the traditional stereotypes without even realizing it. Our views have been revolutionized. Nurses were our teachers. They have explained their work to us, and expressed their insights about health and illness. We are profoundly in their debt. If we could be educated in this way, so can others.

Endnotes

1. Bernice Buresh, Suzanne Gordon, and Nica Bell, "Who Counts in News Coverage of Health Care?" *Nursing Outlook,* 39 no. 5 (1991): pp. 204–208.

2. Bernice Buresh, Suzanne Gordon, and eds., *A Journalist's Guide to Nursing Sources* (Women, Press & Politics Project, 1994).

3. Genevieve E. Chandler, "Taking the Private Voice Public: Sharing Nursing Knowledge," *Revolution: The Journal of Nurse Empowerment,* spring 1995, pp. 80–83.

SECTION I
SILENT
NO MORE

Chapter 1

ENDING
THE SILENCE

Envision how things would be if the voice and visibility of nursing were commensurate with the size and importance of nursing in health care.

The typical health care journalist's Rolodex™ would contain contact information on a full range of nursing sources. These sources would include not only the major nursing organizations and unions, but the names of individual nurses with expertise in various aspects of health care. The journalist would have many names of nurse researchers, public health nurses, nurse administrators, staff nurses, nurses with clinical subspecialties, nursing scholars, home-care nurses, nurse practitioners, and hospice nurses, among others.

Journalists would routinely contact nurses when they have questions about current health care topics, and, as a result, nurses would frequently appear as expert sources in news reports. Nurses would be quoted on all aspects of health care in newspapers and magazines, on radio and television, and on health Web sites. Nurses would be regular guests on such influential programs as "Nightline," the "Lehrer NewsHour" and "This Morning" as well as on local news and talk shows to discuss developments in health care.

No longer would medical research be perceived as the only scientific endeavor leading to health improvements. Health experts, journalists, policymakers, and the public would know about nursing research and would see it as a dynamic, evolving field that expands our knowledge about health care and the human condition. In fact, public support would lead to vastly increased governmental and private funding for nursing research.

The visibility of nurses in the mass media would reflect the expanded presence of nursing everywhere in the ongoing public discussion about health care. Nurses would participate in a broad spectrum of forums on health care in community centers, town meetings, state capitals, provincial/territorial legislatures, churches, schools, universities, consumers' and patients' organizations, economic conferences, the Canadian House of Commons and the US Congress.

Physicians' responses to health coverage would no longer dominate the letters-to-the-editor sections of influential newspapers in North America. Nursing perspectives expressed in letters written by hundreds of nurses would expand the knowledge and point of view of journalists and the public. Nurses would also contribute guest columns to the opinion sections of newspapers and magazines. Their articles and essays in, for example, "My Turn" in *Newsweek,* or on the op-ed pages of the *Boston Globe* and the the *Globe and Mail,* would include personal and ethical reflections, anecdotal accounts of their care of the sick and vulnerable, descriptions of their innovations in clinical practice, analyses of major health care issues, and recommendations addressing either the treatment of individual illnesses or broader system problems.

Nurses would not just sit at the tables of power where top echelon governmental, corporate, or academic experts make policy, they would be full-fledged vocal and assertive decision makers who would be listened to and respected for their views.

Because nurses would educate patients and their families, friends and relatives, neighbors, and community members about nursing work, patients would be fully cognizant of the fact that nurses are key to their survival and recovery. Just as people recognize that it takes someone with education and expertise to do brain surgery, they would know that it takes someone with education and expertise to care for a patient who has just had brain surgery.

When faced with medical treatments or procedures, patients would do more than inquire about the details of the procedures and their physician's qualifications to perform them. They would seek information about the qualifications of the nurses who would care for them during and after their treatments. They would want to know the nurse-to-patient ratio in the hospital unit to which they would be admitted. They would recognize that nurses are critical to outpatient surgery and would inquire about the availability of nursing at such centers. Patients would also inquire about the extent and type of nursing services available to them in their homes or in other community settings.

Prospective nursing home residents and their families would investigate the extent of nursing services in the facilities they are considering and the qualifications of the nursing staff. Similarly, families would be well aware of the need for and the importance of the health services provided by school nurses, public health nurses, and home-care nurses in their communities. People would understand that many nurses, like physicians, have specialized expertise. They would readily accept and often seek the services of nurse practitioners, nurse midwives, nurse anesthetists, and hospice nurses.

Health care administrators and public officials would be under pressure to provide funds for the actual cost of nursing care. Hospitals could no longer afford to treat nurses as members of a cheap disposable labor force or as interchangeable cogs in an industrial machine. Because the public would clearly understand the important role of nursing in health care, hospitals could no longer rely on reducing nursing staff as a strategy for dealing with budget problems. Attempts to cut nursing staff, substitute aides for RNs, and stretch staff through floating and mandatory overtime would produce public outcry. Nursing salaries would more accurately reflect the expertise and responsibilities of nurses. Through greater investment in nursing, full-time jobs would be readily available.

A more complex and authentic image of the nurse would replace dated or distorted stereotypes such as physician handmaiden, self-sacrificing angel of mercy, lewd sex object, and vituperative harridan.

Everyone would know that nursing requires education and training, not just niceness. It would be common knowledge that nurses are educated not born. This understanding would translate into widespread public support for nursing education at the undergraduate, graduate and post-graduate levels. Nursing education would be fully integrated into higher education systems. Schools of nursing would be viewed as major contributors to the academic enterprise at universities rather than as marginal adjuncts.

The public would understand that medical interns and residents are not the only learners and physicians are not the only teachers in teaching hospitals and other health care institutions. It would be generally known that hospitals are educational institutions for nurses too. Institutional budgets would reflect this fact by allocating money for in-house nursing education. It would be accepted that veteran nurses, like physicians, need mentors to keep up with the latest treatment developments as well as with innovations in disease prevention and health promotion. Health care facilities would be amply staffed so that RNs could participate in the planning and management of services during their workdays and could take time away from the job for continuing education. Budgets, of course, would recognize the need for necessary resources for clinical education and extramural educational programs.

Respect for nursing would mean that young women and men who show an interest in nursing careers would be strongly encouraged, not grilled about why they aren't planning to go to medical school. With the challenges and rewards of nursing more fully appreciated, many intelligent women, with a full range of professional options, would choose nursing. Nursing would be an increasingly attractive career choice for men as well. Just as female enrollment in medical schools gradually increased after it became more acceptable for women to be physicians, the percentage of men who would enroll in nursing schools would also rise.

Nurses would receive the three Rs that foster professional satisfaction—respect, recognition and reward. Indeed the episodic nursing shortages of the 20th century would be a relic of the past. In any event, nursing shortages would not be tolerated because it would be accepted throughout society that human health and well-being depend not only on medically necessary care, but on *necessary nursing care.*

Does this vision of the future seem like science fiction?

It's not. We have not presented a utopian dream. The elements of this scenario are attainable through incremental changes. By starting today, nurses can transform the way nursing is regarded.

The vehicle for such change is effective public communication and action. All areas of nursing—clinical practice, education, research, and policy—depend upon public understanding of how and why nursing is indispensable to health care. This means that the public and opinion makers must have a good idea of what nurses really do today. If the work of contemporary nurses is unknown or misunderstood, then nurses cannot be appreciated or supported and cannot exert appropriate influence in health care. If nurses do not take public action to secure their goals, those goals will not be realized.

Throughout this book, and especially in the chapter on campaigns, we will show how nurses and nursing groups have achieved important goals by communicating effectively with the public and policy makers. These nursing campaigns are described in detail so that other nurses can see what it means to "go public," and can employ methods that have proven effective. Nurses can use these campaigns as models for broader communications efforts.

Being silent and unknown is a persistent problem in nursing. Studies on nursing presence in the news media at the beginning of the 1990s and at the end of the decade found remarkably similar results—the largest health care profession is still largely invisible.[1,2] One way this plays out is that nursing is simply overlooked, even in its most obvious and familiar form—hospital nursing.

A disturbing example is a 1999 *New York Times* article on the refusal of managed care and insurance companies to pay hospitals for patient days during which no surgeries, diagnostic tests, or other medical procedures occur.[3] The article was pegged to the Greater New York Hospital Association contesting this practice. However, nursing was never mentioned. If the hospital association recognized that patients are in hospitals because they need nursing care (whether or not they have procedures) and that insurers must pay for necessary nursing care, there was no evidence of it in the story. Instead the distorted view of the insurers prevailed—patients should just go home when they don't have a scheduled procedure.

This article is a textbook case of how patient care is misrepresented when nursing is omitted. If the public is deprived of information showing that nursing is essential to patient care, particularly in a newspaper as influential as the *New York Times*, then how can the public support resources for nursing care? For starters, nurses must respond with letters and phone calls whenever an omission like this occurs.

Another aspect of the public communication dilemma for nurses is the lack of public understanding of nursing work.

Even though medical practice is quite diverse, most people feel they know what physicians do. Some people may idealize physicians, while others may mistrust medical treatment or question the motives of physicians. Still, physicians are so dominant that medical practice is often equated with health care. Even if they have qualms about physicians, most people do not regard physician care as optional. Doctors are considered to be repositories of the kind of knowledge and skills that make them irreplaceable. (In fact, many people think that the definition of being really sick is that you have to go to the doctor.) Indeed, periodic attempts to reduce the number of physicians, at least in the United States, provoke public anxiety and are met with organized and influential opposition.

The paradox is that the public holds nurses in the highest regard, but has little idea of what nurses really do. The nursing profession lacks the kind of identity that would lead the public to insist that nurses are also irreplaceable.

In examining the issue of identity, it is useful to look at public attitudes toward nurses. In 1999, when, for the first time, the Gallup Organization included nurses in its honesty and ethics poll, nurses displaced pharmacists as the most highly rated profession. Almost three-quarters of the respondents (73 percent) rated nurses as high or very high in honesty and ethical standards, significantly above the next highest rated groups: druggists/pharmacists 69 percent, veterinarians 63 percent, medical doctors 58 percent, and grade and high school teachers 57 percent.[4]

In an older, more comprehensive survey by Peter D. Hart Research Associates on public attitudes toward health care and nurses, nurses were far and away the most respected health care providers.[5] Seventy-seven percent of respondents said that nurses played a constructive role in health care, 81 percent characterized their professional contact with nurses as favorable, and 59 percent thought registered nurses were underpaid. Results for physicians were more mixed. A clear majority of respondents had favorable attitudes toward their own doctors, and 42 percent said doctors played a constructive role in health care, but 30 percent saw doctors as pursuing their own selfish interests, and 25 percent thought doctors were selfish but still constructive in the health system.

Nurses, heartened by periodic surveys, such as those by Pollara Research in Canada, documenting the public's trust in them, may not want to probe these findings further. But it is critical to do so to find out the basis for these favorability ratings. Nurses must know whether people like nurses because they understand what nurses actually contribute to health care or because they have an "apple pie and motherhood" view of nurses. High regard based on knowledge of nursing can be developed into public support for nursing initiatives, while good feelings coming from a sentimentalized image are unlikely to have much substance or staying power. The public's expression of trust does not necessarily imply recognition of nurses' knowledge, competence and expertise. The Hart survey, commissioned in 1989 to assist planning for a nursing recruitment campaign, stated that the public has a limited professional concept of nursing: "When people think of nurses, they are significantly more inclined to dwell on either their caregiving and comforting aspect or their customary role (such as in a hospital) than they are to focus on nurses' professionalism or qualifications." The survey report asserted that successful recruitment and the willingness of the public to entrust nurses with more sophisticated duties "lies in elevating the stature of and professional respect accorded to RNs. The [public relations recruitment] campaign must increase people's awareness of nurses' professionalism and trustworthiness by highlighting RNs' health care training, experience, skills, and expertise."

To attract high level recruits into nursing, a communications campaign was launched emphasizing nurses' education and their mastery of sophisticated technological skills. However, there was a tendency in nursing public relations activities at that time to diminish, or even jettison, the care and comforting aspects of nursing. Ignoring Hart's recommendation, the view that caring had to be repudiated in order to elevate professionalism prevailed in a public service announcement slogan widely broadcast in the early 1990s: "If caring were enough, anyone could be a nurse."[6] The implied message was that since anyone can "care," there is nothing special about nurses' "caring," even though the public seemed to think there was.

In fact, caring and comforting was the basis for what the Hart report called "the impressive goodwill nurses enjoy." The report suggested that in communicating with the public, nurses should *build on* the high regard they already had, implying that it was valuable no matter what its basis.

In the rush to promote advanced practice nursing, "caring" was sometimes seen as antithetical to professionalism, and even as an embarrassment. Some advisers seemed to think that the very word "nurse" was tainted. One widely known expert on communication and public policy even suggested to the board of trustees of a leading nursing school that "nurse" be dropped from the title "nurse practitioner" in favor of something "new" that would sound "more professional."

The fatal flaw in this strategy is that it strips nurses of the image that the public favors without adding a more compelling *nursing* identity. It tears down, rather than builds upon, nursing's foundation in caregiving work. Any discomfort that nurses may feel about the traditional nurse image seems to stimulate efforts to cast nurses as anything but nurses. If nurses convey that there is nothing special about the way that nurses care for and comfort patients, however, then those activities—as well as a lot of other so-called routine tasks—can be turned over to assistive personnel, or dropped altogether. On the other hand, if the professional advancement of nurses relies on nurses taking over responsibilities traditionally associated with physicians, or physicians' assistants, then nurses are vulnerable to being cast as junior or cheaper doctors, or, once again, as assistants to doctors.

There may be nothing wrong with a little competition and, in reality, health care services do overlap. But for nurses, it is important not to echo other professions. The job at hand for nurses is to help the public construct an authentic meaning for the word "nurse" that conveys the richness, uniqueness and indispensability of nursing across the spectrum of nursing work. This means not repudiating caring by misconstruing it as simple intuition or as something commonplace, but deepening the public comprehension of caring as a complex, skilled and inherent part of nursing that is essential to patient care.

Of course, some people base their favorable impression of nurses upon their first-hand experiences. But individual experiences do not automatically translate into broad public support for nursing. Many individuals will praise their nurses yet not express any public concern when nursing is threatened. Unless nurses help them to relate nursing to the larger health care picture, they are likely to regard their nursing care as a private transaction whose sufficient reward is privately expressed gratitude.

For these reasons the general public needs to know what nurses do today and why their work is essential. Those in a position to influence legislation, policy making and funding must know that health care environments rich in nurses promote high levels of health whereas understaffed settings put patients at risk. They need to be aware of the incipient tragedies awaiting patients when nurses are not available to prevent falls, complications, errors in treatment and care, or to "rescue" patients in need. They need to be told the myriad ways in which nurses save the lives and health of patients at risk.[7–17]

They need to be party to discussions in which simplistic stereotypes about nurses are challenged. The general public and those in positions of influence need to know that when nurses are overworked and under stress all aspects of quality care are inevitably compromised. They must understand that tens of thousands of nurses today in the United States and Canada work under conditions that threaten the health of patients and nurses alike. It must be generally understood that the aging of our society and the increase in chronic illness demand a larger nursing workforce, but that both the financial and human resources for building that workforce are currently lacking.

Evidence that nursing is little known and misunderstood is all around us. We see it when hospital administrators and consultants persist in arguing that parceling out nursing "tasks" to a variety of workers is the equivalent of placing patient care in the hands of registered nurses. We see it almost everyday in the news media and in other public discussions of health care.

For example, in 1999, the news media covered extensively the problem of "medical" errors in the US. The impetus for this coverage was a report by the National Academy of Sciences' Institute of Medicine stating that medical errors may be responsible for as many as 98,000 deaths in US hospitals per year.[18] This report, which called for the establishment of a new federal agency to deal with the problem, prompted an unusually long cycle of news coverage.

In addition to covering the main points of the report, news stories, analyses and features explored the kinds of mistakes that lead to deaths and injuries in hospitals and what can be done to reduce their incidence. Any number of stories focused on specific problems—the confusion that results when different medications have similar names or packaging, the mistakes that occur in operating rooms, the flaws in hospital procedures, the weak links in hospital oversight, and even the errors stemming from physicians' indecipherable handwriting. Most of those interviewed about these problems were physicians.

It seemed inconceivable that the news media could produce story after story on this topic without substantial input from nurses. Yet, except for occasional references, nurses were "missing in action" in this important media discussion. In the coverage we monitored, nurses were not among the expert sources describing systemic and organizational practices that led to errors. Nursing organizations were not among the groups cited as working to correct this problem. Nurses were not visible making a connection between staffing shortages and the likelihood of injurious errors. Nurses, for the most part, were not even quoted as being concerned about the problem. Nor did we see a rash of letters to the editor or op-ed essays written by nurses on this problem.

Some nurses we spoke with were relieved that nurses were so little noticed. They felt fortunate, for a change, that physicians were depicted as the hub of the hospital wheel, and nurses as just a minor cog. They reasoned that if journalists knew the true role that nurses play in hospitals, nurses would get a commensurate share of the blame for mistakes. Some nurses felt that being invisible was a benefit.

In fact, it is a serious liability. A health issue that becomes this public offers nurses and nursing organizations a chance to show that nursing *matters*. In the sustained coverage given to "medical" errors, the erroneous notion that physicians are the only *significant* health care professionals was reinforced. What they do *has significance*, this coverage implied. What they do *matters*. They are indispensable. They are so important that their mistakes, as well as their successes, are a public issue deserving the most serious scrutiny.

No one proposed that since physicians seem to be involved in so many of the errors, they should be dismissed from the hospitals and their jobs turned over to someone else. Indeed, the Institute of Medicine report went out of its way to avoid the conclusion that doctors, either as individuals or as a group, were the culprits. "The majority of medical errors do not result from individual recklessness, but from basic flaws in the way the health care system is organized," the report stated.

By casting the problem this way, the Institute left the door open for doctors to be seen as part of the solution rather than as the problem. In subsequent news stories, any number of people with "MD" after their names were offering their insights and opinions about how to fix things. People with "RN" after their names were not.

The irony is that even though nursing was a very minor part of the coverage of medical errors, nurses, as a group, did not entirely escape blame. For example, one proposed way to reduce medication errors was to give pharmacists, not nurses, the responsibility for mixing all drug ingredients. This implied that nurses are responsible for many medication errors. In anecdotal accounts, nurses were also shown as parties to cases that had gone wrong. However, even though nurses have pertinent expertise on hospital errors and their prevention, nurses did not appear as expert sources or commentators on this subject.

By being silent in the media discussion, nurses missed the opportunity to show themselves as *consequential* in the delivery of health care. At the moment, physicians are the only ones who truly own this image in health care. When they are involved in a high rate of medical errors, they become more rather than less consequential. This is why a prestigious group—made up almost exclusively of physicians—made sweeping recommendations to lessen the likelihood of medical mistakes.

This proves once again that nursing needs a bigger public presence as a profession of *consequence*. One way to enlarge nursing's presence is for nursing organizations and individual nurses to take advantage of openings provided by media interest in health issues. In this particular case, medical errors offered a public platform for nurses to describe how nurse staffing is critical to this issue. Coverage would have been enhanced by nurses talking about what protocols could prevent the tragic medication and surgical errors so gruesomely described in the media. A discussion of how nurses keep patients safe by checking the five Rs—right patient, right medication, right dose, right route, right time—and what happens when units are so short-staffed that nurses can't spend the necessary time with patients would have added realistic detail to these stories. An analysis of what happens to fail-safe procedures when perioperative nurses are cut from surgical units would certainly make very interesting reading in the press.

Nurses cannot afford to be omitted from public discussions of this or any other broad patient care issues. Nursing cannot be seen as a *significant* health care profession unless it is visible and vocal in connection with all the major health care issues of our time.

How can nurses end the silence about nursing?

The first step is to realize that no one but nurses can truly inform the public about nursing.

The second step is for every nurse to make public communication and education about nursing an integral part of her or his nursing work.

The third step is for nurses to overcome the internal obstacles that silence them.

If nurses were committed to these three steps, nurses would, we believe, quickly heighten their visibility and see improvements in the way their profession is regarded. Of course, we can't guarantee that these actions will give nurses everything they want. We can, however, guarantee that nurses will get very little of what they want without such action.

This may seem like a tall order, and in some ways it is. Fortunately, at this pivotal time, nurses have the *means, motivation and opportunity* to make it happen.

The Means

Nursing leaders sometimes lament that they lack the money medicine has available for promotional purposes. While it is true that financial resources are needed to run public relations campaigns, nursing has an advantage that compensates for limited funds and makes its power potential unique among health care professions. That advantage is its numbers. In the US and Canada, nursing is far and away the largest health care profession.

In the US, nurses outnumber physicians more than three to one, and, according to the latest available figures, some 2,161,700 registered nurses (of the nation's 2.6 million nurses) were employed in nursing in 1996. In that year 238,244 students were enrolled in nursing programs.[19]

In Canada, comparable statistics for 1998 indicate that 227,651 registered nurses of a total of 254,964 were employed in nursing.[20] In the same year, there were some 22,100 students seeking nursing diplomas or university degrees.[21]

Imagine what the impact of these numbers would be if nurses decided that public communication about their work is a fundamental part of their nursing mission. The potential impact of millions of nurses educating the public about nursing is mind boggling. Certainly physicians did not have the advantage of such numbers when they began to transform the image of their profession early in the 20th century.

We are so accustomed to seeing physicians depicted as the dominant—and sometimes the only—health care professionals, that we forget that physicians did not always enjoy such status and had to create it. Physicians achieved their public prominence through well-planned communication campaigns that used the media in creative and innovative ways. In image enhancing efforts (that continue to this day), medical groups used their clout with the entertainment industry to influence how doctors were portrayed in movies and in television series. Other dedicated efforts were pursued to convince journalists to report on the research studies published in medical journals.

Not every physician is an enthusiastic participant in such campaigns. Physicians, however, dominate the public discussion of health simply because a large enough number of them and their organizations actively use the media to present their expertise and views on whatever issues are topical.

Not every nurse has to be seen or heard in the mass media to be a successful public communicator. In this book, we discuss many ways for nurses to communicate with various kinds of publics. Day in and day out, however, a large enough number of nurses and nursing organizations must be actively communicating via the mass media. For all the efforts that are being made, far too few nurses are taking advantage of the power that only the media can offer. Thousands more must be seen and heard via the media if nursing is to acquire public *significance* commensurate with its role in health care.

Let's say that only ten percent of nurses and nursing students actively promote nursing by participating in a rally, calling up a state, provincial/ territorial or national legislator, telephoning a radio or television talk show, writing a letter to the editor, talking to a television producer about doing a feature on a nurse, meeting with the editorial board of a newspaper, sending out news releases on timely research in nursing journals, testifying at a hearing on health care delivery, speaking to a journalist about a nursing innovation, or engaging in outreach in any of the myriad ways available. That would mean conscious activism by a quarter of a million nurses in the US and some 27,000 nurses in Canada. This indeed would constitute a critical mass.

By using their numbers, nurses could succeed without huge budgets. It only takes a few callers to get the attention of most editors. A legislator who gets 100 faxes (or sometimes only ten) on an issue is most likely to pay attention.

One might reasonably ask why so many individual nurses are required to take on this role. Isn't that the job of organizations?

Yes, it is the responsibility of nursing organizations, associations, unions, and research and academic institutions. Without deprecating what they have accomplished, they can and must do much more. It is essential for every nursing group not only to engage vigorously in public communication activities but to regard public communication as an inseparable part of its core mission. However, not even assertive spokespeople for professional organizations and institutions can be substitutes for the authentic voices of nurses in the field. Organized attempts to promote nursing are often defeated when nurses are afraid to participate in public discussions of even non-controversial health care topics. If rank and file nurses don't tell the public what it is they do, their work will remain hidden.

The Motivation

One of the best reasons for explaining nursing to others is that it helps nurses to appreciate their work. When nurses or any other professionals do their work, they aren't necessarily thinking about all the knowledge and experience that goes into it. Expert practitioners usually just concentrate on doing their work not describing what they do. This is especially true of busy nurses.

If nurses do not examine their work from time to time, they can become discouraged about it, particularly if bean counters and others are diminishing nursing for financial reasons. In that kind of atmosphere, it's easy to lose confidence. But as we learned from participants in our workshops, and as Patricia Benner and her colleagues have documented in their work, even a nurse's understanding of nursing can be heightened by dispassionately looking at what goes into it.[22, 23]

Nurses often complain that nurses are too hard on each other, that "nurses are their own worst enemies," or that "nurses eat their young." To counter that negativism, we ask nurses at our workshops to regularly compliment their nurse colleagues for something they have done in their work. Nurses who do this as a conscious daily exercise often report that their colleagues are at first startled because compliments are so rare, and then are heartened by the experience. The nurse who compliments others also feels buoyed.

But there is an additional benefit, as Maureen Renaud, a nurse who does IV therapy at Rhode Island Hospital in Providence, explained to us. "In order to compliment another nurse, I had to actually stop and look at what she was doing," she said. "I had to make a conscious effort to do this. But it made me more observant. I saw what nurses do that's positive. Normally we are so rushed we don't see that."

Nurses, in their busy lives, do not always get a chance to reflect upon just how far nursing has come. To nurses, shortcomings are perhaps more obvious. But regardless of the problems nurses confront, their work and progress as a profession is truly extraordinary.

Just think of what nurses have accomplished in the last half century alone. Nurses took control of nursing and established practice and educational standards. By being assertive and vocal, staff nurses developed primary nursing and gained more of a voice in patient care and institutional policies. Nurses developed the field of critical care. Nurse practitioners gained prescriptive authority. Nurse midwives changed the modern birthing experience. Hospice nurses made it possible for patients to die in comfort and with dignity. Nurse researchers created viable university programs, national nursing research agendas and, in the US, a national institute for nursing research. Today nurses are in the forefront of the struggle to guarantee that hospitals have sufficient nursing staff to provide patients with necessary nursing care.

All of this happened because of the willingness of nurses to go public, talk about their work, and explain their value and their contributions to health care. The struggle for recognition, respect and reward is hardly over. Today many of nursing's accomplishments are being attacked. New challenges continue to arise and require nurses to communicate to gain public support.

The Opportunity

As we write this, the health care systems of both Canada and the United States are in a state of turmoil. On an almost daily basis, the press details their deficiencies. Although Canada has a single-payer system, and the United States has a multi-payer private insurance system, cuts in funding and changes in structure have put great stress on those who deliver health care in both countries, and have created public anxiety over the kind of health care that is and will be available.

Even if immediate systemic pressures are alleviated, we live in a time in which health care decision making is dependent upon public information. Public demand for useful information on health and health care seems almost insatiable. People want answers to their health-related questions. Should they have surgery to alleviate their back pain? Will an herb improve their mental functioning? Should they go to an emergency department if they have chest pains? Who will pay for it if they do? Will hospital care be available if they become seriously ill? What about home health care and long-term care for a population that lives longer but with many chronic illnesses?

Today, to use health care services effectively, people must have information on which to base choices and actions. Hence the importance of the mass media in the current health care environment. Recent studies find that Americans no longer get most of their health and health care information from doctors and nurses. Instead, they rely upon the media as their *primary* source of health information.[24] The same is increasingly true for Canadians.

This climate creates unprecedented opportunity for nurses to communicate with the public. It also places unprecedented responsibility upon nurses to do so. Nurses have valuable information and insight to contribute to the most pressing health issues of our time and to the public debate over what kind of health care systems will be effective. Indeed, the very future of the profession depends upon nurses becoming more vocal now.

Another opportunity for nurses lies in the increasing willingness of journalists to pay attention to nurses. Journalists who cover health and health care have space and air time to fill. They need good stories. They need informed and reliable sources. They can't afford to maintain a bias against an entire health care profession. This doesn't mean that nursing stories are no longer a hard sell. It does mean that they are not automatically a "no sale."

Understandably, being treated like health care window dressing for so long may have dampened nurses' enthusiasm for dealing with the media. But the major problem now is that demand for health care information from nurses is greater than the supply. To put it very simply: once the problem was that nurses were not being heard; now it is that they are not speaking.

Health care journalists who are interested in covering nursing say they don't really know whether nurses and nursing organizations are involved with health care policy and delivery issues because that information is not getting to them. "Nursing groups don't pitch stories to reporters—I heard that again and again," said Madge Kaplan, senior health editor for US public radio's nightly business show, "Marketplace," after surveying her colleagues through an Internet listserve for a talk to a nursing group.[25]

Nurses may be surprised to hear this given that nursing organizations and some nursing schools have media relations specialists on staff. But in the context of the voluminous materials and personal contact that medical professionals and health care suppliers lavish on the media, nursing's outreach seems minuscule.

Most of the approximately 40 journalists who responded to Kaplan's query expressed interest in covering nursing more. But they were quick to point out that they don't get the information they need. The journalists said that nursing groups or their public relations representatives don't reach out enough to reporters. Journalists are at a loss to know which nursing groups to pay attention to. They don't know if there is an equivalent to the *Journal of the American Medical Association* or the *New England Journal of Medicine* that would be an authoritative source on the latest nursing research. Reporters either don't know who the nursing spokespeople are, or find them difficult to track down when stories break. They find that individual nurses are fearful of talking with the press. In contrast with nurses, reporters find doctors to be "very organized and media savvy." They are willing to talk, return calls expeditiously, and will discuss in general terms broad areas of medical practice that are beyond their immediate expertise.

The disconnect between nursing and media deprives nursing of influence both in the larger public sphere and within health care.

Nurses have an opportunity to advance the public understanding of health issues that touch individuals and families. For example, nurses have been innovators in the field of pain management for post-operative or terminally ill patients. They have been pioneers in the kind of palliative care that is the only alternative to physician-assisted suicide. Emergency nurses have organized programs to permit family members to be with their loved ones while physicians and nurses try to save their lives. Geriatric nurses are bringing care into the homes of the growing number of elderly patients, thus helping seniors maintain their independence and avoid nursing home placement. AIDS nurses are helping to keep patients alive and functioning for far longer than anyone once imagined possible. Nurses are experts on how those with chronic illnesses can maintain their functioning and well-being. Nurses are also more familiar than physicians about the kind of health care team and interdisciplinary collaborations that insurers and policy makers are calling for.

Another opportunity awaiting nurses lies in the yearning that people have to hear rational and humane discussion about the kind of health care systems that will work in the future. In the US, patients express their doubts about the ability of managed care to care for patients and families. In Canada, many patients are alarmed by hospital overcrowding and long waits for care, but are worried about adopting a two-tiered, privatized, American-style health care system. In surveys, even those who are generally satisfied with their health care say they are anxious about the future and wonder how they will be cared for in the event of catastrophic illness. Their doubt is reinforced by the continued emphasis on cutting health care costs. Under managed care in the US, the rules about what services are available through public and private programs, how one gets them, what they cost, and who will pay for them seem to shift on a weekly basis.

In Canada (and many other countries in the world), relentless budget cutting by governments is creating an appeal for the very market mechanisms that some Americans see as an impediment to health care. Government cuts in one system and market reforms in another have reduced the amount of time clinicians can spend with patients. The shift of care from the hospital to the home has led to major concern about the adequacy of community-based services. Cuts in nursing staff and changes in employment patterns have eroded care. In both countries, a serious nursing shortage is occurring and may worsen.

As quality of care declines, American consultants continue to sell their market-based health care ideology in Canada, and proponents of privatized health care in both countries strengthen their assault on Canada's health care system known as Medicare. Canadian nurses have responded by campaigning to save Medicare. In both countries, nurses have engaged in highly publicized job actions and strikes to protect the integrity of their profession and patient care.

In North America, turmoil over the shape of the health care system raises serious issues for all of us. The central issues of the health care debate are how to finance and deliver expensive high-tech treatments and nursing care to expanding vulnerable populations. Both clearly involve nurses. In recent years, however, these issues have been appropriated by health care consultants who claim to have not only the key to cost savings, but the recipe for delivering "patient-focused" services.

Administrators of health care institutions from hospitals to hospices are seeking the advice of these "experts." Do these business consultants know more than nurses about how to attend to, engage with, and care for human beings? Do patients yearn for "customer service" or for care and attention? Should health care institutions consistently go to the corporate sector to find out how to focus on the patient? Should they enlist doctors exclusively in their efforts to enhance collaboration among those who work in health care? Who can teach us more about the care of the sick and vulnerable? Nightingale, Henderson, Benner, and other developers of nursing practice, or corporate consultants from the Disney Institute and Ernst and Young?

The answer is nurses.

If nurses fully appreciate the relevance of their knowledge not only to the patient in the bed but to ailing health care systems, and if they exert the power that comes from their compassion and their sheer numbers, they can transform both their public image and the health systems in which they work.

Only nurses can tell patients what to do to make sure there is enough expert nursing care available in the nation's hospitals, clinics, nursing homes, community health centers, and in the home. Only nurses can tell the public what expert nursing care consists of and what is necessary to protect and defend it.

Today's nurses have a critical opportunity to affect the future of nursing. Both Canada and the US face another serious nursing shortage. It is beyond the scope of this book to analyze the reasons for the latest shortage, but the conditions that have demoralized many nurses play a part.

Nursing is a word-of-mouth profession. Many of those who go into nursing are introduced to it by family members or friends who are nurses. As lay-offs of hospital nurses increase, patient loads escalate, working conditions deteriorate, salaries lag, and part-time and per-diem jobs replace full-time work, many RNs are spreading a new message about nursing: "Don't go into the profession. You won't be well treated, and you won't be able to give good care to patients." This is not an enticing message for any young woman or man considering a nursing career.

Today's nurses will have an impact on this problem. What kind of impact is up to them. They can shut up and leave in droves, or stand up for nursing so that nursing begins to get the support it needs. They can say to potential recruits, "Don't go into nursing." Or they can say, "Yes, we have problems and that's why we need assertive people to go into nursing so we can fight to protect the profession and patients."

The struggle for public visibility can be won. But it will not be won with public relations techniques alone. It is true that nurses must learn to craft effective messages about nursing that convey understanding and respect for nursing philosophy, theory and practice. There won't be enough people willing to deliver these messages, though, unless nurses come to terms with the motivational ambivalence that can inhibit even the most basic efforts in this area.

We asked nurses who attended some of our media seminars to describe their inhibitions about "going public."

"I have trouble articulating my thoughts clearly and precisely, and feel this hinders my arguments," one nurse wrote.

"I fear having to explain myself," another wrote. "I feel as though I cannot do that correctly and confidently."

Many nurses described themselves as "not articulate." Others were more specific: "I'm afraid of saying the wrong thing." "I have a fear of sounding uneducated." "I'm afraid of sounding stupid."

"What if someone asks a question I cannot answer?" many nurses asked.

Several nurses asserted that they "weren't knowledgeable enough to speak out." "I'm afraid of not knowing enough about my topic," one said. "I'm afraid my knowledge base is not broad enough," another stated.

There were concerns about accuracy. "I may be unaware of all the facts," one nurse explained. "I'm not sure I have the correct facts," said another.

"I'm just a nurse, how can I speak for the profession?" a nurse asked.

It's no wonder nurses feel this way. There is a world of difference between communicating within one's culture where there are shared assumptions and communicating to others. As linguist Deborah Tannen suggests, communication styles are influenced by culture. Since nursing was largely created by women, the style of communication within nursing often reflects what is standard in women's cultures. Mainstream public communication reflects, on the other hand, a pattern that Tannen sees as being common among men.

In her popular book, *You Just Don't Understand*, Tannen asserts that men tend to be more comfortable doing "public speaking," while women are more comfortable with a style of "private" speaking.[26]

Men, Tannen explains, tend to engage in "report-talk," in which they exhibit their knowledge by telling stories, joking and imparting information. This "report-talk" style serves to maintain their independence, assert their status and help them gain attention.

In contrast, women tend to use language for purposes that are important to them—establishing connection or rapport and negotiating relationships. As many social scientists have noted, women are taught from early on to empathize with others. Thus, rather than emphasizing status or function, women's "rapport-talk" is aimed at displaying similarities and matching experiences. This is why women can feel uncomfortable when they see another woman trying to make herself look distinct, or "better," than others. Within a woman's culture, such a woman can be seen as distancing herself from the intimacy of the group. These generalizations don't apply to everyone. But they do help to explain why women may be most comfortable talking with one or a few people in settings where they feel at home, and why nurses are particularly adept at conversing within the intimacy of the patient-nurse relationship.

For nurses and physicians, the concept of gendered communication styles seems particularly apt. According to Tannen's theory, communication in the hospital, at least when it involves patients, would be parallel to the kind of communication that goes on in the home, where women tend to reign supreme in talking and interacting, and men are quieter. Although there are numerous women physicians, medicine can be seen as a "male" institution because it was developed by men according to male professional standards. That's true of most professions since women have had very little opportunity to influence their culture, values or standards. Nursing, of course, is the premier exception. Not only was it developed by women, it came, as we will discuss in the next chapter, out of the domestic sphere. Although there are men in nursing, they are part of a "female" profession.

These cultural antecedents play out in full force in communication practices in hospitals. Nurses frequently comment on (and even privately ridicule) the awkwardness and discomfort many physicians display in talking with patients. At the same time, doctors do not reward nurses' ability to use language to establish affiliation. Indeed women's mastery of the private realm is often seen as making them unfit for functioning in the public world. And they begin to believe it.

Our hope is that this book will correct these misconceptions. We know that nurses can synthesize "rapport" and "report" talk. Nurses can articulate their thoughts, find the right words to describe their work, do so in a confident way that doesn't sound boastful or self-aggrandizing, believe in their own knowledge and ability to acquire more, answer tough questions, and tolerate making the occasional mistake. In doing so, nurses will reveal what it really means to be "just a nurse."

By developing what we call a "voice and persona of agency," nurses can do this. This "voice of agency" can help strengthen bonds between nurses so that individual advocates will be supported by a culture of collaborative and collective advocacy. In such a culture, nursing will be far more likely to develop supports outside of the profession so that nurses can finally get the recognition, respect and rewards they have so long deserved.

Endnotes

1. B. Buresh, S. Gordon, and N. Bell, "Who Counts in News Coverage of Health Care?" *Nursing Outlook,* 39 no. 5 (1991): pp. 204–208.

2. *The Woodhull Study on Nursing and the Media: Health Care's Invisible Partner,* (Sigma Theta Tau International, 1998).

3. J. Steinhauer, "Hospitals Battle Insurers over Refusal to Pay for Portions of Patient Stays," *New York Times,* 19 October 1999, p. A19.

4. *Honesty and Ethics Poll,* (Princeton, NJ: Gallup Organization, 1999).

5. *A Nationwide Survey of Attitudes toward Health Care and Nurses,* (Peter D. Hart Research Associates, Inc., 1990).

6. National Advertising Council, *If Caring Were Enough…*, television public service announcement developed under the auspices of the National Commission on Nursing Implementation Project (NCNIP), 1990.

7. L.H. Aiken, H.L. Smith, and E.T. Lake, "Lower Medicare Mortality among a Set of Hospitals Known for Good Nursing Care," *Medical Care,* 32 no. 8 (1994): pp. 771–787.

8. L.H. Aiken, D.M. Sloane, and J. Sochalski, "Hospital Organization and Outcomes," *Quality in Health Care,* no. 7 (1998): pp. 222–226.

9. L.H. Aiken *et al.,* "Organization and Outcomes of Inpatient AIDS Care," *Medical Care,* 37 no. 8 (1999): pp. 760–772.

10. J.G. Scott, J. Sochalski, and L.H. Aiken, "Review of Magnet Hospital Research: Findings and Implications for Professional Nursing Practice," *Journal of Nursing Administration,* 29 no. 1 (1999).

11. M.A. Blegan, C.J. Goode, and L. Reed, "Nurse Staffing and Patient Outcomes," *Nursing Research,* 47 no. 8 (1998): pp. 43–50.

12. C. Czaplinski and D. Diers, "The Effect of Staff Nursing on Length of Stay and Mortality," *Medical Care,* 36 no. 12 (1998)3: pp. 1626–1638.

13. S.D. Flood and D. Diers, "Nurse Staffing, Patient Outcome and Cost," *Nursing Management,* 19 (1988): pp. 34–43.

14. A.J. Hartz, *et al.,* "Hospital Characteristics and Mortality Rates," *New England Journal of Medicine,* 321 no. 25 (1989): pp. 1720–1725.

15. W.A. Knaus, *et al.,* "An Evaluation of Outcomes from Intensive Care in Major Medical Centers," *Annals of Internal Medicine,* 104 no. 3 (1986): pp. 410–418.

16. W.R. Scott, W.H.J. Forrest and B.W.J. Brown, "Hospital Structure and Postoperative Mortality and Morbidity," *Inquiry: Organizational Research in Hospitals,* S. Shortell and M. Brown, Eds., (Chicago: Blue Cross Association, 1976).

17. J.-B. Thorens *et. al.,* "Influence of the Quality of Nursing on the Duration of Weaning from Mechanical Ventilation in Patients with Chronic Obstructive Pulmonary Disease," *Clinical Care Medicine,* no. 11 (1995).

18. L.T. Kohn, *et al., To Err Is Human: Building a Safer Health System* (Washington, D.C.: Institute of Medicine, National Academy Press, 1999).

19. Division of Nursing, *The Registered Nurse Population: Findings from the National Sample Survey of Registered Nurses,* (US Department of Health and Human Services, Bureau of Health Professions, 1996).

20. Statistics Canada, *Registered Nurse Management Data* (Ottawa: Health Statistics Division, 1998).

21. Canadian Nurses Association, *Enrollment in Registered Nursing,* (Policy Regulation and Research Division, 1998).

22. P. Benner, *From Novice to Expert* (Reading, Massachusetts: Addison-Wesley, 1984).

23. P. Benner, C.A. Tanner, and C.A. Chesla, *Expertise in Nursing Practice* (New York: Springer, 1996).

24. Roper Starch, *Americans Talk about Science and Medical News* (The National Health Council, 1997).

25. Madge Kaplan, Speech to the American Academy of Nursing, 1999.

26. D. Tannen, *You Just Don't Understand: Women and Men in Conversation* (New York: William Morrow and Company, Inc., 1990).

Chapter 2

CREATING
A VOICE OF AGENCY

The nursing professor is adamant that nurses should not call attention to themselves. For emphasis, she beats her fists against her chest and shakes her head vigorously. "No me, me, me," she says. Nurses who seek attention, she insists, are violating a sacred trust.

This scene occurs in a reception room following a lecture by Suzanne Gordon on nursing and public communication. The nursing professor is upset because the lecture urged nurses to actively increase nursing's public visibility. The speech encouraged nurses to talk about their work in a variety of settings— at home, in the community, at social events, in professional settings as well as at meetings on health care attended by opinion makers such as politicians and journalists. The lecture suggested specific ways that nurses might be more visible and vocal both as individuals and as members of organizations.

During the question-and-answer period, Gordon asked nurses in the audience to explain why nurses so often remain silent about their work.

"I worked all day and when I came home I had to take care of my family," one nurse volunteered. "I made dinner, did the laundry and cleaned. I did the same thing on weekends. It seems like I never had time to talk to my family about my work. Now my kids are grown up." She paused and asked, "Is it too late?"

The audience was moved by her poignant statement. This nurse seemed to feel that her silence wasn't just a product of exhaustion. She felt that perhaps she had been reluctant to reveal a facet of herself that was critical to her identity—her work as a nurse. She now felt that she could have used some of these busy moments at home to talk about her work, and that perhaps she would have liked to. She wanted now to be more forthcoming about her work. Gordon assured her that it was not, in fact, too late to do so.

The nursing professor's angry response to the lecture and the nurse's dilemma suggest that there is a widespread belief in nursing that caring work can be accomplished only in the context of silence. The professor is an unabashed representative of the "virtuous silence" school of nursing. She profoundly disagrees with the suggestion that nurses should speak more about their work in public. Perhaps, she allows, they might talk about their work with each other. But surely not with patients or with the wider public. She is certain such public communication will lead to narcissistic self-aggrandizement. She worries that nurses will boast about their accomplishments and reveal intimate details about themselves and patients.

"But how will people know what nurses do and understand the complexity of their work, if nurses don't tell them?" Gordon asked.

The professor retorted that patients and families will "know that naturally, just from watching what the nurse is doing."

Really?

What most people "naturally" assume about nurses' work is that doctors order every one of their interventions and stand behind every nursing action.

Consider a typical incident, Gordon suggested. A nurse on the oncology floor at a major teaching hospital spends hours trying to get an intern to order a narcotic for a patient suffering from pancreatic cancer. The nurse has informed the intern that the patient is in excruciating pain. Far more familiar with cancer patients and their pain management than the intern, she recommends a course of IV morphine.

The intern refuses to order the narcotic. He simply will not listen to the nurse. Over a period of several hours, she repeatedly engages with him, trying, to no avail, to teach him about cancer pain management. Finally, she corners a resident who agrees with her and directs the intern to write the order. In the patient's chart—the contemporary and historical record of the case—the nurse's struggle with the young doctor is absent. Reading the chart, one would never know that the nurse was responsible for easing the patient's pain and that the intern resisted her attempts to provide appropriate care for the patient to the very end. In this chart the new physician receives the credit for reducing the patient's suffering.

Not surprisingly, the patient and her family believed the doctor was her savior. Several days later, the patient wrote letters thanking her caregivers. She expressed her heartfelt gratitude to her attending physician who, during her hospitalization, rarely saw her when she was awake. She specifically thanked the intern who she thought relieved her pain. She did not thank her primary and associate nurses by name. She included only a general thank you to "the nurses."

Even after hearing this story, the professor still argued for nurses' silence. The exchange with the professor took place in Tokyo. But we have had similar discussions with nurses in the US, Canada and other countries. Some nurses strongly resist any suggestion that they take credit for their work or even that they might want acknowledgment for it. They resist encouragement to explicitly explain their work to patients and families in a way that highlights the *nurse's*, rather than others', clinical knowledge and judgment. Similarly, they feel uneasy about, and sometimes even respond angrily to, the suggestion that they introduce themselves with their first and last names and credentials as a registered nurse to establish their professional identity.

For example, several months, ago we were speaking about nursing on a National Public Radio talk show in the Midwest. Our mission was to explain the importance of nursing, and to explore why our society does not acknowledge, respect and reward nurses' work. We argued that nurses need societal respect and recognition if they are to get the resources they need to deliver quality care to the sick.

A hospital bedside nurse called in and vigorously refuted these assertions. "I don't need credit for my work," she said. "Working with patients is reward enough."

She continued with a lengthy statement in which she shifted attention from nurses to physicians. She told the audience that physicians are hard working, highly educated, and very intelligent. Her remarks diminished nursing, reinforced the stereotypical notion that the nurse exists to support the physician, and legitimized the traditional allocation of resources to medicine. We were stunned by her response and concerned that as a working nurse, her opinion would take precedence over those of non-nurses. In an effort to control the damage, we politely noted: "It's a shame you're taking up so much air time telling the listeners what doctors do instead of what nurses do."

Nurses such as the professor and the caller to the radio station give various explanations for their commitment to nurses' silence. But one theme central to their argument is that virtue is its own reward. They seem to suggest that if a nurse must call attention to her own acts of goodness—or to the acts of goodness of other nurses—then she is tainting the very nature of the act. This belief has its origins in the religious antecedents of nursing as well as in the traditional socialization of women. Central to this belief is the idea that to talk about the good things one does transforms altruism into narcissism and thus nullifies whatever good acts one has performed. In this view, goodness is cultivated and fertilized by silence and is threatened by voice.

This is clearly a very emotional issue. In one form or another, it resonates with many nurses. Even some of the most expert, highly educated and most visible nursing leaders worry that advocacy for the profession will be perceived as "self-serving" and thus will threaten the legitimacy of nursing. They are comfortable when nurses speak out only on behalf of others. Some nurses have very elaborate rationalizations for their position. Others are less articulate. Underlying their arguments, however, is a real fear that increasing the "voice" and "visibility" of nurses and nursing will bring harm.

Whether nurses consciously subscribe to this idea or not, this deep belief within nursing threatens efforts to defend and promote nursing work. Whenever a plan is initiated to make nursing more noticeable, some nurses may directly or indirectly resist, or even fight, such an effort.

It's tempting to dismiss those who express such beliefs as old-fashioned, out-of-touch, or secretly jealous of the nurses who dare to speak out. One can't, however, effectively deal with this attitude by attacking the nurses who hold it. These nurses undoubtedly believe that they are acting to protect nurses and nursing. Their response comes out of a moral concern for the integrity of the profession and a fear of the consequences of what they interpret as self-aggrandizement.

When one looks at modern culture, their concern is not unreasonable. Contemporary culture and the mass media encourage self-involved, indiscreet exhibitionism. The mainstream media have adopted some of the sensationalism of the tabloid media. Nothing appears to be off limits. Nothing is private. In this context, public visibility becomes synonymous with inappropriate revelations distorting human experience and debasing relationships. Too many people in the news are visible not for their service to others or contributions to society, but for their expertise at getting noticed or being notorious. Thus, it becomes easy to equate visibility with meaningless display, lack of standards and invasion of privacy. No wonder many nurses fear that if they cross the line from "silence" to "voice" they will violate patient confidentiality and corrupt rather than serve the profession.

Yet nurses do not have to sink to this low level to enter the public dialogue over health care. The public debate is in great need of articulate voices that can focus discussion on the public good. Entering the "public" realm does not mean that a nurse automatically loses her restraint, her values and her true self.

Voice is not a threat to nursing. Quite the contrary, silence is the threat to caregiving. Caregiving needs voice, not the voice that the nursing professor and many other nurses fear—but a strong and authentic voice that accurately represents and honors the experience of illness as well as the experience of those who care for the sick and vulnerable.

We call this the "voice of agency."

Currently, many nurses seem caught between their fear of self-aggrandizement and their daily practice of self-effacement. Conceptualizing and developing a voice of agency is a route out of this impasse. It is a way of allowing nurses the freedom to talk about their work with honesty and integrity. It is a tool for helping others to understand what caring is and what resources are needed to support it.

What do we mean by a "voice of agency?" According to the dictionary definition, the word "agency" comes from the Latin verb *agere* meaning to drive, lead, act or do. Agency is the capacity for acting or the condition of acting or exerting power. An agent is a person "through whom power is exerted."

For nurses, expressing agency depends not only on recognizing the importance of nursing work but their own importance. It means knowing that nurses can and do act on clinical knowledge and the exercise of clinical judgment. The inner voice of agency dares to say, "I'm here. I am doing something important."

To speak with a voice of agency is to admit the incontrovertible fact that the 79-year-old patient did not teach himself how to take his diabetes medication; that the 61-year-old stroke patient did not read her own EKG, interpret its meaning and act on it; and that the demented man did not assess his own skin, discover the beginning of a decubitus ulcer and prevent further skin breakdown. Patients do not monitor and evaluate their own conditions themselves. When they are most vulnerable, they do not have the ability or the responsibility for preventing catastrophes or educating themselves about their conditions, treatments and medication regimens. Nor can patients always effectively negotiate the complexities of the system and advocate for themselves. This is what nurses do for them.

Agency involves being able to speak for one's self. In her book, *Silencing the Self: Women and Depression*, psychotherapist Dana Crowley Jack asserts that a strong, first-person voice represents the authentic self. "The first-person voice is the self that speaks from experience, that knows from observation," she writes.

"This voice says, 'I want, I know, I feel, I see, I think.' The bases for its values and beliefs are empirical; they come from personal experience and observation. In this sense, the first-person voice is authentic; I will call it the 'I,' the authentic self." This true self, Jack explains, knows what she thinks from her own experience rather than being at the mercy of what she *should* think.[1]

All the classic definitions of nursing, starting with Florence Nightingale's definition and continuing with Virginia Henderson's and Patricia Benner's, emphasize the importance of the nurse making her own observations and acting on them. These nursing theorists see a nurse's mastery coming from her or his own informed experiences. Mastery is developed. It is not present just because one is a "good" woman. It is active, not passive, and thus leads to agency.

Without using the term, Nightingale saw agency as necessary for nursing and was derisive about the trivialization of the qualifications needed for nursing. In *Notes on Nursing* she wrote:

> It seems a commonly received idea among men and even some women themselves that it requires nothing but a disappointment in love, the want of an object, a general disgust, or incapacity for other things, to turn a woman into a good nurse. This reminds one of the parish where a stupid old man was set to be schoolmaster because he was "past keeping the pigs."
>
> The everyday management of a large ward, let alone of a hospital—the knowing what are the laws of life and death for men, and what the laws of health for wards—(and wards are healthy or unhealthy, mainly according to the knowledge or ignorance of the nurse)—are not these matters of sufficient importance and difficulty to require learning by experience and careful inquiry, just as much as any other art? They do not come by inspiration to the lady disappointed in love, nor to the poor workhouse drudge hard up for a livelihood.[2]

In her famous definition of nursing, Virginia Henderson emphasized the mastery, or agency, of the nurse: "The unique function of the nurse is to assist the individual, sick or well, in the performance of those activities contributing to health or its recovery (or to a peaceful death) that he would perform unaided if he had the necessary strength, will or knowledge. And to do this in such a way as to help him gain independence as rapidly as possible. This aspect of her work, that part of her function, she initiates and controls; of this she is master."[3]

Patricia Benner's more recent analysis of nursing practice in *From Novice to Expert*, is grounded in the daily reality of agency. One can't possibly move from novice to expert without being an agent. Even such seemingly inactive nursing work like "being with the patient," and "maximizing the patient's participation in his or her recovery," according to Benner's analysis, requires skill and knowledge and action.[4]

Ironically, while leading nurse theorists emphasize agency as the heart of nursing work, some nurses seem not to have been taught to recognize the agency involved in their work. For example, nurses at a workshop in Montreal objected to the idea that nurses are agents. "But we were taught in nursing school that nurses are facilitators. We facilitate healing and we help people to get better but we don't do it for them," they said. These nurses construed the act of facilitating as counterposed to agency.

Nurses sometimes say they are "behind-the-scenes" players. Marian Phipps, a clinical nurse specialist at the Beth Israel Hospital in Boston, described herself this way. Her teacher had asked the nurses in a class to write a narrative describing how they made a difference to a patient. Phipps wrote how she had helped a patient die in peace and with dignity, and how she worked with his family so that they could cope with his dying process. She painted a vivid portrait of nurses helping patients and families deal with terminal illness. Any reader of this compelling narrative would be moved by the power of the nursing model and the activities of this particular nurse.

In the final paragraph, however, Nurse Phipps suddenly got stage fright. Instead of summing up her accomplishments, she obliterated them. In the ending, she disavowed her actions. Essentially she said that the family did everything that was worthwhile.

As Phipps read this in class, her teacher pointed out that by retreating into the background at the end, the nurse erased the point of her story which was to show the important work *nurses* do. The instructor was curious about why Phipps dragged the nurse from the center of the action to the periphery.

"My role as a clinical nurse specialist is to support the primary nurse, and to do that, I tend to pull back," she explained. "I feel very good about my work, but I don't talk much about it. I see my work as supporting others. I'm a sort of a behind-the-scenes person. I don't step forward. There are many people in the hospital like this. We're the ones who hold the place together and we don't stay very much in the forefront."

An oncology nurse we'll call Ruth Jones similarly placed herself in the background in her description of her work with a cancer patient. Nurse Jones had cared for a young woman with breast cancer for several years. During this time, as the woman grappled with cancer and chemotherapy, she was being beaten by her husband. As her nurse, Jones not only administered, monitored and managed the many side effects of the young woman's chemotherapy, she helped the patient to bring an end to the abuse.

The physician in this case supported the nurse's efforts to help the patient resolve the emotional and relational problems in her life. But the physician focused on the patient's disease not her emotional issues. It was the nurse who enabled the patient to identify her problem, enter counseling with a social worker, and, over time, feel confident enough about herself so that she could leave her husband.

When Nurse Jones told us about her work with this patient, she added that the patient had filed for divorce. "Terrific," we said. "You helped her get away from a person who was harming her."

Rather than acknowledge her accomplishment, she demurred. "Oh no, I didn't really do that much," Jones protested. "The patient's doctor helped a lot."

When we suggested that the doctor's contribution sounded minimal, she agreed. But then she attributed the pivotal role to others—the social worker, the patient, the patient's family. After a full ten minutes of discussion, the nurse finally owned up to her essential work. Then she described in detail exactly what she did and how she did it.

Why do many nurses counterpose facilitation and agency?

Why do nurses seem to believe that backstage players should not be allowed to come to center stage and take a bow?

Why do many nurses resist taking credit for their accomplishments even when the credit is given to them?

The answer lies, we believe, in the legacy of patriarchal culture and in the religious origins of nursing. Nursing grew out of women's domestic labor. Its mission depended upon "women's self sacrificing service to others," as women's studies professor Susan M. Reverby has written in *Ordered to Care*.[5]

Wherever nursing occurred—in the home, the convent or the community—it was seen as women's work. Although such work can be critical, exciting and dynamic, these are not characteristics acknowledged in patriarchal culture. Patriarchal culture places women's work under the control of men and conceptualizes it as an extension of male agency. Women are seen as being men's possessions. In patriarchal culture, when the man leaves the home, he temporarily assigns his agency to his wife, but reclaims it when he returns. In such a culture, exciting, dynamic work is reserved for men.

Women's caregiving work, as sociologist Diane Rothbard Margolis points out in her book, *The Fabric of the Self*, is critical to human and social survival: "Societies without strangers may get on without markets; but no society not even one dominated by market exchange, can get on without a system of obligation that assigns caregiving responsibilities." But this system of obligation ties women to caregiving, while simultaneously disempowering them as caregivers. It also sentimentalizes, devalues or trivializes this work.[6]

Caregiving is not primarily defined as an opportunity for self-assertion or self-fulfillment, but as self-sacrifice. As Reverby wrote: "The responsibility for nursing went beyond a woman's duty toward her children, husband, or aging parents. It fell to all available female family members. At any time the family's long arm might reach out to a daughter working in a distant city or mill, bringing her home to care for the sick, infirm or newborn. No form of women's labor, paid or unpaid, protected her from this homeward pull."[7]

The notion that caregiving relationships within the family are grounded in the denial of women's full identity is not a relic of the distant past. Today, as Dana Crowley Jack and other feminist writers point out, many women believe that to be in a relationship, they must subordinate their concerns, obliterate their identity and deny their feelings—particularly any anger they have over their self-abnegation.

This connection between caregiving and self-sacrifice, and the assignment of social work to the female, has been justified as being God's will or nature's command. The notion that women are "naturally" nurturing conceals the complexity of caregiving and the agency of the caregiver. "Women's work" is said to rely on instinct rather than knowledge, intelligence or judgment. The complex caregiving that is described by such feminist scholars as Sara Ruddick,[8] Laurel Thatcher Ulrich,[9] and Patricia Benner, is missing from the patriarchal conceptualization of "women's work." Most importantly, the traditional definitions of "women's work" deny women belief in their own agency. The female caregiver isn't an actor, she is the container for the hormonal or genetic engine that drives her actions.

Religious interpretations of female caregiving are part of the patriarchal legacy that denies nurses a sense of agency. When nurses are depicted as saints or angels—which they often are to this day—they become the agents of a higher being to whom they are eternally subordinate.

The myth of the nurse as saint or angel serves purposes and interests that must be understood. As Australian nursing historian Sioban Nelson points out, in the 19th century the religious calling opened possibilities for women. The call to serve transcended the father's authority and empowered women to leave the home and go out into the world.

"The religious vocation allowed women to move beyond patriarchal authority and follow a calling to care for the sick in the community," Nelson explains. "It even permitted them to travel all over the world establishing hospitals and pioneering health services. These religious women opened up the space. Pious, secular women, such as Nightingale, followed them into that new territory."[10]

When women entered nursing, they were moving into dangerous moral territory. They were taking care of strangers' bodies—many of which were male. Nursing could be respectable only if it were desexualized. The call to do God's work provided the proper context. Their calling permitted these women to develop their skills. They acquired administrative expertise and created training programs and professional organizations to raise standards for nursing and hospital care. Piety and religion gave these women courage and power to move beyond traditional expectations and to withstand opposition to their mission. The cloak of God's agency allowed them to develop their own, but not to claim it as their own.

Today, thanks in part to these nurses, women have far more freedom to exercise their own agency. Ironically, however, it is the angelic, saccarine interpretation of the work of the religious nurse that lives on in popular stereotypes of the contemporary nurse while her tough-mindedness and enterprise are ignored.

Her appeal still lies in her selflessness. The angel or saint must be there when needed without making any inconvenient demands. She has few needs of her own. She needs no education, and she has no ambitions or personal goals apart from her angelic mission. The concept of a too-heavy workload or the need for a bathroom or lunch break doesn't exist for the angel-nurse. She doesn't need a four-week vacation to recharge her batteries because she has unlimited energy. She may be disappointed by the foolish actions of human beings, but she doesn't complain when she receives a pink slip.

The angel-nurse can't be humiliated or demeaned by the proverbial patient from hell because personal humiliation and anger for herself are not in her emotional repertoire. She exhibits righteous anger only over injustice and mistreatment of others, but she doesn't express "petty" anger over the way she is treated. She takes it on the chin.

The myth of saintly or angelic behavior in the real world is that it will be recognized and rewarded. Many nurses have told us they believe their patients will respond positively to their sacrifices and understand the value of nursing not from what nurses say but from their example. Staff nurses have told us they believe patients will value them because of their good deeds and hospital administrators will ultimately recognize their contributions and fight to protect them. In this distorted view of nursing, rewards come to those who do *not* ask for them. As Michael Traynor points out, in his essay, "Morality and Self-Sacrifice in Nursing Talk," talk of their self-sacrificing role may even allow nurses to assert a higher moral value than managers and administrators who are concerned only with the bottom-line. Nurses use this traditional pose to claim a "moral high ground" and to capture public support.[11]

While asserting a moral position can help nurses and their patients, the heady mix of the social good and self-sacrifice is problematic to nurses, nursing and the public. Without consciously recognizing it, nurses may expect themselves to be superhuman. This assumption discourages the public from providing nurses with adequate resources and working conditions. After all, if self-sacrifice is the ground of nursing work, then to improve working conditions is to actually harm, rather than help, nurses.

The image of the all-suffering nurse also discourages mutual support and may turn nurses against one another. One of the most divisive issues in the profession has to do with nurses taking assertive public action for safer patient care and better wages and working conditions. One can hear the echoes of traditional assumptions in comments some nurses make about colleagues who go public, who organize workplaces, or who engage in conflict around their concerns. "Oh those angry nurses," was all one nurse had to say about nurses at another hospital who waged a successful campaign to control delegation of unlicensed personnel.

"Those nurses are so selfish. They're fighting for themselves, not their patients," a young nurse said of the unionized nurses in her workplace, just moments after complaining about the inability or unwillingness of nurses to fight for themselves in another non-unionized hospital where she had worked.

In such a judgmental atmosphere, even activist nurses may not act until they are pushed to the absolute brink. For example, a union nurse in Rhode Island told us: "I didn't object when they took away my coffee break, I didn't object when they took away my lunch break, I didn't object when they didn't give me time to go to the bathroom, I didn't object when I had nobody to help me turn a patient, but I am objecting now because I can't get the supplies I need." She seemed to expect praise for not making a fuss earlier. But she might have been more effective and she certainly would have been less burnt out, if she had started objecting the moment her hospital began rescinding hard-won protections.

If the identity of nurses is linked too closely to angelic or saintly stereotypes, then nurses are hobbled in their attempts to expand their own agency and risk public displeasure when they act "out of character" by taking assertive public action.

In many ways, hospital and medical institutions replicate patriarchal and religious structures. In fact, nursing historian Joan Lynaugh calls the developmental phase of hospitals in the 19th century "the domestic era." In those early days, hospitals, most of which were run by religious orders or denominations, were seen as an extension of the home. According to Lynaugh, "The nurse superintendent acted as mother in charge and the board of trustees acted as father, responsible for finances and over-all decision making." The nurse superintendent and the nurses under her acted as agents of the hospital trustees. Physicians at the time were staff appointees who "received respectful attention but were not in a position to control internal events in the hospital."[12]

In the last half of the 20th century, the role and power of physicians grew as hospitals relied more heavily on them to bring in business. Physicians, because they supplied the hospital with patients, became the "captain of the ship." Increasingly they took charge of nurses, who instead of reporting to nursing supervisors, now served more as handmaidens to physicians. So clear was the military metaphor that nurses were expected to rise when a physician entered the room and all but salute.

Today, some nurses joke that physicians believe MD means minor— or even major—deity. Whether or not they assume the role of God, physicians have been acculturated to claim proprietorship over health care. Either implicitly or explicitly they give the impression that they are the only health care participants with respectable knowledge and intelligence. Too often they act as though nurses are poorly educated women who would put patients in harm's way if left to their own knowledge and judgment. Many insist that nurses are the physician's agent.

In this context, nursing's caring activities are drained of intelligence and depicted as trivial—hand-holding, pillow-fluffing, and delivering defuse doses of TLC—things any nice, kind person could do. In his book *Health Against Wealth, Wall Street Journal* reporter George Anders quotes a cardiac surgeon who minimizes the nursing care given to elderly post-operative patients. "Most of them are scared to go home after four days," she says. "But they end up doing fine when they go home. There's nothing else we really do for them at that stage of recovery. It's just babysitting and helping them walk up and down the hall a few times."[13]

This statement articulates a common medical view of caregiving—one that sadly permeates much of our culture. The difficult work of helping an elderly post-operative cardiac patient perform the activities of daily living and of monitoring, evaluating, and educating the patient is described as baby-sitting. Although there is a lot more to babysitting than the term implies, it is used to diminish the requirements of the caregiver as well as the needs of the one cared for.

Not surprisingly, physicians seem willing, even eager, to cede such "unimportant" activities to nurses. However, when physicians think the work requires education and knowledge, or when it is lucrative or enhances the image of doctors, then physicians assert their superiority. They will insist that these are "medical" activities. If nurses are permitted to execute them they must do so under medical supervision.

Like the father in the home, the doctor, when he will be away, can temporarily assign his agency to the nurse/mother. But he reclaims it when he returns. When the doctor finds certain patient populations unprofitable or unappealing, the nurse can become a permanent agent *in situ*. When doctors have good working relationships with RNs, they may also bend the rules stipulated in medical and nurse practice acts by allowing nurses to make "medical decisions" that they ratify after the fact.[14] The unstated agreement between physicians and nurses is that nurses' performance of "medical" tasks remain publicly unacknowledged.

The medical system conceals nurses' contributions even when they are uncontested. When a nurse suggests a course of action to the doctor, it is rarely documented or revealed to the patients and families who benefit from it. The young intern who resisted the oncology nurse's suggestion did not contritely acknowledge her contribution to either the patient or family. He wrote the morphine order in the patient's chart with no accompanying note explaining that it was the nurse's recommendation. The medical system prevailed upon the nurse to collude in and reinforce the myth of the doctor's agency and to become its victim.

Denial of nurses' agency is expressed not only in operating procedures but in organizational rhetoric. In numerous practice and policy papers the American Medical Association categorizes nurses as "mid-level professionals," "physician-extenders," and "non-physician providers." Informally doctors often describe nurses as "their eyes and ears." Routinely they compliment nurses by telling them they are so smart, they "could be doctors."

This medico-centric view of nursing not only permeates nurses' lives in their workplaces, it influences mainstream culture's conception of nursing. In Western societies there has been an erosion of the patriarchal model. But it is alive and well within health care. The dominant paradigm is a twist on the Freudian concept of penis envy—the nurse is a person without an MD, a person who didn't have the brains or ambition to get an MD, or who, endowed with the requisite intelligence, made the wrong choice and should take the first opportunity to get an MD.

Nurses tell us that they are "put in their place" on a daily basis, not only by doctors and administrators, but by friends, acquaintances, and even strangers.

"My friends say to me, 'You mean you can do anything, like be a doctor, and you want to be a nurse?'" a first-year master's student at McGill University reported with dismay. She had left a well-paid career in business to do something she felt was useful. She had hoped to receive support for her choice. Instead she encountered only shock.

A Canadian nursing student with a background in biochemistry told us a similar story. "When I told a family friend I was going to nursing school, he said: 'Don't worry, the world is your oyster. When you finish nursing school you can still go to medical school.'"

Another student at a prestigious American east coast university told us: "My friends gave me the cold shoulder and no longer treated me as colleague," when she announced her decision to enter a nursing program. She didn't even have to get her degree to be treated like a "mere" nurse.

Continuing devaluation of nursing is costly in this "post-feminist" era when women have more choices about their careers. When women's options were limited to nursing, teaching, social work, or secretarial work, choosing nursing didn't signal a lack of intelligence or ambition. But today it may seem an inexplicable choice to some when a woman can have higher-paying, higher-status jobs.

The same attitude plagues nurses who become doctors—doctors of nursing that is. Nurses pursuing doctorates in nursing and related disciplines say some friends and relatives want to know why they aren't going to medical school to become "real doctors." They don't understand that advanced education enhances *nursing*. They can't grasp that getting a PhD is as difficult, if not more so, than getting an MD.

These attitudes have seeped into nursing. Student nurses we talk to are shocked when veteran nurses reinforce the public denigration of nursing. Young women and men say nurses ask: "Why are you becoming a nurse?" or "You could be anything and you're choosing nursing?" Nurses sometimes actively discourage them with remarks like, "Oh my God, don't become a nurse."

All of this has a marked effect on the confidence of nurses and nursing students. "I feel inferior to them," a nursing student said about students in the sciences.

"It took me a long time to feel that I wasn't settling for less by becoming a nurse" another reported.

"When they ask me why I'm becoming a nurse not a doctor," another confessed, "I tell them I'm becoming an advanced-practice nurse not a regular nurse."

"You begin to wonder, is everybody really right? Are doctors really smarter than we are?" another student asked her classmates during a discussion of public attitudes toward nursing. We learned that this student later dropped out of nursing school.

Rifts among nurses often stem from these early and repeated experiences. As they come up against persistent denigration of their work, some nurses may seek positions that offer more autonomy in administration or academia because this work seems more insulated from such disrespect. Or, they may seek "legitimacy" from another profession or activity by advertising themselves as say, nurse attorneys or nurse entrepreneurs. These factors may also be part of the motivation to move into nursing roles that look more "medical." As funding pressures destabilize health care systems, managerial models seem to offer relief from both the realities of the workplace and from traditional societal stereotyping. The professional identity of the nurse is supposed to be enhanced if she is a "manager of care" who supervises those who give direct care.

Devaluation is what makes oppressive systems oppressive. Autocratic systems rely not only on physical coercion and economic blackmail to prevail. They function by undermining agency and creating doubt about whether one's work is important and one's choices wise. Doubt leads to confusion about who one is, what one deserves, and how one should regard others who have made the same "wrong choices."

Devaluation is the road to frustration, anger, depression, and back-biting. Susan Jo Roberts, among other writers, has described "horizontal violence" within nursing as an expression of "oppressed group behavior."[15]

Two nurses who have studied anger said in an *American Journal of Nursing* article that nurses tend to express their anger over their powerlessness in the workplace in extremely unhealthy ways. Two such expressions are self-disparagement, which produces hyper-critical attitudes and perfectionism, and disparagement of others in the form of back-biting, fault-finding, name-calling, and subtle sabotage of colleagues and superiors.[16] This kind of behavior not only silences the self, it effectively discourages voice in others.

"What is paralyzing and leads to a sense of hopelessness is the belief that if one were heard, one would not be understood and accepted but would be judged negatively and abandoned," Dana Crowley Jack writes. "Thus, the authentic self goes into hiding and feels angry, resentful, hopeless."[17]

The only way nurses can work through this dilemma and override negative messages is to take the risk of standing up for themselves, each other, and for the nursing work they know is important by describing what they do and by demanding resources to support it. Nurses can do this by understanding and believing in their own agency.

How does the voice of agency sound? The following article by Nurse Jean Chaisson is an eloquent example. When you read it, you can decide if Nurse Chaisson is trying to shine a spotlight on herself or attempting to articulate the essence of expert nursing care.

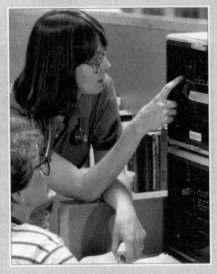

Asking the Right Questions
JEANNIE CHAISSON

As an experienced nurse, I am often called upon to assess a person's ability to function. Last year, a woman I'll call "Mrs. A" was denied Social Security disability benefits, and her attorney asked me to review her appeal. When I agreed, I received a file of paperwork that told me almost nothing. Mrs. A was in her early 60s, an immigrant who spoke little English and had found a job in a cafeteria. For several years she had worked diligently, but she had been fired when a new manager refused to let her co-workers assist her with the heavy lifting inherent in the job. The application for benefits, filled out by an intake worker who did not speak Mrs. A's language, stated that she did not fit into the bureaucratic pigeonholes defining disability. Letters from physicians detailing her currently stable medical condition did little to bolster her cause. They said her breast cancer, for which she had undergone surgery, showed no signs of recurrence.

With physicians as the lens and disease as the definition of the field, fragments of a life were examined. The questions asked had little relevance to her ability to function. Would it be possible for me to meet this woman and do a brief nursing assessment? I asked the lawyer.

Two days later, I met Mrs. A and her son, who served as translator. She was small and slim, smiling anxiously as she shook my hand. Her son, a man in his early 30s, was a graduate student at a local college and spoke English

well. I explained that I was a nurse, and that my questions might be different than those she had already answered. Addressing me in hesitant English, or in rapid-fire phrases to her son, she talked for over an hour.

I learned that Mrs. A's comfortable, middle-class life had been blown apart by revolution in her native country. One son had been killed, and she had managed to escape with the other. In the United States, her lack of English had disqualified her from the managerial work she had formerly done. And she had been happy to take any job. Only when her pain had become intolerable had she asked her fellow kitchen workers to help her with lifting. They had agreed willingly, but her boss had quickly intervened.

I asked her to tell me about

the pain: How severe was it? Where was it located? What made it worse? What could she do to help make it better?

Mrs. A's pain, which so many others had dismissed, turned out to be a relic of 11 operations for breast cancer that she had undergone before coming to this country. One by one, each new lump and node had been removed, and each time the cancer had reappeared. Terrified to permit the doctors to cut her chest muscles out and "take everything," she had lost both breasts bit by bit. A disfigured body and horrible pain that started in her scarified chest tissue and knifed its way up through her right arm and shoulder was her reward. Nothing could banish this pain—not heat, cold, or medications.

Any activity was difficult.

Moving the right arm, or even moving the hand to write or turn the pages of a book, was excruciating. She couldn't lie on that side at all. She had some pain in her other arm, and sometimes her knees hurt from arthritis, but it was the pain in her right arm and chest that cut her off from life. She said that she didn't blame her boss for firing her. After all, she admitted sadly, she had been able to do less and less of her work.

Mrs. A went on to recount a "typical day," and I saw that the feints and parries of a few years ago, when she had gone to work, to English classes, and to doctors for help, had given way to total defeat. She could achieve an uneasy truce with her pain only by giving up her job, her intellectual pursuits, her relationships with others. As my questions uncovered this tale of overwhelming loss, she became animated, then tearful. "Nobody has ever asked her about these things before," her son explained. "Nobody has cared what it is like for her."

I filed my report, and three weeks later, when Mrs. A's attorney informed me that she had been granted disability benefits, I could only wonder at the "health" of a health care system that had provided regular scrutiny of her body for recurrent disease yet had utterly failed to listen to the story of her illness, to bear witness to her pain. Other health care professionals had talked about her disease; I had asked about her life. ∎

JEANNIE CHAISSON, who has a master's in nursing, is a nurse at Beth Israel Hospital in Boston.

Reprinted by permission from *Technology Review*, October 1992.

Endnotes

1.   D.C. Jack, *Silencing the Self: Women and Depression* (New York: Harper Perennial, 1993), pp. 94–95.

2.   F. Nightingale, *Notes on Nursing: What It Is and Is Not* (New York: Dover, 1969), pp. 133–134.

3.   V. Henderson, *The Nature of Nursing* (New York: Macmillan, 1967).

4.   P. Benner, *From Novice to Expert* (Reading, Massachusetts: Addison-Wesley, 1984).

5.   S.M. Reverby, *Ordered to Care: The Dilemma of American Nursing,* 1850-1945 (Cambridge: Cambridge University Press, 1987).

6.   D. R. Margolis, *The Fabric of Self: A Theory of Ethics and Emotions* (New Haven: Yale University Press, 1998).

7.   Reverby, *Ordered to Care.*

8.   S. Ruddick, *Maternal Thinking: Toward a Politics of Peace* (Boston: Beacon Press, 1989).

9.   L.T. Ulrich, *A Midwife's Tale: The Life of Martha Ballard, Based on Her Diary, 1785-1812* (New York: Vintage, 1990).

10. S. Nelson, Interview with the authors, 1999.

11. M. Traynor, "Morality and Self-Sacrifice in Nursing Talk," *Interdisciplinary Perspectives on Health Policy and Practice: Competing Interests or Complementary Interpretations?* J. Robinson *et al.,* Eds. (Churchill Livingston: Edinburgh, 1999).

12. J.E. Lynaugh, "Narrow Passageways: Nurses and Physicians in Conflict and Concert since 1875," *The Physician as Captain of the Ship: A Critical Reappraisal,* N.M.P. King, L.R. Churchill and A.W. Cross, Eds. (Boston: D. Reidel Publishing Co., 1988), pp. 23–37.

13. G. Anders, *Health Against Wealth* (Boston: Houghton Mifflin Co., 1996).

14. J. Fairman and J. Lynaugh, "Critical Care Nursing: A History," *Studies in Health, Illness and Caregiving,* J.E. Lynaugh, Ed. (Philadelphia: University of Pennsylvania Press, 1998).

15. S.J. Roberts, "Oppressed Group Behavior: Implications for Nursing," *Advances in Nursing Science,* 1983: pp. 21–30.

16. P.G. Droppleman and S.P. Thomas, "Anger in Nurses: Don't Lose It, Use It," *American Journal of Nursing,* 1996: pp. 26–31.

17. Jack, *Silencing the Self.*

Chapter 3
PRESENTING YOURSELF AS A NURSE

Not so long ago everyone knew who was a nurse. First, the nurse was a woman in a world of male medical doctors. She wore a starched white dress, white hosiery, white shoes, and a stiff white cap bearing her nursing school insignia. Her appearance left no doubt about her professional identity. Nor did her title, "Nurse," or "Miss," or "Mrs." Nurses' roles and responsibilities were limited, but their dress and etiquette emphasized professionalism.

Today nursing is complex and far more autonomous, but contemporary behavior and dress tend to downplay professionalism, blur the identity of nurses and make the "place" of nursing in health care more ambiguous. Now patients and staff alike are not always sure who is a nurse, what nurses do, or how nurses should be treated. Without a protocol to provide clarity, it is up to individual nurses to convey that information through their appearance, language and behavior.

Nurses have choices about how they present themselves to patients and families, physicians, other clinicians and health care workers, administrators, and the general public.

They can present themselves and insist upon naming practices that assert their personal and professional identity. Or they can appear as part of an undifferentiated mass.

They can highlight their clinical knowledge and competence. Or they can conceal it.

They can affirm their professional individuality. Or they can appear to be institutional property.

They can present themselves as mature adults. Or they can infantilize themselves and their colleagues.

Each day in the workplace, nurses are performing as "public" communicators and educators. What they say and do can elicit the respect and collegial treatment their professional standing deserves, or undermine it. While caring for patients and families and interacting with other nurses, physicians, social workers, administrators, and health care workers, nurses convey messages to these "publics" about nursing's status and importance. Some of the messages are explicit. Others are more implicit—delivered through presentation, body language, tone of voice, and conversational style. These communications can convey precisely the right—or the wrong thing—about nursing.

For example, if a nurse thinks it is advisable to speak to a patient's physician, she can inform the patient by saying, "I'll consult with the doctor about this." This language indicates that she has clinical knowledge and judgment herself and sees herself as a colleague of the physician. Or she can establish herself as a supplicant by saying: "I have to ask the doctor."

When she calls the physician, the nurse can establish collegiality by beginning the conversation: "Hello Dr. Richards, this is Joan Adams, (or preferably, Nurse Adams), Mrs. Smith's nurse. She is experiencing some pain and I think…" Or she can place the physician above the nurse by starting: "This is Joan, Mrs. Smith's nurse. I'm sorry to bother you…"

Nurses can be conscious of the impression they are making without being self-conscious or artificial. Since the health of patients depends upon nursing as much as upon medicine, nurses can reaffirm this important fact by presenting themselves as experts and equals in the health care setting.

The most immediate way to educate the public about nursing work is to begin with those members of the public—patients, families and colleagues— with whom nurses are in the closest daily contact.

Introducing Yourself

Your introduction to the patient and to his or her family is an important moment that has lasting consequences for you as an individual professional and for nursing as a whole.

You can give a firm handshake, introduce yourself with your first and last name, inform the patient or family member that you are a registered nurse, and explain your role in the patient's care. Or you can say: "Hello, my name is Joan," and leave it at that.

Many patients meeting you for the first time have few visual cues as to your identity and role. Your introduction is your best opportunity to let people know that you are a nurse—a serious professional with important clinical knowledge. Being serious and professional is not synonymous with being distant and aloof. It simply means presenting yourself as a knowledgable, expert caregiver. This is a presentation that tends to reassure patients rather than alienate them.

What's in a Name?

Nurses have told us that as recently as 30 years ago, many institutions discouraged them from using their first names with patients. It was strictly "Miss Jones," or "Mrs. Jones." Today the tables have turned completely. Many nurses introduce themselves with *only* a first name. They might say: "Hi, I'm Sally. I'm your nurse." Sometimes the N word might not get mentioned, as in, "Hello, I'm Sally. I'll be taking care of you today," or "Hello, this is Jane from the VNA."

Sometimes it seems that when a nurse graduates from nursing school she substitutes a blank space for where her last name should be. The assignment board in a hospital may list the patient as "Mrs. Smith," "Mary Smith," or "Smith;" the physician as "Dr. Jones," or "Jones," and the nurse as "Pat." A name badge may bear only a first name and sometimes not even an RN. In that last-name space a nurse might substitute a health care institution or service by introducing herself or himself as "Mary from Four South," "Jim from the Emergency Department," or "Pat from General Pediatrics." This is how a nurse comes to be viewed as institutional property rather than as an individual. Some nurses construct an image of themselves as physicians' personal property by introducing themselves to patients as, "Janet, Dr. Wilson's nurse," or just Dr. Wilson's nurse.

Lack of parity in the workplace is reinforced when nurses allow or encourage physicians to call them by their first names while they routinely address physicians by title and last name.[1] Some nurses and physicians communicate with each other on a first-name basis. Usually, however, that happens when patients are not present. When the doctor and nurse enter the exam room, the physician who was "Jim" in the hallway becomes "Dr. Smith." The nurse remains "Sally." Many physicians think that the nurses prefer it this way.

It's true that naming practices have changed as our society has become more informal. We've noticed that some younger physicians avoid using the title "Dr." and introduce themselves with just their first and last names. However, in this situation, the patient understands through various other cues that the person presenting himself or herself is a physician. We've noticed that even physicians who present themselves informally rarely leave patients confused about their professional role. So, if one profession insists upon clear identification in front of patients—usually by use of title and last name—and another profession in the same setting uses only first names for identification, then there is an imbalance of status between the professions. If nurses uphold and reinforce these identification practices, it suggests that nurses, as well as physicians and patients, regard physicians as superior in the health care environment.

We know that this is not the intention of nurses who use their first names only. "When nurses use their first names, they are doing it in the hope of showing the patient that they are on their side, that they are equals, on a par with, in the same shoes as the patient," says nursing historian Joan Lynaugh. "Nurses generally are not seeking 'respect' from their patients, but some kind of identification with them. Indeed nurses are often taught to do that."[2]

The problem, Lynaugh says, is that this practice conceals the power and authority nurses actually have and misconstrues what patients need most and want from nurses. "Patients don't want a friend, they want a nurse with knowledge and skill," Lynaugh says. "A really good nurse will establish the context for a relationship. They will communicate to a patient: 'This is what I do. This is what you do. This is what I know. I will make sure everything is all right for you.'"

A nurse can quickly establish this kind of context or agency by introducing herself or himself with *both* a first and last name, explicitly stating that she or he is a registered nurse, briefly explaining her or his role in the patient's care.

This sort of opening: "Hello, this is Ruth Stevens, the nurse practitioner with general pediatrics. I understand you are concerned because your daughter has a high fever. Can you tell me when she began to feel ill?" would establish that context more than: "Hello, this is Ruth from general pediatrics. You called about your child's temperature."

Similarly: "I am Janet Jones, a registered nurse who works with Dr. Wilson," conveys a different message than "I'm Dr. Wilson's nurse."

Resurrecting "Nurse" as a Title

Nurses say that one obstacle to parity with physicians is that they don't have a title like "Dr." But nurses do have a title that was used sporadically in the past. It is "Nurse." To us it's a wonderful word that could and should be used to reassert nurses' professional identity.

Nurses could ask those physicians who prefer to be addressed as "Dr. (Last Name)" in front of patients, to please address them as "Nurse (Last Name)" in the same setting. Likewise, when nurses refer to each other as "Nurse (Last Name)" they show respect for each other and indicate to physicians and patients that they expect respect.

Use of the title, "Nurse," does not have to be stilted, nor need it jeopardize nurses' sense of closeness with their patients. Once the precedent has been set, you can move to first-name communication with a patient or a physician if you choose. Just as a physician might be "Dr. Jones" in one situation and "Joe" in another, nurses can be flexible according to the situation. At the moment, the conventions of many workplaces give nurses no flexibility at all—only a first name. This is why, as nursing educator Elizabeth M. Grady puts it, nurses must insist upon symmetrical titles and naming practices with physicians.[3]

When symmetrical naming practices are the norm in a workplace, nurses already have a professional identity and it becomes easier for nurses to affirm their competence through confident, professional presentations, as Nurse Crystal Lindaman has recommended.

A Canadian nurse who described in an interview how she had approached a resident for pain medication illustrates that the absence of an identity sets nurses up for failure.

The nurse said she began a phone conversation with the resident by saying: "This is Seven North. I need an order of ..." The resident responded angrily to being bothered while he was busy with another patient. He asked for the nurse's name. Diffidently she provided it. He got her name wrong. She did not correct him. He said he'd get to her request later. She did not try to establish a time frame. He never did write the order. She never called him back.

This physician may well have been a difficult case. But the nurse, on the other hand, did not make a professional presentation or stand up for herself or the patient who needed her care. She did not give her name and title. She did not specifically state her patient's condition and what she needed. The nurse became so intimidated she could not negotiate an agreement with the doctor to attend to her patient's need in a reasonable amount of time. She did not, as Lindaman advises, "set a tone that assumes that compliance is inevitable."[4] She did not persist. She did, however, instruct this young physician that he need not accord professional courtesy to nurses.

In workshops, we have sparked some vehement opposition by urging nurses to use both their first and last names, and to adopt the title "Nurse." Some nurses assert that nurses should use *only* their first names for these reasons:

1. First names make patients' feel that nurses are more approachable in general than physicians.
2. Patients don't want to know nurses' last names. In fact, it's too much to ask patients to remember the last names of their nurses.
3. Patients don't need to know nurses' last names to respect nurses and value what nurses do for them.
4. "Nurse Adams" makes people think of "Nurse Ratched."
5. It's dangerous for nurses to have their last names known.
6. Even if it is a good idea to use last names and a title, it is too difficult to change established cultural practices within an institution.

Are any of these assumptions correct? Let's examine them.

1. First names make patients feel that nurses are approachable.

Nurses have good reason to try to counter the distancing or brusqueness that characterizes some physician-patient encounters. Many nurses initiate reciprocal first-name interactions with patients to ease patients' fears, lower their defenses and facilitate communication. This ability to establish closeness within a professional context is one of the great qualities that nurses bring to patient care. As patients ourselves, we have noted the rapport and ease we usually feel when talking with nurses compared with the apprehension and stiffness that often colors conversations with physicians.

Indeed, nurses' may feel that the use of first names helps to create and protect one area where they clearly can claim superiority in any doctor-nurse comparison or competition—the ability to establish intimacy with patients. Nurses may feel that in their struggle for recognition they can't win the knowledge (number of years in school) competition with physicians, and they can't win the status competition, but they can easily win the "intimacy competition." Nurses may feel that a more formal self-presentation will erode their greatest strength.

But does intimacy really depend upon a first-name introduction? Do patients respond more candidly to nurses because they use their first names? Or do they respond to nurses and trust them because nurses spend more time with them than doctors; because nurses really listen to their concerns and respond to them; and because nurses know how to *be with* patients as well as *do things* to them?

In other words, does intimacy reside in a name and title, or does it reside in genuine attentiveness and empathy?

Physicians' use of their last name and title is not the primary way they distance themselves from patients. Those that distance themselves do it by failing to listen and by interrupting patients' "illness narratives," as Arthur Kleinman puts it,[5] by focusing on diseases to the exclusion of the human beings who suffer from them, and by abandoning patients when their illnesses can no longer be cured.

If nurses truly master what Benner calls "the skill of involvement,"[6] using their last names will not compromise their ability to establish trusting relationships with their patients. But consistently appearing without any last name at all will compromise clinical credibility.

2. Patients don't want to know nurses' last names; patients can't be expected to remember the last names of nurses.

Maybe, maybe not. Some patients might be interested in and perfectly capable of remembering a nurse's full name. Others may not care a whit. By the same token, many patients may not be especially interested in, or capable of remembering, the last names of doctors they encounter in a busy health care setting. Nonetheless, it is important for nurses to make the point that they, in fact, have a last name and, like physicians, are individuals rather than a part of an undifferentiated mass. Even the patient or family member who cannot remember the last name will register that their nurse has one.

The famed sociologist Erving Goffman noted that institutions enforce obedience and conformity by ritually stripping inmates or initiates of the clothes, hairstyles and private possessions that give them a sense of identity. But he added, "The most significant of these possessions is not physical at all. [It's] one's full name." More than any other, Goffman asserted, that loss forces the inmate to suffer "a great curtailment of the self."[7] Historically, nurses have been at risk for exactly this kind of institutional depersonalization.

Just as physicians are usually known to nurses by their full names, nurses should be distinguished as individuals by their names, and not, as one physician put it, as "Maureen in the yellow angora sweater." Besides, many patients as well as colleagues want to know a nurse's identity. As the mother of a nine-year-old recently noted, they want to be assured that they are speaking to a qualified professional.

"When I call the pediatrician's office because my child has a fever and the nurse calls back, it is invariably an infuriating experience," she explains. "The nurse always introduces herself with, "Hi, I'm Kim," and gives the name of the practice. The first few times this happened I had no idea whom I was speaking with or whether she was even a nurse. When I asked her to tell me who she was and her role, it was like pulling teeth to get a response. How am I supposed to know that this person actually knows something? She is as anonymous as Patty from MCI calling to sell me new phone service. I don't care if Patty knows anything. But I want to know that the person who's going to advise me about my sick child knows what she's doing. I want to know from the minute I meet or talk to her that she is a credible professional."

The first-name-only convention also makes it harder for individual nurses to receive credit for their work. We recognize that, in some workplaces, nurses become defensive because they anticipate being singled out for blame more than for credit. But lack of a last name rarely protects a nurse from the former and may deprive her or him of the latter.

For example, one woman recently told us how impressed she was with the performance of the nurses at an outpatient surgery center where her mother had a basil-cell carcinoma removed. The nurses identified a potential heart problem that the physicians overlooked and suggested that her mother make an appointment for a cardiac evaluation. When, three weeks later, the cardiologist identified a previously undiagnosed heart condition, the woman was grateful for the nurses' clinical astuteness. She wanted to write a letter to the hospital administration to commend their actions. But who were these nurses? They did not introduce themselves with a last name. Only their first names appeared on their name badges.

The woman felt she could not send a letter with just the first names of these nurses. She would have had to call the hospital personnel office or the department of nursing and ask for the last name of the Maureen or Joan who worked at three o'clock in the out-patient OR four weeks ago. It would be too much trouble. This may be what accounts for "the nurses were wonderful" letters and comments that praise the group but not individuals.

In the world of work, people who receive credit often do so because they make it easy for others to acknowledge their contributions. A businessman we know, whose first name is John, recalled that during his years as an employee in a company, he always made a point of introducing himself with his first and last name when he was speaking with the executive responsible for salaries. "I wanted him to be clear that I was the one who should get the raise, not some other John," he says.

3.   Patients don't need to know nurses' last names to respect nurses and value what nurses do for them.

"They don't care what my last name is. All they need to know is that I'm Susan and I'm there to help them through their delivery," a labor and delivery nurse insisted.

"It doesn't matter what they call us, patients value us for what we do," a student in an advanced practice nursing program argued.

These comments are illuminating. Hopefully patients do value nurses for their contribution to care and recovery. But patients can value their nurses while simultaneously assigning them a lower status in the health care hierarchy.

Respect and value are related not only to what people know but to how people present themselves. If nurses introduce themselves by their first names only, they are asking to be regarded as non-professionals because that is the conventional way that non-professionals present themselves. Waitresses, garage mechanics and others who introduce themselves with their first names only certainly can and should be respected and valued for the work they do. But they do not have the responsibility for defining their work and their place in the workplace in the same way that nurses do.

In most societies, there are conventions that govern how professionals present themselves. When members of the largest health care profession opt out of the standard professional greeting, they risk communicating that they do not regard themselves as professionals or on a par with the other professionals.

4.   Nurse Adams = Nurse Ratched

In many of our seminars, nurses eventually agree that calling themselves "Nurse (Last name)" may be a good idea. But then they argue that patients will automatically associate "Nurse Adams" with one of the most heinous literary portraits of a nurse—Ken Kesey's sadistic Nurse Ratched from the book and movie, *One Flew Over the Cuckoo's Nest.*

Nurse Ratched was a monster. But why assume that juxtaposing the title Nurse with any of the millions of last names nurses have will instantly evoke this evil character? Is this connection in the public imagination or in the minds of nurses?

To find out we asked about a dozen people we know to say what comes into their minds when they hear the words "Nurse Benner, Nurse Smith, Nurse Woo." Not one came up with Nurse Ratched. They did, however, associate the names, with "kindness," "caring," "compassion," "competence," and "trustworthiness."

A number of younger people had never even heard of Nurse Ratched. But let's say someone had immediately associated Nurse Adams with Nurse Ratched. So what? A knee-jerk response does not indicate that this association will permanently taint the title "Nurse." If millions of RNs routinely identified themselves as "Nurse —," it would quickly seem normal and the association with an aberrant nurse character would fade. After all, medicine has its share of evil doctor prototypes such as Dr. Mengele (the death doctor of Auschwitz) and Dr. Kevorkian. But because "Dr. (Last Name)" is such common usage, negative connotations don't prevail.

5.   Potential danger.

"I will not take any more risks," an emergency department nurse declared heatedly when the subject of introductions came up at a workshop. "I'm already in danger. People come in with weapons and sometimes they go berserk and hit us."

"If they know our last names, they might stalk us. They might follow us home," another nurse contended.

Whenever the use of last names is discussed, some nurses argue that the personal safety of nurses depends upon concealing their last names.

We do not take the subject of personal safety lightly. Health care workers *are* sometimes physically attacked. As women, we are aware of the particular vulnerability of women in dealing with strangers. The very nature of nursing work puts nurses into intimate contact with people who may be violent, mentally disturbed or who may misinterpret caring for a sexual invitation.

Because personal safety is so important, it merits a thorough evaluation. Nurses must protect themselves and must be protected from physical danger to the greatest degree possible. The question is, does the use of a nurse's last name subject the nurse to additional personal risk?

Emergency nurses point out that attempted or actual physical assaults by patients are not unusual. The emergency nurse quoted above indeed is "already in danger." She works in a hospital with inadequate protections. People carrying weapons are able to enter the facility. The protocols for controlling physically aggressive patients apparently are non-existent or not implemented.

We asked this nurse whether nurses and physicians are attacked at random in this facility, or whether attackers deliberately single out a particular clinician. She said that physical violence was directed against anyone who was around. She said it made no difference whether the staff member's last name was known or not. Still, she was adamant. She would never use her last name at work because she was already vulnerable to diseases and to physical attack, just by working there. Her last name would add one more layer of vulnerability, she insisted.

This nurse was so terrified, she couldn't perceive the illogic of her position. She was hoping for some kind of magic to protect her—if they don't know who I am, maybe I'm safe.

We're concerned that some nurses are relying on an ineffective measure for protection. If a nurse works in a situation in which disclosing her last name to certain persons could be dangerous, of course she must behave accordingly. But nurses and other health care workers must go to the source of the problem when their institution is failing to provide proper security. They must find out from their professional associations and other institutions what systems are effective, and require their own institutions to adopt such measures.

One serious question raised by this debate is whether nurses belong to a special endangered class that would cause them to hide their last names even when physicians don't. When we've discussed this with nurses, several have suggested that it would be easier for a person to harass or stalk a nurse if her last name is known.

But just how much safety does last-name anonymity confer? If a patient is disturbed enough to harass or harm a nurse, couldn't he just follow her home after work? How do women physicians, who usually use their last names, handle this problem? Are they not also vulnerable? Or are they in another special category as far as risk is concerned?

That's a question worth pondering. We live in violent times. In the US especially, we have been inundated with killing sprees by heavily armed individuals who go after people they deem responsible for their misery. It's true that people have been slaughtered because they were a member of a certain race, religion or profession, or merely because they were nearby.

As female reporters we have covered volatile situations and violent people. We've experienced our share of danger. For those who deal with the public, irate customers or clients come with the territory. But lawyers, journalists or stock brokers simply do not have the option of jettisoning their last names as a protective measure. As a professional, it's standard practice to use one's whole name. Other precautions to reduce the risk of danger must be taken. It might be prudent to limit the amount of personal information given to a client. An unlisted home phone number might be wise. Employing a firm tone of voice, and assertive body language will help dissuade anyone who becomes overly familiar.

We have found no studies that suggest nurses in general constitute a special class where violence is concerned. Except in very special cases, the kind of anonymity that comes from using only a first name provides minimal physical protection, but considerably lessens nurses' agency and status. For nurses, who have fought long for professional legitimacy, demoting themselves to non-professional status is a big price to pay for something that has little value.

6. It's just too difficult to change cultural practices within an institution.

It certainly is difficult to change cultural practices if nurses unwittingly reinforce them. That's why it's important to start deconstructing deferential naming practices right now.

Many nurses say they would like more recognition and egalitarian treatment in the workplace. But they may still be acting out of habit by unwittingly enforcing an atmosphere of reverence and subordination to physicians.

Consider the nurse who works at a major teaching hospital, has a masters degree in nursing, and generally behaves in an autonomous and assertive manner—except when it comes to naming practices. Privately she calls her doctor colleagues by their first names, but in front of patients, she always uses Dr. (Last Name). When she talks to a nurse in the presence of patients, however, she always calls them by their first names. "Why?" Gordon once asked her.

"Well, the patients should respect their doctors," she replied.

If respect resides in a last name and title, then why, Gordon probed, doesn't she call her colleagues "Ms." or "Nurse (Last name)." The idea startled her so much she was speechless.[8]

Many practices in institutions have become so habitual that no one thinks about them anymore. Because they are so familiar, people sometimes defend conventions that really don't do them justice. This is the case when nurses insist they must use the physician's title and last name so that the patients will know that the person treating them is, in fact, a doctor, but argue that nurses can get along just fine with only first names.

If the term "Dr." indicates function, nurses have to ask themselves why patients don't need to know that the women and men who are RNs also have a function—to serve as their nurses. The importance of nurse identification seems even more urgent when nurses may be replaced with aides who have little nursing education or training. The way that patients will know who is a nurse is by hearing the word "nurse" applied repeatedly. They will hear that word if a nurse introduces herself as Nurse (Last name), if the physician refers to Nurse (Last name), and if a nurse refers to her colleague as Nurse (Last name). Workplace conventions will change when nurses ask physicians to address them this way in front of patients and when they give one another the same professional respect doctors give each other.

Decoding and altering naming practices ought to be a part of nursing education so that young nurses will treat nursing as a profession that is different from, but on a par with, medicine. To do otherwise is to suggest to young nurses that physicians are better than nurses because they have more years of education than RNs.

This was what a nursing student in Philadelphia essentially said when we counseled student nurses to insist on being called "Ms.," "Mrs." or "Mr." if residents and interns and even medical students want to be referred to as "Dr." in front of patients. "But he's a doctor," she responded, "and I'm just a nursing student."

"So what?" an older African-American student countered. "I do it all the time. I just walk up to them, put out my hand to shake their's and say, 'I'm Mrs. Smith. How are you?'"

We have noticed that African-American nurses often are more sensitive to naming practices than their white colleagues. There is a reason. It wasn't so long ago that African Americans were purposefully addressed only by first names, by nicknames, or by insulting titles such as "boy" for an adult man or "auntie" for an older woman. This naming system was used to keep an identified population in a subordinate social and economic position. One of the explicit goals of the civil rights movement in the 1960s was to stop this practice. There was great resistance in some areas to adopting a more respectful form of address, namely honorific titles and last names, because the change would prompt and symbolize an elevation in status. We should not forget the courage it took to press this issue and the significance of the change.

To apply these hard-won rights to nurses might not be as daunting as some nurses fear. This was illustrated in a seminar on nursing and feminism that nurse educator Elizabeth Grady and Suzanne Gordon conducted at Tufts New England Medical Center some years ago.

One of the older nurses in the group explained that she would like to be on a first-name basis with the physicians she worked with. Although most were much younger than her, she was fearful that she would offend them by calling them by their first names. After all, she stammered, they were doctors weren't they? The instructors suggested that she rehearse. They told her to pretend that she was arriving at work, and when she sees the doctor she says, "Hi, Tom, how are you?"

She said she was terrified that Tom would chastise her for stepping out of line. The instructors suggested that if "Tom" responded that way, the nurse should continue to use his title, but ask him to call her "Mrs. (Last name)."

Over the next week, she practiced at home until she felt more confident. One morning she went into work and said, "Hi Tom, how are you?" Without batting an eye, Tom replied cheerfully, "Fine, how are you?"

The system of deferring to doctors, even when they may not want such treatment, can be quite entrenched. "I keep telling the nurses I work with to call me Emily," one physician says. "Some nurses say they can't bring themselves to call me by my first name. So then they call me Dr. Emily."

At a health care service in the Boston area, the convention was that physicians, nurses, pharmacists, secretaries, clerks—all the personnel—referred to doctors by title and last name. The nurse practitioners and the clinical nurses, however, were referred to by their first names. The disparity was most obvious when a patient called for an appointment. The appointment secretaries responded: "Dr. Smith will see you at 3 on Wednesday," or "Janice (a nurse-practitioner) will see you…" Pharmacists routinely asked: "Did Dr. Smith or Janice give you a prescription?" Strikingly, the personnel tended to refer to the physician's assistants as "Mr.," "Ms." or "Mrs." The respect accorded the physicians apparently extended to their assistants as well.

We brought up this disparity with the medical director. Now the appointment secretaries say, "You can see Nurse (Last Name) for your flu shot at 10," etc. The prescription labels now give the names of the nurse practitioners and the proper abbreviation of their credentials.

Nurses are not alone in this issue. Most professional women have had to sort through what would constitute equal treatment with men. Forms of address have been part of that struggle.

We decided some time ago to establish ground rules before participating in panel discussions or radio or television programs. We ask the host or moderator how they will address and refer to other health care experts on the panel who may be physicians, PhDs or nurses. If the hosts or interviewers say they will refer to MDs and PhDs as "Dr.," then we insist that they refer to us as "Ms." and to the nurses as "Nurse" or "Ms." If the hosts plan to call us by our first names, then we tell them that we prefer that they refer to the MDs and PhDs by their first names also. We decided that the risk of appearing odd is far outweighed by the benefits. We know that any disparity of address between us and the doctor in the house cues listeners to take our knowledge and insights less seriously than another expert who has a title. We feel that our message about caregiving is too important to be overshadowed by traditional messages about status and hierarchy.

Looking like a Nurse

On those (all too rare) occasions when a nursing issue is covered in the mainstream media, chances are that a vintage photograph of hospital nurses in uniforms and caps will be among the illustrations. Even though we write about current health care issues and contemporary nursing, we've learned the hard way that editors tend to illustrate our articles with a romantic image of a Victorian-era nurse or with an old hospital-school photo of student nurses lined up like military cadets. Now we inquire about the illustrations well in advance of publication.

There are many reasons the lay public, and often nurses themselves, find nostalgic images compelling. These images are the icons of nursing. If a reader or a viewer sees an image of Florence Nightingale with her lamp or a uniformed hospital nurse, it is instantly understood that the subject matter is nursing. It's hard to broadcast this immediate content with the image of a contemporary nurse at work. A caption or other cues may be needed to effectively identify the subject as nursing.

Now freed from the laborious upkeep of starched uniforms, nurses must provide new visual cues to their identity or continue to face the familiar patient complaint: "You can't tell who the nurses are. You can't tell whether the person coming into the room is a nurse, an aide, a housekeeper, a technician or what."

When patients express these concerns you can be sure that they want to know who the nurses are, and that what they consider to be an un-nurselike appearance makes them anxious. An elderly couple we know wrote a critical letter on this point to the administrator of a Boston teaching hospital. The husband and wife, who had both been inpatients, complained that there was no way to identify the nurses.

Perhaps this couple had antiquated expectations about how nurses ought to look. Nonetheless, the issue is a serious one. While dress conventions vary from workplace to workplace, a significant cultural change has occurred over the years. The formality of the conventional uniform of the past had the effect of making hospital nurses—who often were very young—look older and more professional. In contrast, much of the clothing being marketed for today's nurses—who clearly are adults—is very informal and juvenile, even girlish, in tone. Uniform catalogs are full of smocks and scrubs covered with teddy bears, flowers, or other cutesy patterns. Even more conservative, solid-color scrubs might still be embroidered with hearts or smiley faces on the chest.

Pediatric nurses might consciously choose such clothing to put their young patients at ease. But what impression does this clothing convey in adult settings? Teddy bears, hearts, flowers, and smiley faces create an aura of youth and even childishness in a setting where maturity (irrespective of one's age) is an essential qualification. A nurse in this garb may feel she is telling a patient not to be afraid of her, but she is also suggesting that her patients and colleagues should not take her seriously.

Standardization of dress is not so much the issue. The issue is the need to adopt a style of dress that assists nurses' efforts to be treated more professionally. Some nurses feel that lab coats and solid-color scrubs fit the bill. A name-pin that gives the wearer's full name—minus the hearts and smiley faces—and that clearly identifies her or him as an RN is essential.

Who's a Girl?

There are other commonly used words and phrases that, upon examination, tend to undercut the agency of nurses and place them in a juvenile category. The most ubiquitous in everyday interactions is "girl."

The son of an elderly patient tells the nurse manager that his mother needs help. She wants to assure him that a staff nurse will soon be there by saying, "I'll get one of the girls to help her." In fact, she is undercutting the professional standing of nurses by using this word in a professional setting.

Actually, the word "girl" has various meanings and connotations. Sociolinguist Deborah Tannen, author of the best-selling book, *You Just Don't Understand: Women and Men in Conversation*, told us that "girl" (or "lady") has traditionally been used as a euphemism for "woman" because the latter term, in some cultures, carries the unacceptable suggestion of sexuality and/or age.[9]

So your 80-year-old mother may tell you that she is having lunch with the girls and mean it as a compliment. We might refer to our best friends as "girl friends." An African-American woman might say to her friend, "Girl, let me tell you…" A husband might say to his wife, "How's my girl?" In these settings, the word conveys closeness and affection.

However, in the workplace, the word "girl" connotes the standard dictionary definitions: l) a female infant or child, or young unmarried woman; 2) a maidservant; 3) a sweetheart.

Do patients want a child to take care of them when they are sick? Do nurses want to be thought of as maidservants or sweethearts or young unmarried women? Just as forms of address were a major focus of the civil rights movement, one of the goals of the women's movement was to stop the routine use of the term "girl" to describe grown women.

Some might argue that men use a parallel terminology. But, in fact, they don't. According to Tannen, men use "boy" in a stylized way, as in "old boys' network" (which emphasizes the power of older males) or "night out with the boys" (which conveys the idea that men will temporarily put aside their adult responsibilities). Men don't use the term in a generalized way or in a professional setting.[10] Has anyone ever heard a physician tell a patient: "I'll call neurology and get one of the boys to come down and do a neuro-consult?"

Today a male physician probably wouldn't dare call a female physician a "girl." Nor would a female physician refer to another female physician as a "girl."

When "boy" is used in a professional setting, it is overtly demeaning, and racist if the man in question is African American. Similarly, if a nurse uses "girl" to refer to nurses aides or other health care workers—some of whom may be people of color—they risk sounding not just condescending, but racist.

For all of these reasons it is essential that nurses in the workplace cease using the word "girl" to refer to other nurses or to other adult workers. Instead, when referring to an RN colleague, one could simply say, "I'll ask my colleague for help," or, "I'll ask another nurse for help." And when referring to an aide or other health care worker, "I'll send one of the aides, (or women) in to help you."

Body Language and "Presence"

Just as seemingly innocuous words and phrases can communicate volumes about nursing, so too can gestures, postures, physical arrangements, and actions.

Consider the following examples:

- In one HMO, the physicians, male and female, usually shake hands with patients when they greet them. The nurses rarely do.

- Nurses at one east coast medical center point with pride to their strong nursing department and their collaborative relationships with physician colleagues. At this hospital, nurses round with physicians each morning and insist that they communicate their concerns as equal members of the health care team. Professionals from other facilities frequently visit to examine this collaborative model in action. We notice on one unit, however, the stratified way that nurses and physicians arrange themselves to discuss cases. The interns perch on an air conditioner ledge in front of the windows. The resident stands a little to the side facing them. The nurses fan out behind the resident. With her back to the nurses, the resident speaks to the interns, and they direct responses to her. When the nurses provide information about patients, they tend to speak in deferential tones, and the resident barely turns her head.

- A nurse needs to talk with a physician about a patient. She finds the physician in the waiting room deeply engaged in a conversation with another physician. The nurse stands quietly next to them. The physicians continue to talk without acknowledging her presence. Eventually the nurse shrugs and walks off, muttering that she'll catch the physician later. About an hour later, one of the physicians comes up to the nurses' station where the same nurse is talking with several of her colleagues. Without apologizing, the doctor interrupts the nurses with a question. They immediately stop their conversation and the nurse responds politely.

- A physician does a thoracentesis on an elderly woman with lung cancer while her daughter holds her hand. When the physician finishes, he starts to pick up the debris from the procedure. "Oh, let me do that," the nurse says reaching past him and commandeering the clean-up job.

What do these scenarios communicate? What do they teach physicians, nurses and the public about the status and roles of RNs and MDs?

In the first case, by opting out of the traditional handshake, the nurses are communicating that their role is not as significant as that of the physicians. No matter what the nurses say about themselves in the introduction, their failure to assert their individual presence through physical contact suggests that they prefer to be in the background.

In the second scenario, nurses claim to be equal collaborators in patient care. But, by standing behind the resident, the nurses collaborate in another way entirely. They help to construct a configuration that makes nurses appear to be spectators. The physicians have arranged themselves so that they converse with each other. When a nurse tries to contribute to the conversation, her hesitant speech conveys what she seems to feel, that she does not have a rightful place in this discussion.

In the third example, nurses are undermined in their assertion that what they have to say to physicians about patients is as important as what physicians share with each other. In this case, the physicians' communication not only took precedence, but shut out the nurse. As in the second example, nursing is positioned outside the circle of influence. The nurse assents to this interpretation by shrugging and walking away. And, when the physician interrupts her and her colleagues an hour later, by answering immediately she reaffirms that what the physician needs to know is much more important than what she and her colleagues are discussing.

The fourth scenario goes to the heart of the stereotype of nurses as handmaidens to physicians. In this case, the physician, by cleaning up after himself and the nurse, communicates that he does not see the nurse as a maid. But the nurse, ironically, becomes anxious about collegial treatment and rushes to reaffirm the traditional definition of the nurse as wife or maid—even though she might well have protested, or at least complained later to her peers, if the physician had ordered her to clean up. By taking over the clean-up, this nurse is communicating a stereotypical job description of nursing to the doctor, patient and family member.

Corrective Strategies

A firm but cordial handshake is an essential part of a professional introduction and provides the opening for nurses to state their names and credentials. When meeting a patient a nurse can simply extend her or his hand, shake the patient's hand firmly, make eye contact, and say, "I'm Linda Jones, RN" or "I'm Nurse Jones," or "I'm Linda Jones, your registered nurse."

In the second case, nurses on rounds could simply intersperse themselves among the physicians, and speak up with authority when they have something to say.

In the third example, the nurse could politely interrupt the physicians and state her business. And when the physician barged in on their conversation, the nurses could politely but firmly ask him to wait a moment until they finished consulting about a patient.

Obviously, in the last example, the nurse could just let the physician clean up.

Workplace encounters such as these are both "private" interactions and "public" communications that convey information about the status and agency of nurses. As the sociologist Erving Goffman noted in exploring this issue, how one presents oneself contributes to the construction of social and professional reality. "When an individual plays a part," he wrote in *The Presentation of Self in Everyday Life*, "he implicitly requests his observers to take seriously the impression that is fostered before them."[11]

Paying attention to self-presentation does not require a personality transplant and definitely does not mean that nurses have to turn themselves into unapproachable authoritarian figures. As British sociologist Celia Davies put it, nurses may feel they must choose between two models of behavior in the workplace—one that is self-orienting or one that is self-effacing. But Davies, in her book, *Gender and the Professional Predicament of the Nurse*, suggests that the choice need not be limited to either the autonomous male professional model or the passive/dependent female role. Instead she advocates "reconstructing" a model of professionalism appropriate to both the needs of the sick and of the largely female nurses who care for them. "The professional practitioner of the future needs to avoid the boundedness/connectedness dilemma and to envisage being neither distant nor involved but engaged," she asserts. This new model of professionalism could be constructed around the concept of "meaningful distance" that "acknowledges that there will be a commitment and emotional response, but seeks to avoid over-identification on the one hand and under-involvement on the other."[12]

In other words, by asserting their agency in their self presentation, nurses need not worry that projecting a "professional" image will make them seem distant, or feel self-conscious, false, or stilted. Instead, nurses will be presenting an authentic image of themselves, one that calls forth responses that are respectful of them as nurses and as human beings.

Endnotes

1. S. Gordon and E. M. Grady, "What's In a Name?" *American Journal of Nursing*, 1995: pp. 31–33.

2. J. E. Lynaugh, Interview with the authors, 2000.

3. Gordon and Grady, pp. 31–33.

4. C. Lindaman, "Talking to Physicians about Pain Control," *American Journal of Nursing*, January 1995: pp. 2–3.

5. A. Kleinman, *The Illness Narratives: Suffering, Healing, and the Human Condition* (Basic Books, 1988).

6. P. Benner, C. A. Tanner, and C.A. Chesla, *Expertise in Nursing Practice* (New York: Springer, 1996).

7. E. Goffman, *The Presentation of Self in Everyday Life* (Garden City, N.Y.: Doubleday Anchor Books, 1959).

8. Gordon and Grady, pp. 31–33

9.   D. Tannen, *You Just Don't Understand: Women and Men in Conversation* (New York: William Morrow and Company, Inc., 1990).

10. D. Tannen, Interview with the authors, 1996.

11. Goffman, *Presentation of Self.*

12. C. Davies, *Gender and the Professional Predicament in Nursing* (Buckingham: Open University Press, 1995).

Chapter 4

TELL THE WORLD WHAT YOU DO

A medical-surgical nurse who had just participated in a major nursing conference called the hotel bellhop for help in getting her bags to the airport shuttlebus. As the nurse and bellhop were walking to the elevator, the young man turned to her and remarked, "The people here aren't ordinary nurses, are they?"

Intrigued by the question, the nurse asked what he meant. "Well," he said, "I've been walking through the exhibit area and there are all these fancy medical machines and equipment. Ordinary nurses don't use such complicated equipment," he stated confidently. "This must be a conference for chiefs."

Without skipping a beat, the nurse replied: "This is a conference for ordinary nurses. We use all kinds of sophisticated medical equipment and medications when we take care of you. Ordinary nurses are the chiefs of patient care in hospitals."

Another nurse told us about an incident that occurred when she flew into Rochester, Minnesota, for a conference at the Menninger Clinic. On the way into town, her cab driver proudly boasted about Rochester's medical reputation. "We have some of the best medical care in the world," he said. "The best doctors and researchers are here. People come here from all over the globe just to see them."

She listened and gently pointed out that he forgot an important part of the health care team—nurses. "All of these great doctors," she told him, "wouldn't succeed without great nurses. You must remember to tell your next customer about that too."

Life presents nurses with countless conversational openings to talk about nursing. These openings occur at cocktail parties, backyard barbecues, relatives' weddings, school events, church programs, and most importantly of all, in patients' rooms. Not every nurse will be called by a reporter from the *New York Times* or the *National Post,* but nurses constantly speak with relatives, friends, neighbors, patients, teachers or guidance counselors who ask what they do, or who make a comment about nursing. Sometimes these comments contain erroneous information that needs to be corrected. Other times, the comment may give you an opportunity to advance someone's knowledge about your profession.

Educating the Public in Everyday Life

In great part, because of the media's singular focus on doctors and their failure to cover nurses, what people read in newspapers or magazines or see on television does little to educate them about the content of contemporary nursing. In fact, the media may actually misinform the public and leave them more confused than ever about what nursing is and what nurses do. If nurses don't tell the public about their important work, archaic images of nursing will persist.

Although the second half of this book provides instruction on how to reach out to the news media, speaking to the public about nursing usually does not require extraordinary efforts. You don't have to go into public relations to tell the public about nursing. You can take advantage of the opportunities in ordinary situations to enlighten people with whom you come into daily contact. Practice in these arenas will help when you want expand your audience to the media or political representatives.

Describing Your Work

Most nurses, of course, consciously communicate with patients and families to receive and impart information about the health and care of the patient and to put the patient at ease. But in getting information about patients' problems and in giving information to the patient and family, you are also imparting information about yourself as a professional and about nursing's work and status. You can consciously influence what people know about nursing in this setting.

In conversations with patients and others, you can educate people about the scope of nursing by being more specific about the kind of nursing you do. Instead of saying only that you're a nurse, you might say a bit more, such as, "I'm an oncology nurse, I work with children with cancer," or "I'm a psychiatric nurse, I work with patients with…"

When the opportunity presents itself, you can also describe in more detail what you are doing and why you are doing it. For example, say you are taking care of a patient who has just had a stroke. His daughter comes to visit while you are feeding the patient. You can do your work silently. Or, while you are feeding the patient, you can explain to him and to his daughter the significant aspects of what you are doing. It isn't necessary to deliver a dissertation on the four phases of swallowing. But it may be useful to explain that you are assessing the patient's gag reflex and why that is important. In describing all this, you are not only teaching the patient and his daughter how to feed safely, you are teaching them that nurses have special, life-saving knowledge.

To many people the more domestic activities of nursing seem simple or even trivial. In fact, they may even wonder why it takes an educated person to do them. This is an opportunity to enlighten them. Explain why activities like feeding, bathing, toileting, walking, or turning patients can be some of the most important things a nurse does.

You might assume that a patient and family understand your work—even its most high-tech aspects—just because they see you do it. Like the bellhop we introduced you to at the beginning of this chapter, they may think that what you do as a nurse is the exception, not the rule. "You're an extraordinary nurse," they might think, not an "ordinary" nurse doing extraordinary things. That is why when you are caring for a patient using high-tech devices, teaching the patient how to master drug regimens at home and answering questions about the patient's disease, or helping educate the patient about health promotion, it is important to point out in some way during the conversation that "these are things registered nurses do."

Making the Agency of Nurses Known

Nurses are too seldom given credit for relying on their own knowledge and judgment. Many people believe that everyone in health care—including the nurse—follows the doctor's orders. They believe that a sort of invisible line runs from the doctor's brain to yours, and that you are acting on his knowledge, not your own. That's why many patients thank their doctor for the good work that nurses have done or even thank doctors for "training their nurses so well."

To convey the content of nursing, nurses must describe the complexity of the care *they* give and the clinical judgments *they* use. They must take care in their discussions with patients and families, with the broader public, and with media and political representatives not to depict themselves as extensions of the doctor's agency.

For example, in a seminar we conducted in Canada, a nurse discussed with some dismay an experience she had with a hospitalized diabetic patient. She had worked long and hard with this patient to teach him about his complicated drug regimen. She thought they had established a good rapport and was sure he trusted her expertise. As she was walking past his room, however, she overheard a conversation between the patient and his doctor that she found disheartening. The patient was checking up on the information she had just given him. "The nurse said this. Was she right?" was the gist of the conversation.

"Why was he verifying the information I'd just given him," she wondered, with real sadness in her voice.

The group asked her how she had presented the information to the patient. "I told him the doctor wanted him to take this medicine, and the doctor wanted him to follow this diet," she responded.

"Ah," her fellow nurses commented. "No wonder he's checking up on you." The group explained that she had presented herself as a handmaiden to the doctor—a kind of human medical tape recorder repeating his instructions—rather than as a partner in care. The other nurses thought it was perfectly rational, indeed even wise, for a patient to ask the proverbial horse if the horse's mouth got it right.

What would have happened, they suggested, if the nurse had spoken from her own agency along these lines: "Let's review what diabetes is about. Here is what has happened to you. Here's what makes your blood sugar go up. Here's what makes it come down. What diabetes means is that your body no longer corrects for these things. And here's the role of the medication in helping to prevent damage. Here's how you need to take the medicine."

The oncology nurse we described in chapter two faced a similar problem. Her patient and the patient's family needed to know her role in getting much needed pain medication. If she had used conventional terms, she would have told the patient that the doctor "ordered" her morphine. This, however, would conceal her contribution. She couldn't tell the patient she'd fought with the doctor to get the morphine, so she negotiated the dilemma by saying: "I've consulted with the doctor and he agreed with my recommendation to give you IV morphine. You'll be feeling better soon."

Even innocuous remarks offer an opportunity to present your agency. A nursing student at McGill University says that when patients remark, "It's so nice you're studying nursing," or that nursing is such a "nice" profession, "I'm never sure if they're really just blowing nursing off."

So we recommended that the next time a patient says that to her, she respond with: "You know, you're so right. Nurses do such important work to keep patients safe in the hospital. That's why I wanted to be a nurse."

If the patient is healthy enough to comment on your choice of profession, they're healthy enough to hear about the contribution of nurses to their safety and well-being.

Dealing with the Fear of Making Doctors Angry

Many RNs report that they are worried about making doctors angry and thus don't voice their opinions or talk about their work. Sometimes doctors act very aggressively to silence nurses and put them in their place. At other times nurses silence themselves even when doctors might not complain or might be supportive. There could be any number of reasons why a physician might respond defensively, aggressively or abusively to nurses. We believe nurses should deal directly with physicians who try to silence them by discussing the aspects of their behavior related to gender, patient care, collegiality, and etiquette. Abuse from physicians must never be tolerated. Nurses who make such abuse public will be surprised by the social support they will receive. Today, after decades of struggle by women, this kind of behavior is not socially or legally sanctioned.

What's most distressing about some doctors' behavior towards nurses is that it elicits the expectation that all doctors might behave this way whenever nurses express their opinions or talk about their work.

For example, an officer of a nursing organization who was practicing speaking on camera during a media training session, reacted with fright when she realized she was favorably comparing nurses to physicians. She had explained that nurses are in frequent and ongoing contact with patients, and remarked that "physicians see patients for only a few minutes a day." Then she clapped her hands over her mouth.

Everyone in the room, including her, laughed at her dramatic gesture. She explained that her gut reaction was that she had disclosed something bad about doctors and that they would be angry. Upon reviewing that tape, however, she decided that she was not criticizing physicians, but stating a fact.

Making your work visible in a way that distinguishes the roles of nursing and medicine is not bad mouthing either physicians or their profession, or revealing shameful family secrets. Even the most egregious behavior of physicians toward nurses or patients can be described accurately and placed in its historical context. This allows nurses to frame the issue as a system problem rather than a personal attack.

At times nurses have an obligation to clarify their professional responsibilities for the benefit of patients, physicians and the public. Psychiatric nurse Beth Halusan fulfilled this obligation while working with a teenaged patient in a short-term psychiatric hospital in Wisconsin.

"Samantha" had been admitted to the facility for treatment for drug abuse and depression. She was a high school dropout and the mother of one-year-old twins. She was considering placing them in foster care because she couldn't handle her parenting responsibilities.

"How are things going for you?" Nurse Halusan asked when she met Samantha.

"Not really good," Samantha replied. "I don't like my doctor."

"You don't like your doctor?" Halusan inquired.

"No, I don't think he understands me," Samantha said.

Samantha explained that she felt she would fall into severe depression and start using drugs again unless she had ongoing treatment and "a place to stay." However, the physician recommended that she go home after one week of treatment.

"You need to tell the doctor that you have been down this path before," Halusan advised Samantha. "Maybe he doesn't understand how serious you are about this."

"But he doesn't listen to me," Samantha complained.

Nurse Halusan counseled the patient on how to articulate the issues and her needs. She also advised Samantha that if she and the physician could not reach a meeting of the minds, then "I would ask the doctor if he could recommend a doctor who would be a better match."

When Halusan returned to work two days later she learned that the physician was opposed to a residential placement. She was about to contact him to ask him about "his line of thinking," when he burst onto the scene interrupting a conversation Halusan was having with a colleague.

"There is something very serious going on on this unit," the physician said heatedly.

"What's that?" Halusan asked.

"Patients are instructing their doctors about what's best for them," he replied.

"Are you talking about Samantha?" Halusan asked.

"Yes, and I don't think you understand how serious it is to encourage patients to fire their doctors," the physician said.

"That is not what transpired between Samantha and me," Halusan said, and explained that she encouraged the patient to discuss her concerns openly with the physician. Halusan reported that she also told the patient that she has "other options."

"It's not your job to determine what's best for the patient," the doctor replied.

"It is my job to give the patients all their options," Halusan stated firmly. She went on to discuss the case in detail, and then pointed out that no physician can be a perfect match for every patient.

Samantha was placed in a residential treatment facility after a treatment team—the physician, Nurse Halusan and a social worker—evaluated the situation with her. The physician never did concur with the recommendation. But the anger about the disagreement has faded and the physician's behavior is collegial.

"He listens to me," Halusan says of their relationship. "He knows that my job is to take care of patients."

Kathleen Connors, President of the Canadian Federation of Nurses Unions agrees that when nurses stand firm with physicians, the doctor may not like it, but may actually learn to give nurses greater respect.

When she was working in a 75-bed acute care referral hospital in northern Manitoba, Connors reported a doctor who refused to come to the ER to care for a critically ill patient. "Other nurses put up with this difficult physician for a long time, but when I was confronted with his behavior, I wouldn't. I told him he needed to come and see this patient. He refused.

"To clarify his position, I said, 'So I take it you're not coming in.'

"I got another physician to come in and we evacuated the patient from northern Manitoba to Winnipeg where she subsequently died on the OR table."

Connors said the patient would have had to have been flown to Winnipeg even if the doctor had come to the ER. But two precious hours—hours that may have meant the difference between life and death—wouldn't have been lost.

Connors documented what had happened and delivered both a written and oral report to the director of nursing and the chief of staff at the hospital. "I told them his clinical judgment was lacking and I wasn't going to be part of situations like that. His performance was reviewed, his admitting privileges were suspended, and he had to prove he would respond to emergency situations in the future. The result was that he showed me a great deal more respect from that point on and was more respectful to the other nurses in the department."

Another doctor once told Connors that she should not take care of one of his patients who was in the labor and delivery room. "I told him that when he started paying my salary and employed me as his nurse, he could determine who worked with him or not. I was an employee of the facility and if he didn't want me to look after his patient in established labor he'd better be prepared to put on his nurse's uniform and care for her. So of course I stayed."

Learn to Accept Thanks

Nurses also have the opportunity to explain their work when a patient expresses gratitude for excellent nursing care. Think about the last time a patient thanked you. How did you respond? Did you accept their acknowledgment? Or did you say, "Oh, it was nothing." "Oh, I didn't do very much." "Oh, it was just my job."

A lot of us rely on this conversational tack when we are complimented. But for nurses it has consequences.

Studies show that patients trust nurses. So when nurses consistently repeat, "Oh, it was nothing," or "I didn't do much," the danger is that people will believe them. And if "it"—nursing work—is "just a job," or "not very much of anything," the logical conclusion one draws is that nurses are nothing special. Why then should the public worry about replacing nurses with aides, or as so frequently happens today, with untrained family members who are asked to act as surrogate professional nurses in the home? If nurses do little or nothing, why should the public be in favor of increasing resources for nursing staffing, education and research?

An alternative approach can reveal the content of nursing care. A woman tells you: "God you were so great. You helped my husband learn to cope with his diabetes." This is your opportunity to respond: "Thank you. It was a privilege to take care of your husband, to teach him how to take his medication and to help him learn how to alter his diet. If you have any further questions or needs, please talk to me about them."

We talked with oncology nurses in Rhode Island about the tendency of nurses to trivialize their own work. Phoebe Fernald, an oncology clinical nurse specialist, approached us afterward. She said nurses' difficulty in saying "Thank you," and "You're welcome," in response to compliments and thanks struck a cord with her. "It's scary how automatically pat answers come out of our mouths," she said.

Fernald gave an illustration. She had recently helped family friends navigate their father's illness and death from cancer. At the calling hours before the funeral, the family thanked her and told her how much they appreciated what she had done. And what did she say? "Oh, I didn't do very much at all."

"But when I think about it," Fernald told us, "I did a lot. What I did was take time and listen to them. They needed to talk about their pain and hurt. They needed to talk about their concerns—whether they were doing the right thing, choosing the right treatments, and, when he no longer wanted more treatment, they needed to know that was okay too. They needed confirmation that they were making the right choices. And they needed it from someone who was an expert. [Fernald, initially said, "from someone who they perceived to be an expert," but changed her wording when we reminded her that she is one.] When patients thank us they are thanking us for our expertise and our skill in caring. When we say 'Oh, it was nothing,' we're denying that expertise and skill."

When we suggested that Fernald could have said, "You're welcome. It was a privilege to be able to help you," she responded, "That would not be a dishonest answer. It was a privilege."

Be Prepared to Take Advantage of Openings

If you were asked to do a presentation on nursing at your church, or to go on a local television show and talk about health care, you would take time to prepare your remarks. The more spontaneous communication opportunities that regularly come your way also require preparation. Although they don't come in the form of an invitation, these openings are nevertheless quite predictable. At times, conversational openings may even appear to be put-downs.

For example, someone at a party asks you what you do. You respond, "I'm a nurse." The other person doesn't know what to say. "Oh, how nice," she mutters politely and then goes on to a different subject.

Or, upon hearing that you are a pediatric nurse, an oncology nurse or a hospice nurse, an acquaintance responds: "That must be so depressing. How can you stand working with sick children—cancer patients—dying people?" To someone outside of health care anything that has to do with sickness, vulnerability and death may appear to be totally draining and unbearably depressing rather than enriching and rewarding.

Other conversational openings may come in the form of jibes that seem to overtly devalue nursing. One nurse recounted that she was talking to a businessman about her work as a nurse practitioner. "So you've gotten out of the bedpan business," he retorted.

Another told of a man at a cocktail party who asked: "Why did you become a nurse when someone as obviously intelligent as you could have been a doctor?"

And of course, student nurses are often queried—rather than applauded—about their decision to go into nursing rather than to medical school.

In another situation, the nurse may be left entirely out of the picture even when it seemed she was included. A nurse described her participation in a conference on the ethics of the care of the dying. One of the members of her panel described a study on hospital culture that was designed to help clinicians transform the experience of death and dying. The panelist reported that the study revealed three cultures in hospitals—the overall culture of the institution, the physician culture and the patient culture. Our friend was astonished listening to this. Whatever happened to the nurse culture? she wondered.

A student nurse told us she often goes out with a group of friends that includes medical students. Over dinner, those friends who are in business or law address their questions or comments to the medical students and never ask her questions about what she's learning and doing in nursing school. "What about me?" she wonders. "What about nursing?"

Obviously such experiences are enormously demoralizing. Their frequency can leave nurses speechless, so angry they want to scream, or worse still, so inured to it all that they just shrug.

Being prepared to respond constructively is a better approach. To be prepared, you must be willing to acknowledge that situations like this are not going to miraculously disappear. Indeed, you can be really effective if you embrace even the most negative comments as educational opportunities. Be glad that someone has mentioned nursing. Consider your friends, relatives or acquaintances as people requiring instruction and try to evince sympathy for people who are ill informed. Even the most disheartening comments about nursing usually stem from ignorance rather than malice. We live in a culture, after all, that systematically undervalues and misconstrues caregiving.

Thus, a person who sees a psychogeriatric nurse holding the hand of an elderly person in a hospital as she listens and speaks to the patient might think of the nurse, "What a nice lady." The observer is probably unacquainted with both the complex physical and psychological condition of the elderly patient, and the education and training the nurse brings to her. He or she is most likely unaware of the fact that the nurse is mentally compiling a list of the patient's depressive symptoms, thinking about what recommendations to make for treatment, finding out what kind of family support the patient has, and calming the patient's agitation, all at the same time.

Once you do appreciate the fact that most members of the public are largely ignorant of the content of nursing work, you can prepare yourself to grasp the opportunity concealed in comments that seem to ignore or denigrate that work. In this sense, the public is also your patient. By taking on the exciting challenge of educating the public about nursing, you can give new meaning to the term "patient educator."

Responding

When someone says to you, "How depressing it must be to deal with sick children or dying patients all the time," you can respond: "Sometimes it's very sad, but it's not depressing. Let me tell you what I did yesterday so you'll understand." Then you can describe your work and the difference it made to those who benefited from your care.

For example, Susan Sweeney, an emergency nurse at a level one trauma center in Rhode Island, recently told us a very moving story. A beautiful, 19-year-old man was brought into the emergency department following a car accident. He was dead on arrival. But the injuries that killed him were all internal. He looked perfect on the outside.

When his mother saw him, she refused to believe he was dead. He was just sleeping, she insisted. See, she said, calling to him to awaken him, his hand is moving. He's in a coma. He'll recover.

Sweeney and her colleague, a trauma physician, recognized that the woman was in shock and denial and needed a great deal of attention. Sweeney assessed the situation and recommended against medicating the mother because it would only delay what she inevitably had to recognize—that her son was dead. Sweeney knew she had to work with the woman until she was able to go home. Nurse Sweeney spent more than an hour with the woman trying to help her deal with her denial and grief.

This is what nurses do. Yes, it's terribly sad. But it's also extraordinarily rewarding to help people cope at times like this.

If someone makes a crack about bedpans, you can respond the way the nurse practitioner did. Without exhibiting the slightest anger, she said, "Let me tell you about bedpans..." and explained how the contents of a bedpan reveal a great deal about a patient's condition.

If an expert on your panel treats nurses as though they didn't exist, when it's your turn to speak, you can preface your remarks with a comment to the other panelist: "It was interesting to hear the results of your study. But I wonder why nursing culture—the largest culture in the hospital—was overlooked. I think it's a serious omission since hospitals are nursing institutions. You might consider rectifying this omission." Then make your presentation.

Perhaps the most infuriating question you'll get is: "Why did someone as intelligent as you become a nurse?" Or for students: "Why aren't you in medical school instead of nursing school?"

We have thought a lot about this question. We used to advise nurses to explain their choice and illuminate how nursing differs from medicine. We still believe that is an essential part of any response. Now we also feel that the erroneous assumptions embedded in the question must themselves be challenged.

This question "why did you become a nurse, why didn't you become a doctor" is simply illegitimate. When we tell people we're journalists, no one asks us why we didn't become poets. When doctors tell people what they do, no one asks them why they didn't go into bio-engineering instead. They ask them what their work is like. When a bright young man says he is in medical school, he's asked what he wants to specialize in, not, why isn't he going into a different health profession altogether. Today, when a woman announces her decision to become a doctor, she's viewed as a representative of the advancement of women.

Not so with nurses. An interesting social disconnect takes place when an intelligent woman or man is a nurse, or announces an intention to become one. We want nurses to be there when we're sick. We get angry—at them or the system—when they don't have time to answer our buzzer or give us the empathic attention we need. At the same time, when we're healthy, we neither applaud their career choices nor reward them with respect and admiration when we learn they are nurses. Rather than being viewed as pioneers expanding the definition of masculinity, men who are nurses or nursing students are often viewed as peculiar, while women who are nurses or nursing students may be viewed as having made the wrong choice.

These attitudes must change. Nurses can help to change them by the way they respond to questions.

Instead of telling people "I became a nurse because I want to care for people," you might calmly reply: "You know, if you asked me what I do as a nurse, and let me describe it to you, then you would understand why I didn't become a doctor."

Or, if you're a student, you might say brightly: "Why don't you ask me what I want to do as a nurse, then you'll understand why I'm going to nursing school and not medical school."

Or this: "Don't you want someone as intelligent as I am at your bedside when you're in the hospital (clinic, hospice, at home, or nursing home)? Think about it for a minute—if all the bright young women and men became doctors, who would be left to provide expert, knowledgeable care of the sick?" Then you can add: "When you, or a member of your family, is in the hospital you'll be glad so many intelligent, ambitious women and men decided to become nurses rather than doctors."

Finally, in social situations, when people find out you're a nurse and say nothing, or mutter "Oh how nice," that too can be an opening. You can direct the conversation with a few engaging questions and comments, such as: "It doesn't sound like you know much about nursing. But today, with a looming nursing shortage, public awareness of the profession is really important."

Stories and Anecdotes

People can begin to understand the nature of nursing through the stories that nurses tell about their work. Story telling allows a broader public to enter into the fabric of your work and appreciate its value.

To begin constructing your anecdotes, pretend you're a reporter planning to describe nursing work. Set the scene. Tell us about the situation/patient/family/system. What did *you* do? What kind of clinical knowledge and judgment did *you* bring to the encounter? Why did *you* do what *you* did? Why did it make a difference? What role did *you* play with the other members of the health care team? Identify for yourself and then for others the components of your agency. Whether or not any one else has given value to your activities, your job here is to identify and assert their value.

Silence that internal voice that takes your actions for granted. You may think, "Oh, no one would be interested in hearing about this," or "They would think it's ordinary." Banish that echo. Describe why these ostensibly ordinary actions are important. What would have happened to the patient or system or society if you hadn't taken this action? You may not look like you're "doing something" when you're sitting with a dying patient or witnessing a family's grief. But you can reveal the hard work involved in *being with* other human beings in a time of need.

An excellent example of how to do this is Jean Chaisson's description of her agency in getting disability insurance for a woman with breast cancer. First she introduced herself and established her credentials. Then she introduced us to the patient. She told us the patient's story and was not afraid to highlight the failings of some other health care professionals. She told us how she discovered the patient's needs. Then she explained what she did to help. Finally, she took full possession of her agency, not in a way that was self-aggrandizing but simply and matter-of-factly by identifying why her nursing expertise was essential. Even though she acknowledged the failures of medicine, she never claimed superiority. She simply stated the facts.

When you tell your stories, don't submerge your "I" into the "we" of the health care team. As nurse organizational consultant Elizabeth Grady has explained, nurses seem to have great difficulty acknowledging the "I" in the "we." Nurses will regularly highlight the contributions of other health care professionals while obscuring their own. Physicians, on the other hand, often exhibit the opposite behavior. Although physicians will admit that patient care is a collaborative affair, in public, they often give the impression that patient survival or recovery depends upon their efforts alone. As Nurse Grady put it, "physicians can't find the 'we' in the 'I.'"[1]

When Susan Sweeney initially told us about her care of the accident victim's mother, she recounted the story as if it were entirely a group effort. We asked her to clarify who did what. Did both she and the physician she worked with spend an hour with the mother?

No, she explained that early on the physician left to do other work and that she was the one who stayed and worked with the distraught mother.

Nurses often think that when they use the "we," people will understand that they made discrete contributions based on their clinical knowledge and judgment. In fact, given the prevalent stereotypes of nursing in our culture, the automatic assumption could be that everything was the doctor's idea and the nurse acted on the doctor's orders. This is why nurses must make their actions and judgments explicit.

Although your anecdotes will sound spontaneous when you tell them, they will be more effective if you prepare them in advance.

Making the details count

In your work you can be on the lookout for the "telling detail" that allows a lay person to get a sense of the complexity and tone of what you do and the environment in which you do it. Listen to how Nurse Paddy Connelly, an oncology nurse, brings us into her world: "I am taking care of a 25-year-old breast cancer patient who will have a bone marrow transplant. My patient will lose her breast, will probably lose her hair, and perhaps lose her ability to have a child. When my patient hears all this, she is overwhelmed. You have to realize that she is processing everything and nothing at all. So I, as a nurse, am aware that I need to be available to her to probe the questions she couldn't ask initially when she was essentially in a state of shock. In fact, over time, I may even have to help her formulate the questions to ask. No one else but a nurse is there to do that."

In telling this story, Nurse Connelly gave listeners the kind of detail they needed to imagine the scene. She also allowed others to see the patient as a human being, not as a case. She did this by using everyday language instead of the hospital jargon and technical terms that many health care professionals automatically use.

Avoid using jargon

While working on nursing anecdotes at a media seminar for nurses, we asked a volunteer to come to the podium and pretend she was being interviewed about her work by a television reporter.

"What do you do?" we asked.

"I'm a nurse practitioner," she said enthusiastically. "I deliver primary health care services. I do skilled assessment. I'm a patient educator and a patient advocate."

An oncology nurse stepped up next. She described her work with women on high-dose chemotherapy who experience premature menopause: "I do symptom assessment, I monitor the effect of chemotherapy on ovulatory function, and I do patient education."

Other nurses undoubtedly would know what this means, but would a non-nurse hearing these phrases, be able to see these nurses in action and grasp the kinds of problems their patients have?

Despite the obvious commitment of these nurses to their work, neither really brought her listeners into the daily world of nursing practice. In communicating with the public, nurses need to mobilize the words to do the job. This means making a distinction between what one says to other health care professionals and what one says to lay people.

How, for example, would a non-nurse react to the following statement? "My patient suffered from a short run of ventricular tachycardia and my intervention saved him from the ultimate negative patient outcome."

Or imagine what your neighbor would say if you told him this: "My patient was admitted from the ED with fulminating pulmonary edema. Opening PA pressures were 58 over 28, with a wedge of 30. O2 sat was 84 percent and his ABGs showed a PO2 of 82. He was in sinus tech with frequent runs of multiform PVCs and his SVR was 2400."

If you used this much hospital-speak, you may as well stay silent.

"My patient had an irregular heart rhythm and my quick action saved him from dying," is obviously much clearer to the non-nurse.

So is: "My patient had too much fluid in his lungs. His oxygen levels were low, and he had many irregular heartbeats. He had difficulty breathing and could have died suddenly. So I acted quickly to reduce his fluid volume and gave him morphine to help him relax."

Getting prepared ahead of time

We advocate that each nurse develop three anecdotes about her or his work that can be used in a variety of settings whenever an opening occurs. It may help to try writing them out in a conversational style.

Paint a picture infusing the story with human-interest details. That's what Jean Chaisson did when she described her care of the elderly stroke patient to a reporter who didn't understand how the so-called simple tasks of nursing are extremely complex.

Use facts and statistics. A great way to bolster your arguments and descriptions is to use a few choice facts and statistics. This enhances your credibility. A medical nurse speaking to someone she wants to influence about nursing might add something like this to her anecdote:

This kind of nursing is at the heart of health care. In fact, hospitals are nursing institutions. Nurses make up approximately one-quarter of hospital staff. Today no one is in a hospital if they don't need nursing care. They can get procedures and many kinds of surgery on an outpatient basis. Patients stay in the hospital because they need 24-hour-a-day monitoring from skilled nurses. However, lengths of hospital stays are shorter and shorter meaning that patients in the hospital are sicker than they have ever been before and there's no margin of error in their care. Expert nurses can represent the difference between life and death to such patients.

Judith Shindul-Rothschild, a psychiatric clinical specialist and professor of nursing at Boston College, describes some of the things psychiatric nurses do this way:

> Many patients on anti-depressant medication have a problem with sex. Men can't get erections and women can't reach orgasm. We have ways to help patients deal with this. For example, we can give patients a drug holiday. Over a weekend, when they may be more sexually active, they can skip their medication and this won't lower the drug level significantly or reduce its therapeutic effect.
>
> The problem is that patients don't want to admit that they're having trouble with sex. It's awkward for them to talk about it. So it's hard to help them. That's why it's so important for them to establish a trusting relationship with someone they know well. In most instances, this will be a nurse. A nurse who takes the time to talk to them, to register their subtle signals, and to respond is pivotal in dealing with this sort of problem.

When you're talking about your role at the bedside you might explain the consequences of nurses not being available to attend to the "small" things. For example, you might explain that when a nurse bathes a patient he looks for skin breakdown. He knows that the little red spot on the hip or heel can turn into a crater-sized decubitus ulcer that could eat all the way down to the bone. The care needed to heal this type of bedsore can cost several thousand dollars. Bedsores are 100 percent preventable with good nursing care.

Another anecdote could be about the danger of deep vein thrombosis. If a patient isn't helped to walk or move his legs, he can develop a pulmonary embolus, a blood clot to the lung. This catastrophic consequence of surgery or prolonged bedrest kills thousands of people a year. An expert nurse can help prevent DVT and pulmonary emboli.

Preventing aspiration pneumonia is another nursing job. So is preventing hospital-acquired infections. In these ways nurses not only save lives, but money as well.

Reflecting clinical judgment

An anecdote told to us by critical care nurse Judith Donnelly illustrates how veteran nurses employ clinical judgment and experience in situations that call for swift action.

Donnelly, who works in a telemetry unit at a New England hospital, was taking care of a heart patient scheduled for surgery the next morning. That night the patient called for the nurse because he was experiencing shortness of breath. As Donnelly checked him, she found what she had expected: he had fluid building up in his lungs and was sitting up to breathe more easily. His condition was stable but his heart rate was somewhat elevated. Donnelly asked the secretary to get a med order and began preparing the appropriate medication.

Then the patient said urgently: "Can you help me? I have to have a bowel movement."

Donnelly turned to the secretary and said quietly, "Call a code."

"Code?" the secretary replied.

"Now," Donnelly said.

When the code team and the resident arrived, the patient was still "normal." Suddenly his heart rate dropped to 30 and he began losing consciousness. The code team went to work. After the patient was stabilized, the resident asked Donnelly, "How did you know?"

She told the resident the patient needed to move his bowels.

The resident understood, but we didn't. Donnelly explained that the patient would not have had that urge under the circumstances unless something was happening with the vagus nerve. This nerve affects both the heart rate and stimulates the bowels. The patient's urgency was the tip off that his heart rate was about to drop.

When Donnelly described this, she said she acted on her own "gut feeling" about what this patient needed. In fact, as Patricia Benner has pointed out, for an expert, a "gut feeling" is the distillation of knowledge, skill and experience.

Another kind of clinical judgment became apparent in the story a pediatric nurse told us about her work with a three-year-old leukemia patient. She said she watched "Barney" with the little girl every morning. When we prodded, she explained that she used this time watching television to establish trust on the part of the child so that the child would view the nurse as a source of comfort during painful tests and procedures.

Her ability to articulate this last detail was critical. She wasn't just a tender loving person who sat with the child watching TV; she was an expert who recognized that relationship is a powerful therapeutic tool. Because of her clinical experience, the nurse understood the procedures and treatments the child had to face and knew that if surrounded by strangers, the child would be terrified. She could endure her medical treatment only if a source of comfort and reassurance was available to her.

Patricia Benner put this idea into wonderfully direct and vivid language: "Among other things," she said, "a nurse's job is to make sure hospitals don't scare patients to death."

Don't suppress your enthusiasm

As every nurse knows, affect is important in establishing a connection with patients. It is no less so when talking with members of the public. Don't be afraid of appearing engaged or emotional when you tell your stories. Let your eagerness, enthusiasm and commitment to nursing be reflected in your voice and body language. When nurses do so, they are in the foreground, not the background and, when nurses speak with passion and conviction—rather than in cautious, passive and neutral tones, they convince the public that nurses are important professionals who cannot easily be replaced.

When you are discussing changes in the health care system that cause harm, don't be afraid to express your moral outrage. As long as you're not shrill or out of control, expressing profound concern is appropriate and justified. Similarly, don't be afraid to show your sorrow or grief. If you are telling a story about patient care that brings tears to your eyes and a catch in your throat, don't be embarrassed. Those who listen to you will be impressed with the depth of your feelings and your commitment to your work and patients.

Highlight the implications of your actions and connect your work with pressing contemporary issues

Some years ago, nurse manager Karen Kline told us about her successful efforts to prevent a novice physician from prolonging the agony of a dying patient.

A 74-year-old woman had come into the intensive care unit suffering from renal failure and overwhelming infection. Because of the patient's deteriorating condition, the resident on duty knew he had to act quickly. Hastily, he approached the woman's husband. "Do you want us to make your wife comfortable?" he asked the old man.

Without a moment's hesitation, the man pleaded," Yes, please, please do everything to make her comfortable."

"Fine," the resident said. Turning away from the patient's husband, he told the nurse, "We'll start mechanical ventilation and put her on dialysis."

Karen Kline said that when she overheard this conversation, she asked the woman's primary nurse several questions about this new patient. She learned the woman's age and condition and the most salient fact of all—the woman would never get off the ventilator and leave the unit alive. She also discovered that the family had come to Boston from a hospital in Maine. Strangers to this city and this hospital, the patient had no doctor or nurse who was acquainted with the previous details of her case, or who knew her wishes or her family's values.

Nurse Kline knew that translation was the order of the day. She recognized that the words "please do everything to make her comfortable," hardly had the same meaning for the family and the medical team. To the resident, they clearly meant he should keep the woman alive using all means available. But did those words mean the same thing to the woman's husband and to the brother who arrived on the scene? That was not at all certain. "Please do everything to keep her comfortable" might easily mean just the opposite—keep her off machines; use all the pain medication possible to prevent suffering; do something to stop her agitated gasping for air.

Kline told us that when she talked with the woman's husband, he was shocked to learn that "everything to make her comfortable," meant artificial life support. "I don't want any machines to keep her alive, I don't want any machines," he repeated.

Reassuring the husband that the staff would make sure the woman did not suffer, Kline relayed this information to the resident. Without questioning her intervention, the physician agreed and stopped aggressive treatment. The nurse administered morphine and the woman's breathing immediately quieted. Several hours later she died peacefully.

Reflecting on this experience—one she lived daily—Karen Kline explained, "Nurses are interpreters who are aware that the patient and the physician may be speaking two different languages. If we are to make sure that the patient's needs are met, and that the patient and the family do not suffer needlessly, we must do a lot of this kind of interpretation. In this instance, my work saved the patient and her family months of useless agony and the health care system thousands of dollars on futile heroic care."

Respecting patient confidentiality

Nurses are understandably very concerned about violating their patients' privacy when they talk about their work. Unfortunately, concerns about patient confidentiality can paralyze nurses and serve to completely silence them. Because it is difficult to talk about what nurses do for patients without mentioning their patients, some nurses feel there is no way around the patient confidentiality problem and, therefore, refuse to talk at all.

Consider this example: A nurse at a major hospital had been interviewed for a story about the emergency room. A photographer from the magazine in which the article was appearing called to arrange a photo shoot. The photographer wanted the nurse to appear in the article with patients. The nurse's manager told the photographer that the nurse would have to ask the patients if they would agree to be photographed, and the manager reminded the nurse to ask the patients for permission before allowing the photographer in.

But the manager didn't leave it at that. She kept harping on the need to prevent any violation of patient confidentiality. The photographer said the manager made the nurse so nervous that he didn't even want to approach patients to ask their permission. Finally, after much prodding from the photographer, the nurse approached several patients. Like many people, they were delighted that they might have their picture in the paper and agreed instantly. By this time, however, the nurse had become so anxious about the photo shoot he was stiff and looked uncomfortable every time the camera clicked. None of the pictures was usable. The photographer was extremely frustrated. She said she had never had such a bad experience on a photo shoot. Much to the chagrin of the hospital administrators who were courting good publicity, this hospital and all the people in it never appeared in the article.

Nurses can make their work with patients public without violating patient privacy and confidentiality. This issue can be dealt with by changing details that might reveal the identity of patients or by talking about a general group of patients without mentioning the details of particular cases.

When you use a particular case as an example of your work, you can explain that you've altered certain facts to protect your patient's privacy, but that the essence of the story remains. Your listeners aren't concerned with the name, age or address of a particular patient. They're interested in your experience.

In many instances, patients have similar problems and experiences and unless you give specific identifying details, there will be no way that anyone could possibly determine who your patients are.

Some nurses fear that talking about their work might mean that they're exploiting their patients. Nothing could be further from the truth. You don't just owe it to yourself to tell your stories. It's a moral imperative to talk about nursing and a contribution to better health care.

Dealing with your fears

Many nurses have told us they are afraid that they will make mistakes if they talk about their work. They say they fear being misinterpreted or getting an angry response. Some are worried about generating conflict or controversy, being fired or viewed as disloyal to their institutions. Perhaps a nurse's worst fear is that nobody will care.

These are serious concerns. Despite good efforts to be knowledgeable, we are all vulnerable to making mistakes when we speak or write. When using facts and statistics, it is important to make sure they are correct. If you are concerned about an argument or tone, run it by a trusted colleague who is knowledgeable about the issue.

At the same time, be realistic. Many mistakes can be rectified. Some points may be debatable rather than right or wrong. Indeed, much of the information about nursing that you might convey to individuals and groups will represent your perspective as a nurse. Others nurses will have different perspectives, but it doesn't mean that yours is "wrong" or "mistaken." Your experiences and ideas are just as valid as anyone else's.

It is also important to recognize that no matter how much you learn, no one ever has perfect knowledge. Try as you might, you can never reach a point where it is guaranteed that you won't make a mistake. If you are waiting for that day before you can speak up, you will be silent forever.

Worrying about how others will respond to one's comments is normal. But the fact is, none of us can control the responses of others. The moment one opens one's mouth to tell a story, share a feeling or express an opinion, one loses control over how it will be received. The more people you speak to, the more you can be sure that someone will misunderstand, misinterpret, misconstrue, disagree, feel betrayed, or just turn off. This is a fact of life. Just as it does not deter most of us from talking to our friends, acquaintances or co-workers, so too it should not deter us from speaking to a wider audience in person or through the media.

Your remarks will sometimes generate conflict and controversy. That may be difficult for some nurses to cope with. After all, for decades the mandate of nurses has been to conceal conflict within health care institutions, or to try to manage and smooth over conflict with patients and families. This is reflected in the comments nurses have made at our workshops. "I'm afraid of getting into a situation of 'one side against the other,'" one nurse said. One nurse indicated just how dangerous she believes conflict is: "I'm afraid of causing conflict/chaos."

Seeing controversy and conflict solely as stations on the road to chaos obliterates the constructive role of disagreement. Reluctance to risk disagreement hampers intellectual and professional development, not only for individuals but for a whole profession. One editor of a nursing journal feels that "conflict phobia" among nurses is curtailing rigorous intellectual debate about nursing. She says that she solicits critiques of articles in her journal to enlarge the discussion of important issues. But instead of critiques, she mostly receives innocuous commentary that fails to engage the issues.

"I think even highly educated nurses are too afraid that they might offend someone," she says. "So they just give a very tame response."

In fact, the oft-stated yearning that nurses should "speak with one voice," can be interpreted as a wish for total safety. In one voice there is no disagreement, thus no risk, and ultimately no story. Waiting for all 2.6 million American and

255,000 Canadian nurses to speak with one voice is the perfect recipe for self-silencing. Self-silencing is also the result of the fear that exposing unpleasant facts will cost nurses their jobs. This fear is hardly unrealistic. But it is important to do a reality check and find out what kind of public speaking or advocacy might result in a nurse losing her job.

Even if an institution would prefer that nurses be seen and not heard, RNs can and should talk about their practice and the important work that they do. This is unlikely to result in the termination of employment.

Taking controversial positions or exposing serious problems within an institution in particular or health care in general is not, however, without risks. To minimize the risks it's important to know state, provincial/territorial or federal labor laws and recognize that you're on a much stronger legal footing if you act in concert with others rather than alone.

In the US, for example, labor law only protects workers who act in a group, i.e., with two or more fellow workers, to discuss conditions of work. If nurses are concerned about patient care, in order to receive protection under the National Labor Relations Act, their concerns must be related to working conditions. Before taking action, therefore, it's important to document concerns and try to raise them within the institution involved. If nurses are not represented by a union, they can try to consult with the staff of a local or national union that represents nurses, or they may want to consult with an attorney who specializes in employment law (see chapter eight).

Kathleen Connors advises that nurses should always try to work together to expose system problems. "The fear of being fired is a fear that's expressed everyday by nurses who are in unions as well as those who aren't. The first thing people have to realize is that they're showing the highest regard for their professional nursing judgment by indicating when situations need to be changed and steps need to be taken." She says, "If nurses are afraid to do this on their own, they are supported and protected by their union if they have one, and hopefully by fellow nurses.

"In situations where a union is not present," Connors says, "nurses should make sure they document their case or concerns and have accurate information. Depending on the situation, they can enlist the help of nursing colleagues, management or perhaps physicians. I've said to doctors: Are you guys satisfied with this? If you're not, let's get together so we can talk about this, and we have. It takes a lot of courage and trust in your own professional judgment to do this."

Some nurses are afraid to expose system problems not because they fear job loss but because they do not want to be disloyal to their institution. Nurses have told us they don't want to publicly discuss serious problems because they don't want to harm an institution whose mission, if not its actions, is a worthy one. They worry that public exposure will rupture relationships in their workplace, a community they value, and harm their hospital or clinic.

Claire Fagin, Dean Emerita of the University of Pennsylvania School of Nursing, is sympathetic to this dilemma. Fagin and others point out that institutions are far more resilient than nurses believe, and exposing serious problems may strengthen institutions, rather than weaken them. "I always advise nurses to go through channels before they expose any serious system problems," Fagin says. "But if you get absolutely nowhere, it's important to determine your bottom line. Is your bottom line loyalty to your institution or is it to protect patients? The bottom line has to be to protect patients."

When courageous nurses take controversial positions to protect their patients and the public, this sends a very powerful message about the value of professional nursing.

Perhaps nurses' worst fear is that no one will pay attention or care what they say.

"I'm afraid people won't listen," one nurse told us.

"People are not interested in what we do," another nurse said. "They say it's too depressing. They don't want to hear about illness."

"It can be very frustrating talking with people who are not in nursing as they don't really understand what you are experiencing. Unless you are a nurse, you can never really know what it means to be a nurse," another offered.

When nurses express these feelings, we're always surprised. We are not nurses. What we know about nursing we have learned from nurses. We have found that when nurses talk about their experiences with confidence and conviction, it can be stimulating, sad, moving, anxiety provoking, funny, terrible, informative—anything but uninteresting. Of course other people can understand what it's like and what it means to be a nurse, if you are willing to tell them.

Endnote

1. Suzanne Gordon and Bernice Buresh, "Finding the 'I' in the 'We,'" *American Journal of Nursing,* January 1996.

SECTION II
COMMUNICATING WITH THE MEDIA AND THE PUBLIC

Chapter 5
HOW THE NEWS MEDIA WORK

This chapter examines the scope of health care reportage. It describes how reporters decide what is news, how they cover health care, and who and what they regard as expert sources of information. It analyzes why health care coverage has been increasing, and looks at opportunities for nurses to be a more integral part of health care news.

The Increase in Health Care News

Look at a newspaper, open a popular magazine, turn on the television news, or log onto the Internet and inevitably you will encounter health care information and news. While people have always been interested in information that might spare them from illness and death, North Americans have only recently begun to rely upon the news media as their *primary* source of such information.

As this chapter will detail, many cultural, political and economic factors have contributed to giving the media unprecedented power to inform and influence people about their personal health and health care. Nurses cannot afford to ignore or underestimate the role of the media in shaping the public credibility and prestige of nursing.

A Brief History of Health News

For most of human history, people have been at the mercy of deadly diseases and epidemics. It's not surprising that public health was front-page news in the first North American newspaper, "*Publick Occurrences. Both Forreign and Domestick,*" whose first and only issue appeared on September 25, 1690. "Epidemical Fevers and Agues grow very common, in some parts of the country ..." the newspaper reported and followed with another, more reassuring item: "The Small-pox which has been raging in Boston, after a manner very Extraordinary, is now very much abated."[1]

The power of the press to influence health care policy is hardly a recent phenomenon. In 1721, half of Boston's 10,500 inhabitants were infected with "the Small-pox" and hundreds were dying. Convinced that the theory of immunization was sound, Dr. Zabdiel Boylston began inoculating residents, including his own children. Despite positive results, many citizens, including physicians, were outraged that someone would intentionally infect people who might then become carriers. James Franklin (whose brother Benjamin worked for him as a printer-apprentice) was the brash publisher of the newly launched *New-England Courant*, and he crusaded against the practice by printing diatribes against the Puritan leaders who supported Boylston. No one will ever know whether Boylston's vaccine would have stopped the smallpox onslaught because the public frenzy Franklin helped to unleash curtailed the experiment. It took another 75 years before Edward Jenner's development of a safe cowpox-based vaccine in England laid the foundation for widespread immunization.[2]

In recent decades, dramatic medical and surgical breakthroughs such as antibiotics and organ transplants have stimulated media and popular interest in medicine. The first heart transplant surgeons, for example, received so much publicity they became household names. Publishers of medical journals also grew more sophisticated about how to present new medical interventions to the media and the public.

A parallel development fueling health coverage was the rise of the women's movement and its revolt against medical paternalism. It may be hard to believe now, but when the Boston Women's Health Book Collective published its first version of *Our Bodies, Ourselves* in 1969, the book was considered a radical, underground document because it urged women to investigate how their own bodies function. In the 1980s, people with AIDS proved the power of patient activism when they confronted medical, research and governmental institutions and demanded information and a greater commitment to fighting the disease. Since then, other health activists, notably those concerned with breast cancer, have learned how to get media attention to further their goals. Even the US government seemed to put its imprimatur on this kind of patient activism when it issued a special stamp to help fund breast cancer research.

In the 1990s, debate over health care policy became such a big story that one journalist declared: "Health care has supplanted once-trendy subjects, such as the environment, to become *the* hot topic for coverage."[3] Conflicts over how to finance health care, problems with access and delivery, and disputes over the roles of government and business in the health care system still drive this area of coverage. As physicians and nurses have less time to spend with patients and as patients question the motives and morale of their health care providers, the public is demanding more health information from media sources.

Advertisers—not just reporters—are happy to provide that information. Revised US Food and Drug Administration guidelines permitting TV commercials to run with only a "brief summary" of potential negative side effects has given rise to a blitz of prescription drug advertising since the late 1990s. Drug manufacturers now spend more than a billion dollars a year in the US just on consumer ads encouraging patients to ask clinicians for specific prescription drugs (which the latter apparently accede to, at least part of the time).

Advertising on this massive scale not only allows drug manufacturers and other health industry corporations to reach health care "consumers" directly, it provides the financial support for increased news coverage of health care. This chain of events can be observed on television's regular health news segments or features "brought to you" by a drug company. In some cases, a specific amount of time is set aside for health coverage whether reporters think there are good stories that day or not. This is comparable to reserving time in the newscast for weather or sports reports. By providing revenue to media outlets and by calling attention to health products and services, big health-industry advertisers support expanded media coverage of health, which in turn promotes public awareness of health issues.

The advertising-editorial link is very strong in women's magazines like *Chatelaine* or *Vogue*. Although editors generally deny they are producing content to please advertisers, cosmetics ads spawn beauty columns and food ads lead to recipe sections. Articles and columns on cosmetics and food in turn direct readers' attention toward ads for such products. There's nothing like the lure of advertising revenue to create an editorial interest in health. *Better Homes and Gardens*, for example, is a magazine one would think would deal only with the intricacies of designing and decorating homes and gardens. Yet, it carries a hefty health section each month not coincidentally punctuated by prescription and nonprescription drug ads and other health-related advertising. (Cigarette advertising is wisely situated far from the health section.)

While there is more of a firewall between advertising and news departments at newspapers and television stations, health industry advertisers do fuel the demand for health information and indirectly provide the revenue to pay the salaries of reporters, editors and producers, some of whom produce the health reportage their readers, viewers and listeners demand. The bottom line, according to the National Health Council is, "The media have become an integral member of America's health care team."[4]

What People Want from the News Media

Most Americans under the age of 60 regard the media as their primary source of health and medical information, according to a comprehensive survey co-sponsored by the National Health Council and PBS's *Health Week*. More people turn to television (40 percent) as their primary source of health information than they do to physicians (36 percent), according to the survey. Magazines and journals are the primary information source for 35 percent of the respondents. Newspapers serve that purpose for 16 percent.[5]

A different survey of women aged 45 to 54 came up with an even stronger finding about the role of the media. More than 80 percent of 1,000 women surveyed for the National Council on Aging reported that they rely on television, newspapers and magazines for information on health-related issues. Only one in four (26 percent) said they get information on health topics from doctors and/or nurses.[6]

The broader National Health Council survey found that only older people and those with chronic illnesses rely upon physicians as their primary information source. However, both groups still use the media for health information. After physicians, elders turn to magazines and journals, while those with chronic conditions cite television news magazines as their second most-relied-upon resource.

As an indication of just how the information pipeline has reversed, the majority of respondents (53 percent) said they consult their doctors (6 percent consult nurses), when they want to know more about health information they gleaned from the media. The majority of those who had media-inspired conversations with their doctors said that their physician was "happy to talk about it"; and 17 percent said their doctor responded to the conversation by putting the patient on the medication, diet or therapy suggested in the media, by ordering a medical test or by giving the patient more materials to read. One can conclude from these findings (as pharmaceutical companies surely have) that clinicians' responses can be influenced by what appears in the media.

The survey also found that people take specific actions based on information provided by media to improve their health. Eighty-two percent of the respondents believe that health and medical news helps them to lead a healthful life, and 58 percent report changing their behavior or taking some type of action as a result of a health news story. Of this number, 76 percent said they took the advice offered in a news story they heard or read.

Very high percentages of the respondents found physicians (93 percent), nurses (92 percent), pharmacists (92 percent), and patient groups such as cancer or heart associations (93 percent) "completely or somewhat believable." They also said they found print and broadcast media believable. They ranked television news magazine programs such as *20/20* or *60 Minutes* as the most believable (87 percent), along with public service announcements on television or radio (87 percent). This was followed by nightly or morning television news broadcasts (83 percent), daily newspapers (83 percent), news magazines (81 percent), and news on the radio (81 percent), although only 4 percent of the respondents got their health news from the radio.

The implication is that people rely on journalists to select information that is significant and to point them to expert sources that are trustworthy. Indeed, when asked what makes a source of health news "completely believable," 43 percent of those who found at least one source completely believable attributed that to "professional credibility."[7]

In commenting on the survey, Don Riggin, chair of the National Health Council, linked the role of the media to the rise of managed care. "The results of this survey dramatically demonstrate the importance of the media's role at a time when doctors have fewer minutes to spend with each patient," he said. That being the case, he added, "both the media and those who provide them with information, have a responsibility to ensure that the public gets facts that are precise and timely."

The Broad Scope of Health Care Coverage

Every day an immense volume of health care information spews forth from the media. Only a portion of that information, however, is the product of journalism. Much more of it is advertising or other forms of communication produced by the sellers of health products and services.

In this book we are primarily concerned with the news media and how they report on health care. When we speak of the news media, we are referring to the coverage that results from the practice of journalism. Journalism may be disseminated via any of the traditional or new media including print, electronic and digital media. However, whether the specific medium of communication is newspapers, magazines, radio, television, or the World Wide Web, the role of the journalist is "to find, gather, organize, explain, interpret, and disseminate the news, ideas and opinions of the day to an ever-increasing audience,"[8] and to do so with accuracy and fairness. By definition, journalism is a dynamic process. The name itself derives from the old French *journal*, meaning daily. The timeliness of journalism is also captured in the word news—something that is "new." Advances in communication technology have sped up the process even further.

Today, competition for audiences is blurring the line between news and entertainment. As media companies merge into giant conglomerates, there are fewer divisions between the various types of media. Print reporters are on TV.

TV stations have Web pages. The newspaper has a TV broadcasting station on site. Nevertheless, the function of the journalist is to give people the information they need to make informed decisions as citizens and, increasingly, as consumers. Journalists receive an overwhelming amount of material from interested parties. It is up to them along with their editors and producers to decide what is credible and worth passing on to their readers and viewers.

Advertising and public relations communication, on the other hand, is referred to as "controlled" communication because it is under the control of the corporations and organizations that create and pay for it. Their purpose is to influence directly what people buy, do or believe.

Although they represent vested interests, advertising and public relations campaigns can also be helpful to the public. Indeed, in chapter seven, we urge nurses to be more actively engaged in public relations to benefit both nursing and the public welfare. It should be kept in mind, though, that the goals of advertising and public relations are different from those of journalism. This is why pharmaceutical companies, despite spending enormous amounts of money on direct advertising, still make full-fledged efforts to get their products mentioned in the news. A news story that talks about the efficacy of a drug carries the imprimatur of truth, while an ad stating the same thing is expected to be taken with a grain of salt.

News Media Coverage of Health Care

Today, health care reporting has many facets. A major news organization is likely to have several reporters covering various aspects of health care on either a full-time or part-time basis. For example, one reporter might cover health care policy issues out of Washington or Ottawa, while another reporter might cover health care legislation and regulation on a state or provincial/territorial level. A business and economics writer might keep track of corporate activities or labor actions within the health care industry. Someone else might focus on a branch of that industry such as biotechnology or pharmaceuticals. A medical writer is likely to be responsible for reporting on research studies published in medical and other scientific journals. The same writer might also report on problems with patient care. Yet another might do human-interest features on patients' experiences with illness, on health care trends, or on interesting approaches being taken by individual physicians or nurses. Reporters who cover such "beats," as "aging" or "women," might episodically cover health issues affecting these particular groups. A large newspaper is also likely to have an editorial writer who specializes in health care. Columnists with a broad range of interests—like America's Ellen Goodman, or Canada's Allan Fotheringham—might write about health care from time to time.

Television is by far the most popular news medium. Even so, it is important to pay attention to newspapers to understand what constitutes health care news. Because of their larger editorial staffs, major daily newspapers cover a broad range of health topics more regularly and in greater detail than most television news programs. Television news staffs often look to local or national newspapers for direction on what stories to pursue. But television coverage veers toward those events that have a strong visual component and away from issues, like health policy, that require in-depth exploration.

Many of the reporters who end up covering stories on health care are not specialists in the field. One of the conventions of journalism is that reporters with no particular expertise in an area are often assigned to take on complex stories and produce them in a very short time. Even reporters who cover a health beat may venture into unfamiliar territory.

In one of our media projects, we monitored the health care coverage of two major daily newspapers—the *New York Times* and the *Boston Globe*—for a month (January 1997).[9]

It was immediately obvious that the newspapers carried a great deal of health care news. The two newspapers ran a total of 235 health items (including letters to the editor) that month. (We excluded topics that focused more on legal than on health issues, such as liability settlement negotiations with tobacco companies. We also excluded sports sections even though they carry stories on player injuries and treatments.) The amount of health news seemed to have increased substantially since 1990 when we conducted a broader study of health care coverage in three newspapers over a three-month period.[10]

The health care items were found in various sections. For example, of the *Boston Globe's* 138 health-related items, most of these (118) were news stories situated in the national, local or business sections. Sixteen of the items were brief reports on new research studies in the paper's Thursday "Medical Notebook" column. Ten of the items were features or longer articles for the *Globe's* weekly Health/Science section. Another 20 items (14 percent of the sample) were opinion or advice items in the following categories— 8 editorials, 3 op-eds or other opinion pieces, 3 advice columns, and 6 letters to the editor.

The breakdown of the 97 health-related items in the *New York Times* was similar, except that a much larger percentage (28 percent) fell into the opinion category. Eighteen items were letters, seven were op-eds or opinion columns and two were editorials. The *Times* has an unusually large and well-edited letters section. Letters-to-the-editor sections—particularly in this newspaper— elaborate on the news by allowing outside "experts" to comment and illuminate new aspects of an issue.

A Day in the News

By looking at health coverage on one heavy news day, we got an idea of what is newsworthy and why. On Wednesday, January 22, 1997, the two newspapers produced a total of 18 health-related items—ten ran in the *Boston Globe* and eight in the *New York Times*. Most of the news that day was about health care policy (ten articles) or health care research (six articles). There was one health care business article and one article we classified as human interest.

Health care funding, regulation and policy

For at least the last ten years, this has been a vibrant area of health coverage. On our sample day, both newspapers ran front-page stories on the funding of the American Medicare system, which insures those over 65. They were based on an announcement President Clinton made the day before saying that he would consider trimming the growth of Medicare spending by $138 billion over six years. This figure represented a larger cut than he had previously been willing to consider.

A journalist would automatically regard this event as newsworthy because it has several of the factors or "news values" that constitute newsworthiness. These include *timeliness* (the announcement just occurred), *prominence* (the President is a prominent and powerful figure and, therefore, most of what he does is considered news), *currency* (there was an ongoing political debate about Medicare funding), impact (many people would be affected by changes in Medicare), and *conflict* (the level of funding had been a contentious issue for two years).[11] Therefore, the *New York Times* gave this story big play, devoting considerable attention to both the politics of the announcement (a "conciliatory gesture" to Congressional Republicans) and its implications (hospitals would lose $45 billion in payments over six years and HMOs about $46 billion).

However, in the *Boston Globe*, the presidential announcement was only briefly reported. Instead, it ran a different Medicare story—one dissecting a federal commission's recommendations for reducing Medicare spending. It quickly became apparent why the *Globe*, located in the medical center of Boston, took this tack—the commission wanted to reduce funding for medical education and revamp the way hospitals are paid to train doctors. If adopted, these recommendations would have a major impact on Massachusetts's four medical schools and its numerous teaching hospitals. To the *Globe*, the factors of *proximity* and *local impact* made this story more newsworthy for its readers.

Both newspapers covered a report issued by the federal Veterans Affairs department linking the accidental release of toxic chemicals in Iraq in 1991 to Gulf War Syndrome illnesses. The day before, Dr. Kenneth Kizer, the Veterans Affairs Under Secretary for Health Affairs, presented the results of the department's analysis to a House subcommittee. Reports from authoritative bodies constitute a major news source. News organizations would have been notified in advance of Kizer's testimony and might even have had an advance copy of his report.

However, again the *Times* and *Globe* emphasized different aspects of the same material. Although it may have been edited by the *Globe*, the *Globe's* piece came from the Associated Press wire service rather than from a staff member.

The *Boston Globe* ran another Washington datelined piece that it picked up from the *Washington Post*. Individual newspapers often make their material available to other news organizations through a wire service operated by their parent company or a syndicate. The *Globe*, by having access to the *Washington Post's* in-depth governmental reporting, was able to give its readers an article on a complex population-based health study that it would not have produced itself.

The business of health care

The business sections of newspapers frequently carry reports on health care and biotechnology companies. This is also where coverage of employment disputes between nurses and hospitals or government payers usually appears. These sections, along with the US's premier business newspaper, the *Wall Street Journal*, and Canada's *Financial Post*, are aimed primarily at investors.

On our heavy news day, the *Globe* ran a business story reporting a dramatic increase in the price of shares of the Massachusetts company that makes the antihistamine, Allegra. The fortunes of Sepracor, Inc. were improving, the article reported, since Allegra was replacing Seldane, a similar antihistamine that the FDA wanted to get off the market because of a potentially lethal side effect. The article also said that Sepracor "is heading into the home stretch" on development of a new version of Albuterol, a widely used asthma medication. This upbeat article on Sepracor's products was undoubtedly good news for the company, its investors, and potential investors. The fortunes of companies like this one can hang on what is said about it in the news media. This is why the health industry devotes extensive efforts to getting into the news.

Research news

A great deal of health care news comes from studies published in medical journals. Health care news tends to swell mid-week because the biggest medical journals, the *Journal of the American Medical Association* (*JAMA*) and the *New England Journal of Medicine*, publish on Wednesday and Thursday, respectively. *JAMA* studies prompted most of the six research-based articles on our sample day.

JAMA was the source of stories in both newspapers that drug reactions and mistakes in prescribing drugs may account for as many as 140,000 deaths each year, hundreds of thousands of illnesses or injuries, and an extra $4.2 billion in hospital costs. The *Globe* article, written by that paper's veteran medical reporter, Richard A. Knox, led with statistics confirming the scale of the medical error problem. The *Times* piece, by its leading medical reporter, Lawrence K. Altman (an MD), started out in a more subdued manner outlining the problem first and getting into the numbers later. The source for both accounts was a package of three studies and an editorial published in that day's issue of *JAMA*. As medical reporters, both would have had advance copies of the issue as well as news releases calling their attention to these particular studies.

On the same day, the *Globe* ran another *JAMA*-based story that it took off the AP wire on the efficacy of a drug for cardiac by-pass patients.

In addition to appearing as breaking news, medical studies are the basis for comprehensive pieces on illnesses, treatments and preventative health measures. The *New York Times* weekly Personal Health page provides a forum for such pieces. On our sample day the page carried three long articles on illnesses.

One was Jane E. Brody's "Personal Health" column on the origin, transmission, treatment for, and prevention of hepatitis C. Using research studies and interviews with specialists as sources, Brody described hepatitis C as an "insidious and perplexing organism" present in 3.5 million Americans. There was no new study that made this subject timely that week. But reporters like Brody, who write regularly on health issues, "save string" on subjects they think will be newsworthy by keeping a file of journal articles, other materials and the names of experts in the field.

The lead article on the Personal Health page, "Lag Seen in Aid for Depression" by Susan Gilbert, did have a time element in that it was based on a report in that day's *JAMA*. However, we assume that any medical reporter would have a background file on a subject as popular as depression. The news "peg" for this piece was the *JAMA* report by a panel of experts that said depression is underdiagnosed and undertreated. The article provided readers with considerable information on depression.

The third article on the page, with the self-explanatory headline, "A Simple Blood Test Helps Predict Patients' Prospects after Strokes," also came from a research study. The study, by a group of Spanish researchers, had been reported ten days earlier in the British journal *Lancet*.

"Hard" and "Soft" News

Reporters traditionally classify news as being either "hard" or "soft." A timely event or breaking story is "hard" news. It has to be covered right away, and if it isn't, it will cease to be news.

"Soft" news generally lacks a pressing time component and, therefore, has a much longer shelf life. It's considered something that the public doesn't need to know urgently.

These categories are no longer as discrete as they once were. A political campaign produces news in both categories. Reporters will do timely "hard" news stories on who won a political contest and "soft" news features—"sidebars" when they augment the main article—on the candidate's personal history.

News Values

Timeliness—something just occurred.
Prominence—an "important" person, corporation, organization or institution was involved.
Currency—the event is part of a larger continuing debate or discussion.
Impact—the event or issue affects a lot of people.
Conflict—the story contains tension, competition, dissension, war.
Scandal or wrongdoing—the media's job is to report on (or uncover) crime, fraud and abuse.

Human interest/features

Feature articles and human interest pieces that deal with illness, treatment or the experiences of a health professional appear frequently in newspapers. None of these appeared on January 22. But there was a report on the mayor of Boston being hospitalized for severe abdominal pain. While no diagnosis was available at press time, the article did quote a statement from the mayor's office saying that the pain was "consistent with that of kidney stones," a problem the mayor had previously experienced.

These days the illnesses of prominent people are seldom private and offer a peg for medical informational pieces. When actor Christopher Reeve was injured in a riding accident, the media were filled with stories on spinal cord injuries. Similarly, the medical treatment of victims of sensational crimes— such as the "Central Park jogger," a woman who was brutally attacked and left for dead in Manhattan—can stimulate continuing coverage. These stories often cast physicians as heroes working to save the lives of these seriously injured patients. The nurses who care for the patients and sustain their lives, however, are rarely seen.

What Is News?

Journalists don't sit down with a list of news values and refer to it every time they get a phone call or press release. Their training teaches them that some things are "stories" and some aren't. Developing a news sense can help nurses plan successful media strategies.

Consider the following example. One nursing specialty organization, like many today, recognized that its members were having greater difficulty providing quality care because of staff cuts in hospitals and clinics. They were grappling with how to deal with the threat to their patients. A media expert urged them to go public with their concerns by holding a press conference to reveal the breadth of the problem.

Several of the organization's leaders met to plan the press conference. What would be their news peg? They felt it should be their policy statement declaring that every patient had a right to quality care in their field.

The organization had constructed the policy statement to define its commitment to patient care. However, the statement contained no reference to the current problems in the field. Nor did it propose any way to finance that care. The development of this policy statement was significant to those who worked on it, as well as to the members of the organization. But the leaders were dismayed when they were told there was no "story" in it.

What would have been a story?

1. People talking about the problem.

The organization could have asked working nurses to come and talk about the obstacles to giving good care in institutions more concerned with the bottom-line than patient care. The organization could have asked patients to come and talk about the suffering and sense of abandonment they experienced due to cuts in nursing care. Outside policy experts also could have been called upon to provide historical background and suggest appropriate policy approaches to the problem.

2. Documentary evidence.

Studies documenting the link between widespread cuts in nursing care and increasing problems for patients would have helped them make their case. If no specific studies had been done, the nurses could have produced research findings connecting nursing care to better patient outcomes in general. Studies linking adequate staffing and the prevention of decubitus ulcers, falls and urinary tract infections would have been relevant. So would studies demonstrating nurses' ability to help patients cope with the physical and emotional suffering associated with disease and with the side effects of treatment.

They would have been justified in organizing a news conference that incorporated either or both of these elements. It would have provided what many reporters would consider a very good story. It would have attracted attention to the work of the organization's members and given the organization itself a dynamic, courageous and compassionate image.

This kind of media event has attracted coverage in both the United States and Canada. A number of reporters came to a day-long conference held at the University of Pennsylvania School of Nursing in December 1995 with the provocative title, "The Abandonment of the Patient: The Impact of Profit-Driven Care on the Public." Canadian nurses' organizations and unions have held similar events.

Organizations are often fearful that if they expose system problems and take strong positions about them they will alarm and/or alienate the public. But it is also alarming to the public when caregivers don't forcefully advocate for patient care. Moreover, timid approaches like issuing apple pie and motherhood "policy statements" or weak responses to political initiatives won't attract public attention for nurses.

To determine what is news, you have to weigh whether internal organizational actions are relevant to the public. In general, organizational positions are not news. Many nursing organizations produce reams of instant waste paper in the form of news releases saying they are for or against something (for example, the President's proposal to insure all uninsured children, an expert's plan to reduce violence against women) with no other news elements. This sort of release doesn't have a prayer of producing coverage.

News releases with no news values are not necessarily benign interventions. They can harm nursing's public image by depicting nursing organizations—and, by extension, nurses—as standing on the sidelines watching events set in motion by others. Press releases larded with phrases like "we applaud this," "we share these concerns," "we have a long-standing commitment to," "this is congruent with our long-standing goals," "we have a long history of advocating on this issue," positions a group as a spectator rather than as an actor, or tells the world: "We're just nice nurses."

A news release that articulates a stance on an important and timely issue and suggests or announces that the organization is going to mobilize to do something about it (thus containing the news value of impact) casts your group as a participant with influence or power.

Monitoring the News Media

To see what constitutes news and to assess the opportunities to integrate nursing into health care coverage, look at the news media nearest you with a curious eye. As you read newspapers and magazines, listen to the radio and watch television, go to bookstores and libraries, and visit various Web sites, take notes on who is reporting on health care and the way they do it. Even if you are working with public relations professionals, you still need to be familiar with how health care and nursing are reported.

Newspapers

A good place to start is with your newspaper's health page or section. Most larger daily newspapers have some sort of weekly health or health/ science section. What do you see there? Does the section usually lead with a health care feature story? If the section covers both health and science, what is the usual mix of stories? What kinds of health subjects and people are covered? Who writes these stories? Do you see the same bylines repeatedly? The bylines may tell you whether the writers are staff members or free lancers who contribute features. Is there a masthead (usually a small box) in the section which names the reporters who do health reporting?

What other kinds of health items appear in the section? Is there a columnist who specializes in personal health, health and fitness or some other area? Is there a column on research studies that runs in the section or on another day? Who writes it? What are the sources of the reports? Are most from the *New England Journal, JAMA,* and the *Canadian Medical Association Journal* or are other journals cited frequently? Are nursing journals ever cited?

Does the section carry service items? Is there a calendar of health-related events like lectures, support group meetings and schedules of health screenings or immunizations?

Keep in mind that a regular newspaper section *needs* stories to fill it. Yes, there is competition for that space, but there is also a big demand for good stories. This presents nursing with an opportunity.

As you are monitoring the newspaper, look at other features and columns that might reach audiences of specific interest to you. For example, some newspapers, especially those in geographic areas with large older populations, have regular "age beat" features or columns. These might be the ideal place for stories on home care, preventative care and research in geriatric nursing. The Lifestyle section or Sunday magazine could be a good place for a story on a nurse who is doing interesting, unconventional work, who has written a book, or has had an unusual experience.

Monitor the news sections. The first section of a newspaper usually contains a mix of national, international and local "breaking" news. What makes these stories news? Are they based on an announcement, the release of a report, a hearing, a press conference, an event? Does the newspaper have a separate regional, metropolitan or local section? What kinds of health stories appear there? Who writes the health-related news? The business page or section should not be overlooked for health news. How heavily does it cover the health care industry in your area? Is this where stories on nurse staffing or on labor disputes appear?

In major newspapers, the last two pages that face each other in the first section are generally reserved for editorials, letters and opinion columns. The editorial page will be found on the left, and what is known as the "op-ed" page, on the right. Some papers put op-eds, or short opinion essays, on the same page as the editorials. Op-eds may also appear in other parts of the paper like the business or health sections.

An editorial page typically contains a column of editorials that are prominently labeled as such. They are written by editorial writers—staff journalists assigned to the editorial page—or by the editor of the page. Editorials usually have no byline because they are supposed to present the newspaper's opinion and recommendations rather than those of individuals. By concentrating on opinion, the editorial staff has a different function than the reporting staff and is separate from it. On a large newspaper, editorial writers might specialize in certain areas such as health care. Editorial writers have to be alert to breaking news and must understand the elements of complex issues. Their job, after all, is to write timely editorials that both summarize and take stances on these issues.

Newspaper editorials can have an effect in the community particularly when they are well argued and call for specific policy or regulatory actions to deal with pressing problems. It should be borne in mind, however, that when editorial writers make policy recommendations, they do so in accordance with the editorial page's political philosophy. For example, the *Wall Street Journal* is noted for editorials that are among the most conservative in journalism. They differ markedly from those in the *Boston Globe*, which tends to be more liberal. The same disparity is apparent between editorials in the *Financial Post* and those in the Toronto's *Globe and Mail*.

Most newspapers run letters to the editor on the editorial page. Writing a letter to the editor is one of the quickest and most effective ways to draw attention to nursing expertise (see chapter nine).

The op-ed page also bears scrutiny. This is the home of the 500- to 850-word essay. The work of local or syndicated columnists addressing political and public issues often appears on this page. But many newspapers also take op-ed submissions from non-journalists who have a strong point of view. Some newspapers run a "guest" op-ed once a day or several times a week. Although many op-eds are sober considerations of policy, sometimes the form is used for "slice-of-life" pieces in which a person takes you through his or her experience to illuminate a timely topic. (Chapter nine will show you how to write op-eds.)

Also pay attention to your newspaper's Sunday magazine and any health magazine special issues. Feature writers may be open to delving into a particular area of health care. For example, the *Boston Globe*'s Paul Hemp followed one pediatric oncology nurse in her work and produced a substantive Sunday magazine piece on this area of nursing.[12]

Some of the most innovative pieces in the media are done by freelancers. An example is Darcy Frey's vivid account of doctors' and nurses' efforts to save a 26-week-old infant at Boston's Brigham and Women's Hospital and his exploration of the ethical and emotional issues involved in such medical care. His *New York Times Sunday Magazine* article provoked letters from hundreds of readers.[13] Another good example is an article on the Carol Youngson/Winnipeg Children's Hospital case in *Elm Street*.[14]

Don't overlook the work of local or national columnists, some of whom are syndicated throughout the nation. In the summer of 1999, the author Mordecai Richler, devoted several of his weekly Montreal *Gazette* columns to supporting the nurses on strike in Quebec. Other columnists, like Bob Herbert at the *New York Times* and Eileen McNamara at the *Boston Globe*, have built their reputations by writing forcefully about cases of injustice, inequality or abuse of power. Crusading columnists take sides and often revisit issues that capture their attention. By reading various columnists, you can determine if your project or campaign might pique their interest.

While it is important to monitor your local newspaper, it is also useful to take a look at the national newspapers that influence policy makers and the national news agenda. The two largest newspapers in the US are the *Wall Street Journal* and *USA Today*. The *Wall Street Journal* is must reading for investors, business people, policy makers, and anyone following major industries such as health care and communications. Its subject matter is selected to be of interest to its business-oriented audience, but that takes in a lot of territory. It is a readable, well-edited newspaper that carries human interest profiles and features on the people who are making things happen in corporations and government.

USA Today, which rivals the *Wall Street Journal* for the largest circulation, was started by Gannett Co. in 1982 with an intentional television-like appearance emphasizing color, graphics, news summaries, and short news-you-can-use features. Offering the same fare everywhere in the country, it was quickly labeled "McPaper," the epitome of junk-food journalism. However, in recent years its clear presentation and coverage of serious issues has been earning it greater respect in journalism circles. To build its circulation it sells copies at bulk discount rates to airlines, hotels and automobile rental companies, which pass on copies free of charge to business travelers.

The *New York Times* remains the US "paper of record" because of the scope of its coverage and excellent staff. Two other city-based newspapers widely read among policy makers and journalists are the *Washington Post*, the premier political and government news organ, and the *Los Angeles Times*, the paper of record on the west coast.

In Canada, the two national newspapers are the *Globe and Mail* and the newer *National Post*. Both compete with the *Toronto Star* for circulation and upper-income readers. Together they reach millions of readers across the country. The *Financial Post* is the main financial newspaper.

These newspapers are available in most big city libraries. All of them cover health care extensively, but it is useful to compare their styles and approaches.

Newsmagazines

The newsmagazines *Time*, *Newsweek*, *US News & World Report*, and *Maclean's* circulate nationally and internationally. All of these cover health care to a greater or lesser extent. *US News*, for example, does an annual cover story on the "best" hospitals in the US. In general, news weeklies place breaking national and international news in the front of the "book," business news in the middle, and such subjects as education, science, health or medicine, books, sports, theater, and film in the "back-of-the-book." Stories dealing with health care might appear in more than one section.

Another thing to know about newsmagazines is that their correspondents operate out of regional bureaus. Look on the masthead that lists these bureaus and see which one is closest to you. Usually a story in your area will be covered by a correspondent from that bureau. These bureaus also keep up with the major industries in their area.

Wire services *et al.*

Wire services make it possible for news breaking in one place to travel to news outlets throughout the world. Newspapers, news magazines, radio and television stations, and networks all subscribe to one or more of the major wire services such as the Associated Press (AP) and Reuters.

The Associated Press is the biggest wire service in the world. Its own reporters and photographers cover the globe and transmit stories to member news organizations. It also receives and sends out articles and photos that originate with its member news organizations.

When thousands of nurses marched on Washington, DC, on March 31, 1995, in a demonstration organized by Laura Gasparis Vonfrolio, then publisher of *Revolution,* to protest layoffs of RNs and their replacement with unlicensed assistive personnel, some newspapers, such as the *Pittsburgh Post-Gazette,* sent reporters to cover nurses from their areas. But many newspapers that didn't want to incur the expense carried a wire story written by Christopher Connell of the Associated Press. The story was illustrated with an AP photograph of nurses at the march.

Individual newspapers and newspaper chains operate their own smaller wire services. They sell their newspapers' articles and columns to other news organizations. Thanks to wire services, local coverage does not necessarily remain local. Because of wire services, nursing strikes in Ireland and Poland reached audiences in North America, and North American nursing strikes have been reported in other countries.

News organizations also get specialized material—like health care advice columns and features, comic strips, editorial cartoons, and cross-word puzzles—from news syndicates.

Audio and video news stories and features also go to television and radio stations via satellite services. Public relations sources supply their materials to the news media via specialized PR wires and satellite feeds.

Television news

Many local television stations have a reporter who specializes in health care and who does regular reports or features on a current issue. The major broadcast networks and some cable channels have seasoned medical editors and correspondents. Television reports tend to be heavy on health tips and brief interpretations of new studies on popular health subjects like nutrition, heart disease and diabetes. Except for the Canadian Broadcasting Corporation (CBC), the Public Broadcasting System (PBS) in the US, and some cable channels, television tends to do far less on policy issues, financing and in-depth reports on the health industry. Note which experts are featured on the more serious shows.

Television "newsmagazine" shows regularly do mini-dramas based on people's experiences with illness and health care. When you are watching television news, note the kinds of health stories that are covered and who covers them. Another staple of television reporting is the week-long series—

how to lose weight, how to manage seasonal allergies, how to keep fit after 50—designed to be of service to viewers. You might see these series as part of the evening news or as a feature of a morning show.

As you watch television note how visual images dictate the presentation. Simply put, television depends more on pictures than words to convey the news, while newspapers use more words than pictures. A story without many visual possibilities, or one that the local television station has failed to get video on, has less news value to the television news organization than to the newspaper. As Richard Salant, former president of CBS news, has said: "You see more fires on local television than you do in the newspapers because fires look better on television."[15]

In recent years, channel proliferation has fragmented the viewing audience. However, some outlets reach influential audiences and a report on a network or major cable channel like CNN can still reach millions of viewers at once. When a nurse appears on the *Lehrer NewsHour, Good Morning America,* or *Pamela Wallin,* influential or large audiences are guaranteed.

Television relies heavily on interviews to put the story into perspective. Therefore, at least some of the working nurses and academic nursing experts who want to describe nursing practice or expose problems in health care must be willing to speak on the record. A television staple is the expert who, in a few well-chosen words, can provide a snappy "sound bite." Nurses may feel that most television news reports do not give them enough time to develop their position. Television formats are created with the "flighty" viewer in mind. Faced with viewers, who use their remote control to channel surf, television uses tight, dramatic formats to keep the viewer tuned in.

Radio and television call-in shows

Radio and television so shape our understanding of public events that they are central to any media strategy. While radio and television offer many opportunities for nurses to be seen and heard, the ubiquitous call-in show has become an essential tool for those who are trying to influence public opinion and public policy.

Ironically, radio, which was thought to have been eclipsed by television, is now enjoying a new popularity thanks to the call-in talk show. Up and down the AM and FM radio bands, talk radio is available on hundreds of stations in North America. At the same time, the call-in show has emerged as a genre on television, especially on cable stations. Sometimes the same program is carried simultaneously on radio and television.

Instead of debating political issues in their town and city halls, most people now turn on the radio or television to sample political discourse. All political candidates use these shows to make their campaigns visible and viable.

Talk radio does have an advantage over television. It can enter workplaces and automobiles more easily than television. Thanks to the cellular phone, commuters stuck in traffic can join the broadcast conversation.

Talk radio and television are especially influential in mobilizing people against something. As Robert Blendon, professor of health policy at the Harvard School of Public Health, told us: "Talk radio is very important. A large share of people listen to it. And some people who listen to talk radio write letters and take direct action that moves Congress."

Therefore, talk shows are a venue for nurses who want the public to hear their concerns about, and perspectives on, important issues. When call-in shows deal with health care, nurses ought to be on them both as experts and as callers. By working with the producers of these shows, nurses can initiate programs on issues that might otherwise remain invisible. Beware, however, of the rising tide of trash talk shows whose sole mission is to terrify or incite the public.

Radio

Most commercial radio stations offer brief news breaks at the top of the hour from "rip and read" wire copy. Some radio news shows—particularly those at public stations—explore current issues through on-scene features capturing sounds and voices of the setting. Nurses have the opportunity to be interviewed on more substantive nightly and morning news shows and to call producers' attention to topics that should be covered like innovations in nursing practice or developments in nursing research.

There are other radio formats that nurses can use to get their messages across. Many local commercial radio stations have community bulletin boards that can be used for announcing events. In addition, radio stations carry public service announcements (PSAs) gratis for nonprofit organizations. Organizations can contact radio stations for PSA guidelines. During the nursing shortage of the late 1980s, PSAs on radio and television were used to show nursing as an attractive career. While PSAs are aired free (although there may be production costs), sometimes organizations find it useful to go a step further and invest in paid advertising.

Magazines

There is a magazine for practically every subject on earth. Think creatively as you peruse them. City magazines, for example, frequently do health care service pieces such as naming the "best" physicians in the city, or rating HMOs, hospitals and other services in the area. (You might ask editors to do stories on the best nurses or nursing services.) Some of the best monthly and quarterly magazines are published by universities for their alumni. They also venture into health issues particularly if the university has a medical school, a nursing school and a school of public health. Many publications put out by religious groups also carry features on health care.

Women's and self-help magazines offer almost unlimited potential for stories on health care. Women's magazines have dozens of columns on personal health and fitness. Health and self-help magazines target niche audiences— young men, older men, women between the ages of 25 and 40, and, of course, aging baby boomers. There are all sorts of opportunities for nurses to present their perspectives on health and illness in these publications.

Books

Books are critical to informing the public about health care. Every year new books dealing with health care policy, medical practice, specific illnesses and treatments, and other aspects of personal health arrive on the market. Some of these books are written by professional writers who call upon medical expertise and sometimes feature a heroic medical character. Others are written by physicians themselves. These are "trade books," meaning they are marketed to large, popular audiences by commercial presses like Simon and Schuster or McClelland and Stewart. Increasingly, university presses publish trade books and market and distribute them just like commercial presses.

Library catalogs and bookstore shelves reveal a large selection of books on diverse subjects authored by doctors. Physicians have written about their work with particular categories of patients—those with AIDS, cancer or neurological problems, for example. Doctors who have suddenly discovered what it's like to be a patient themselves have written books on their experiences. One of these books, *A Taste of My Own Medicine*, by physician Ed Rosenbaum was adapted into the film *The Doctor* starring William Hurt. Many physicians have described their personal journeys as did Rafael Campo in his memoir of his life as a doctor, poet and homosexual in *The Poetry of Healing*.

As a group, physicians appear to be confident enough about themselves, their profession and their audience to write about the profession's shortcomings. Books like *The Lost Art of Healing*, by the cardiologist and Nobel Peace laureate Bernard Lown, Eric Cassell's *The Nature of Suffering*, and Arthur Kleinman's *The Illness Narratives*, among others, take other doctors to task for their failure to listen to patients and for abandoning the humane roots of their profession.

The public learns about new books through reviews and publicity. Reviews appear in newspapers, and general and specialty magazines, on the Internet, and on TV and radio. Publicists send new books to radio and TV news and talk shows hoping to get a mention or even a whole program devoted to the book. Physicians, and the people who write about them, often appear as guest authors, experts or commentators. Physicians get a lot of mileage out of this kind of public exposure. It reinforces the public perception that medicine *is* health care.

Books about and by doctors are attractive to publishers because there is a large market for them in the medical profession itself and among the general public. "When we go to sign up a book, the first thing we try to figure out is how big the guaranteed market for the book is," says Steve Hubbell, a former senior editor at Henry Holt.

The medical profession has helped to create and maintain a physician market for books by running book reviews on all sorts of topics in its major journals. For example, the largest circulation medical journals in their respective countries, the *New England Journal of Medicine*, the *Journal of the American Medical Association*, and the *Canadian Medical Association Journal*, publish book reviews in every issue. So does the medically dominated health policy publication *Health Affairs*. These reviews are not limited to books on clinical practice. Physician reviewers and others critique a broad spectrum of books related to health care and medicine—including analysis, memoir and fiction. They even review the occasional book about nursing. The *New England Journal* also lists the books it has received that week but could not review.

These journals, knowing that their readers want current information, publish reviews in a timely fashion. They also seem to recognize that trade books have a very short time in which to find an audience. Medical journals thus make it possible for publishers to reach the medical market, which, in turn, makes potential books on doctors and medicine more appealing to publishers.

Nursing in North America offers an even larger potential market than medicine. That potential, so far, has not been realized. With notable exceptions such as *Intensive Care* and *Tending Lives* by Echo Heron, and *Just a Nurse* by Janet Kraegel and Mary Kachoyeanos, too few books by nurses are candidates for publication beyond the nursing press because they are not written for broad audiences even within nursing. When nurses do write books for the mainstream audience—or when other authors write books about nursing or nurses—the nursing profession inadvertently prevents these books from easily reaching the nursing market.

Nursing journals either do not regularly review books, or limit their reviews to books on clinical practice. Few review health policy books, journalistic non-fiction, memoirs, or fiction. Indeed book publicists have told us they have been ignored or rebuffed by editors of nursing publications when they've attempted to bring specific books by or about nurses to their attention. Some nursing journals review books years after their publication. This doesn't help the sales of a worthy book nor deliver timely information to readers.

Nursing journals and other nursing publications rarely run book excerpts, profiles of authors or interviews with either the author or subject of a book. Publishers trying to reach nurses through nursing publications must buy advertisements. Ads are costly and these days mainstream publishers try to spend as little money as possible on promotion. All of this makes nursing an unreachable market.

When considering whether to publish a book by or about a nurse, the first thing a publisher will ask is how many nurses there are. "Any editor would sit up and take notice when an author says that a potential market is three million nurses and nursing students in the US and Canada," Hubbell says. "But the question an editor will ask is 'Can we reach that market?' If it's a market of people who don't read, or if it can't be reached, then it's not a good market. It doesn't matter how large a potential readership is if we can't reach those readers."

An unreachable market of millions has serious consequences for the profession. When nurses don't hear about books of interest to them, they don't buy them. When they don't buy these books, this registers on the sophisticated computer tracking system publishers employ to determine who buys their books, where they buy them and when. The lack of a viable nursing market means it is difficult for a writer to find a publisher for any project on nurses or nursing. It also means that nurses get stereotyped by publishers as nonreaders.

With some concerted strategic thinking, we believe this problem can be remedied. More nurses could be encouraged to write books on a wide variety of subjects and to try to place them with mainstream publishers. But their success will depend on convincing nursing publications to allow mainstream publishers to reach the nursing market. Nursing publications could do this by creating book sections that run timely reviews and excerpts of upcoming books. Journal editors—particularly those of quarterlies—should be aware that publishers will provide them with advance galleys of a book months before its publication date so that they can assign and edit reviews expeditiously. If a book is written by a nurse or about a nurse, interviewing or profiling the authors and subjects will not only make a good human interest story, it will inspire or embolden other nurses to either write themselves or to invite journalists to enter and write about their world. This will, in turn, encourage mainstream publishers to pay attention to nursing, to publicize nursing books and even to solicit nursing manuscripts.

Through the publicity thus generated, the public will learn that nurses are doing exciting work, leading interesting lives and thinking critically about important issues. All of this will improve not just the income of the nurses or writers who have authored these books, but the image of the profession.

The Internet

Hundreds of millions of people throughout the world now have the capacity to access the Internet. Some use it to send and receive e-mail. Some use it to monitor breaking news on the Web pages of newspapers and television stations or through the news services carried by Internet providers or search engines. Millions of people use the Web to get health information and to research specific illnesses. Internet chat rooms provide an alternative to radio and television talk shows for discussing current issues.

Increasingly, the Web is a two-way media street. As more news organizations develop Web outlets, the Internet is a choice medium for publishing the news and commentary on the news. It is also a place where journalists can collect information that will go into news stories. The Web is a 24-hour billboard. Journalists can get news releases, research papers, and other information from the Web, or via e-mail, and can download this material onto their own computers.

In various ways, opportunities for nurses to be heard abound on the Web. Advances in digital telecommunications will offer even more possibilities.

What Journalists Need

To get into the news, though, nurses must know what journalists need to do their work.

1. Journalists need people who will talk to them.

The late Kirk Scharfenberg, editorial page editor of the *Boston Globe*, often pointed out that journalists don't cover disembodied ideas, they cover people and events. They relate even the most complex stories through the voices and images of the human beings involved. Nurses will not get into the media if they do not talk to journalists.

2. Journalists need multiple sources of information.

Even if some of them are not obvious, every news story you see has several sources of information. The story may seem to have one main source or "character," but the writer or producer has undoubtedly talked with many other people about it. Sometimes a story will be centered on one person and additional sources are brought in to comment on what the primary source has said or done. Some sources, such as public relations representatives, may provide "background" and thus never be quoted. On occasion, when sources might lose their jobs or face other penalties, journalists will agree to use their information without naming them. But to do their work, journalists require visible sources who can be quoted or put on camera.

When we've interviewed nurses for an article and even for this book, some have asked us, "Is it important for you to use my name?"

The answer is: Absolutely!

How can we or other journalists capture or convey your reality if you or others aren't willing to present it? How can journalists be credible without some named sources?

3. Journalists need knowledgeable sources.

This doesn't mean that a nurse must have a PhD or be an administrator to be considered knowledgeable. If the story is about the provision of nursing care and you're a caregiver, that makes you an expert. If the story is about research on a particular topic, and you do it, you're in a position to contribute your expertise to coverage.

You can always learn more about issues that concern you. If you are going to approach a reporter or know that a reporter will be talking to you, you can get the information you need to be prepared. You can gather information from organizations like the American Nurses Association, the Canadian Nurses Association, Canadian and American associations of colleges of nursing, Health Canada, the National Institute for Nursing Research, Statistics Canada, the Canadian Federation of Nurses Unions, nursing specialty organizations, nursing schools and libraries, and other nursing unions, as well as governmental and community sources. Most nursing organizations will provide information even if you aren't a member. An increasing number of organizations have Web sites where they post reports and documents and link you to other information sites. Some organizations have automated "fax-on-demand" systems that will immediately send you a fax covering the organization's position on a current issue. Some also respond to e-mail queries.

We suggest that you keep a file on subjects you might want to talk about. If you see a useful statistic or fact in a newspaper report or journal, clip it and use it when needed.

Keep in mind that journalists don't expect sources to be omniscient. Don't silence yourself because you might not know every answer to every question posed to you. When you don't know an answer, one simple response is to say, "I don't know." You can recommend someone else who might know, or you can offer to find out. Then do it.

4. Journalists need events in order to justify coverage.

Something happening at a certain time gives a journalist a "peg" for an issue. Testimony at hearings is a staple of journalistic coverage because whenever an official body investigates serious allegations, journalists have something to cover. Even the release of a report is an "event." Legal and regulatory actions are also events that offer a framework for discussing issues. Journalists also rely on legal actions to tell stories because materials filed with a court may be quoted without fear of libel. Court documents provide a wealth of information about complex transactions. If you know of a relevant court case, bring it to the attention of journalists.

Many groups construct events just to attract media coverage. Marches, rallies, informational pickets, press briefings and conferences, charitable actions, supportive statements from celebrities—these may all be contrived to give the media something to cover.

5. Journalists need sources that respect their deadlines.

Newspapers and magazines go to press at predetermined times and writers have to meet their deadlines to get into print. For those who work for radio and television news outlets, deadlines could occur at several points during the day or night. Wire service and Internet reporters must update so frequently they literally have deadlines around the clock.

If you work with the press, you have to accept the fact that people will call you or e-mail you with requests for material or interviews when it's inconvenient. Even if journalists are working on a magazine or broadcast feature that has considerable lead time, there may be production and scheduling factors that require them to gather certain information quickly. If you want your issue or perspective to be covered, you have to respond expeditiously. If you wait three weeks to return a phone call, you can be sure that your information or point of view will not make it into the story. The journalist will have gathered the facts from someone else, probably from a doctor. Moreover, faced with the journalistic equivalent of patient non-compliance, most reporters won't call you again and may not respond favorably to an overture you might want to make in the future.

The best approach is to return the phone call immediately and find out what the journalist wants. You might be able to deal with it quickly. If you are busy, ask the reporter about his or her deadline and try to arrange a more convenient time to talk. If you have a secretary or assistant, ask him or her to arrange a time for a conversation with the reporter. If you are too busy to deal with it, have your assistant refer the journalist to another nurse who can help.

6. Journalists need sources who will provide them with written documentation.

Nurses must understand that journalists are concerned about making a mistake and wary of going out on a limb without written documentation. Journalists rely on validated information. Although individual accounts are essential to any good story, when a complicated phenomenon arises, data are needed to document the amplitude and effect of the trend.

Organizations can provide such information by sponsoring surveys and other data gathering efforts, by highlighting certain aspects of existing studies and developing stories around them, and by disseminating existing data. Do not assume that just because studies are "out there" in the nursing world, journalists know about them. Make it a point to provide journalists with such studies. If you think you might need to go to the press to make something public, be sure to keep internal memos, correspondence, records of meetings, and any other documentation a journalist might need.

However, don't e-mail massive amounts of material to a journalist and expect her to take the time to read it, print it out or download it. As one journalist told us: "I opened my e-mail one day and found 15 messages on the same subject from someone who wanted me to cover it. Each contained a lengthy document. My heart sank. I e-mailed back and asked them to send me this material through the mail."

If your office has too much documentation to send, you can invite a journalist to your headquarters to look at the data and talk with your experts. The Service Employees International Union (SEIU) gave *San Francisco Chronicle* journalists access to their files for a major investigation on the lack of safe needles in hospitals (see chapter eight).

Don't ever tell a journalist—particularly one on deadline—to go to a medical library to look up material or to do an on-line search. Not only does this make the journalist's work impossible, it signals that you are not sophisticated about dealing with the media.

7.   Journalists need someone who will interpret complex material from a specialized field so that they can understand and write about it.

This means you may have to spend a considerable amount of time explaining what certain data mean or how things work in a certain environment. Journalists need to understand the standard operating procedures in your workplace or field as well the underlying assumptions that guide your work. In others words, you have to be willing to give journalists a crash course on nursing in general and on your work in particular.

8.   Journalists need someone to help them test their interpretations and framing of their stories.

The issue of accuracy is complex. Not only does the journalist want to make sure that the facts, names, titles, and quotes are correct but that the overall framing of the issue makes sense. Journalists worry about whether they are getting it right or not. "Sometimes we really want to do a story, but we just can't figure out how to get a handle on it," public radio editor Madge Kaplan told us. "If a reporter can't figure out how to do the story, the story won't get done."

Journalists rely on trustworthy people who will help them conceptualize an issue and structure their stories. Nurses often complain—and correctly so—that most reporters frame health care stories around medicine or money and ignore care and thus nursing. No journalist can take an unusual approach to a story—i.e. a nursing-centered approach—without first selling the idea to an editor or producer. The journalist has to feel confident about an unusual "frame" and sources to convince an editor that it is the right "take" on the issue.

Often, the testing of the conceptualization occurs on deadline. That's one reason why journalists might put in an urgent call to you at an inconvenient time.

9.   Journalists need sources who can summarize issues briefly and quickly and furnish the quotable quote.

The journalist's job is to reach a wide audience. To do this, journalists need sources who can get to the heart of issues in compelling, concise language. Today, the media, particularly TV and radio, depend on the tight sound bite. Reporters working on deadline often call a source, describe the story they are working on, and ask, "Would you comment on this?" If they are not doing a lengthy, in-depth exploration of the subject and are on a tight deadline, journalists really appreciate someone who will make an immediate, to-the-point comment. This is not the time to tell a journalist that he or she should read all the material you've produced on the subject and then call back with questions.

One of the things that happens when someone becomes a valued source for a journalist is that the reporter feels free to call and say, "I need a quote on this." People who are in the news a lot are there not just because they are experts on their subjects, but because they can provide a good quote at the right time.

Harvard economist John Kenneth Galbraith is one of the great masters of the "good quote." Bernice Buresh recalls how Galbraith made her work at *Newsweek* easier when she was reporting on economic developments:

> We each had our own list of sources and tried to get a variety of voices, including women's, into our stories. But you could always count on Galbraith when you needed him. You'd call him in Cambridge, Switzerland, or somewhere else, tell him what the economic issue was, and ask for his response. In a very genial fashion

he would give you one or two perfectly on-point, elegant quotes that seemed to come with even the correct punctuation. And then he would say, "Anything else?" You'd say, "Thank you very much professor." And that was the end of the phone call.

Not surprisingly Galbraith's voice and opinions permeated economic coverage throughout the world for decades. There are very few sources in this class. But journalists value someone who will take the time and exhibit the willingness to construct quotable quotes for or with them.

10. Journalists, like the rest of us, need people who will treat them cordially and with respect and not talk down to them, belittle them, get defensive and irritable, and act as though talking to them were a terrible imposition.

Being cooperative will generally lead to a better story and greater visibility for nurses. There are media outlets like supermarket tabloids and exploitation shows that you wouldn't want to cooperate with at all. But with the legitimate media, even when you are dealing with difficult people, the best results will come from firmness and courtesy.

Veteran political columnist Mary McGrory cited cooperation as the reason that Senator John McCain became so popular with the press during the US presidential primaries in 2000: "The reason is simple: He talks to the press, returns our calls, says things he shouldn't, takes them back, and doesn't blame anybody else. This is novel. Other Republicans prefer to bash the press. He woos us and wows us and seeks out our company."[16]

Even if you establish an excellent working relationship with members of the media, there will still be mishaps and frustrations. At times you may be misunderstood or misquoted. In simplifying complicated issues, journalists will make errors. You might be quoted out of context. In some instances, you, your specialty, and profession may get negative coverage. That's the risk of voice and of being "consequential."

You may spend an hour talking to a journalist and not even get mentioned in the final report. You might refer journalists to other people in the field who also give them valuable time only to find out that the journalist—or editor or producer—has decided not to do the story. Television documentary or feature producers are notorious for picking a source's brain, implying they will interview them on air, and then going off in a different direction or finding someone else to put on their show. Journalistic demands may prove disruptive to your work and home life. When you try to help and seem to get nothing out of it, this can be infuriating.

But even if your efforts don't produce immediate results, they can have a long-term impact. Most journalists have never talked with a nursing expert. They don't know how to cover nursing, how to think about nursing, or even the first question to ask about nursing. They don't know that nurses can comment intelligently on many health care matters beyond nursing practice. Many don't even know there is anything intelligent to say about nursing practice. When you take the time to talk to a journalist, you're building a foundation for recognition and respect for yourself and your profession.

For example, we recently talked with a television producer who was trying to figure out whether he could do a documentary proving that cutbacks in hospital staff were undermining quality care. The producer knew of an incident that seemed to connect understaffing with serious patient injuries. But was there enough there for a story? he wondered. He didn't have any nursing sources. "I have no idea how to get into nursing," he confessed.

We talked with him repeatedly over the course of a week and gave him the names of several nurses to call. He talked to the nurses and was impressed with their knowledge and accessibility. Two weeks later he told us he wasn't sure he and his colleagues had enough substantiation to go ahead with the project. Whether the project gets on track or not, we know this producer has a more positive view of nursing than he had before. His new knowledge of nursing can lead him to future stories and he can share his knowledge with the journalists he works with. That, in and of itself, is a positive outcome of a nursing intervention.

Endnotes

1. F.L. Mott, *American Journalism: A History 1690–1960*, 3rd ed. (New York: Macmillan, 1962).

2. J. Hohenberg, *Free Press, Free People* (New York: The Free Press, 1973).

3. T. Case, "No Dearth of Health Care Coverage," *Editor & Publisher*, 1 October 1994.

4. National Health Council, *21st Century Housecall: The Link between Medicine and the Media—Key Survey Findings* (National Health Council, 1997).

5. Roper Starch, *Americans Talk about Science and Medical News* (National Health Council, 1997).

6. Wirthlin Worldwide, *Myths and Misperceptions about Aging and Women's Health: Initial Findings* (National Council on the Aging, 1997).

7. Roper Starch, *Americans Talk about Science.*

8. J. Hohenberg, *The Professional Journalist: A Guide to the Practices and Principles of the News Media* (New York: Holt, Rinehart & Winston, 1978), p. 44.

9. B. Buresh, A Month of Health Care News (Unpublished report, 1997).

10. B. Buresh, S. Gordon, and N. Bell, "Who Counts in News Coverage of Health Care?" *Nursing Outlook*, 39 no. 5 (1991): pp. 204-208.

11. M. Mencher, *News Reporting and Writing*, 2nd ed. (Dubuque, Iowa: Wm. C. Brown Company, 1981).

12. P. Hemp, "Witness to Courage," *Boston Globe Magazine*, 5 February 1995.

13. D. Frey, "On the Border of Life," *New York Times Magazine*, 9 July 1995.

14. H. Robertson, "Heartbreak," *Elm Street*, March 1998.

15. Mencher, *News Reporting and Writing*.

16. M. McGrory, "The Secret of McCain's Success Is that He's Fun," *Boston Globe*, 12 February 2000, p. A15.

Chapter 6

REACHING OUT
TO THE NEWS MEDIA

News coverage doesn't happen by accident. With or without public relations help, nurses must reach out and develop ongoing relationships with journalists who cover health care. The process of working with the media is much like nursing itself. It requires monitoring, intervention and maintenance. This chapter shows how to build media relationships step by step.

A lot of people believe that if they are doing something newsworthy, the news media, for better or worse, will discover it. Popular culture supports this misperception by depicting reporters as relentless in their pursuit of good stories.

A notable example is the 1974 book, *All the President's Men*. It offered a spellbinding account of *Washington Post* investigative reporters Bob Woodward and Carl Bernstein doggedly chasing down "Watergate" leads all the way to the White House. The work of these reporters not only led to the resignation of President Richard Nixon, it made journalism seem far more exciting, glamorous and classy than it had ever been, particularly after Robert Redford and Dustin Hoffman played Woodward and Bernstein in the movie. The book and movie created great public awareness of journalism.

Most journalists, however, are not investigative reporters. Most do not spend their time zealously digging through records, relentlessly bird-dogging sources at their workplaces or homes, and initiating major probes into wrongdoing. You will not find most health care reporters prowling through hospital corridors in the dead of night, or sifting through hospital trash looking for evidence of misdeeds. While they are eager for good stories and try to stay on top of newsworthy developments, most of the time journalists aren't looking for scandals.

Reporters are not Lone-Ranger-like figures who independently decide what news to cover. In general, interested parties draw journalists' attention to significant developments and issues. When investigative stories appear (such as the *San Francisco Chronicle's* series on needle-stick injuries described in chapter eight), they've usually been inspired by whistle blowers, individual sources or organizations with enough factual material to convince reporters, editors and producers that the potential story was good enough to justify the time and expense of an in-depth probe. According to public relations professors Todd Hunt and James E. Grunig, an estimated one-half to two-thirds of news stories are "source-originated."[1] Often the source is a public relations professional who works on staff or as a consultant for corporations, government departments and agencies, organizations, or individuals.

While journalists don't want to be tools of promoters and marketers, they also don't want to miss significant stories. "We live in dread that we will miss *the* important development on a given day," Cornelia Dean, editor of the *New York Times* Health Science section, told us. "If we do, we know we will hear about it."

One way journalists might hear about it is to see the story reported by a competing news outlet. Then they may have to scramble to do their own story. Another is when they start getting phone calls from those they consider to be the heavy hitters in a given field.

Journalists operate within a network of relationships. They find out what's going on from people who provide them with critical information. These "sources" reach out to them by sending them press releases, calling them to underscore the significance of a particular event, inviting them to meetings, press conferences, and organizational or professional conferences, furnishing them with reports and studies, arranging discussions with them and their editorial boards, meeting them for lunch or for a drink, and schmoozing with them periodically. Since journalists have cooperative/competitive relationships with their colleagues, they often learn about interesting developments from other reporters.

It's impossible to overestimate the value of developing relationships with members of the media. When the late Barbara Roderick was the executive director of the Massachusetts Nurses Association, she began a conversation with her next door neighbor in the back yard. She knew that he wrote about public affairs and political issues for the *Boston Globe*. So she talked to him about pending state legislation that would permit advanced practice nurses to write prescriptions. A short time later, an op-ed article appeared in the *Globe* strongly advocating that advanced practice nurses be given prescriptive authority. The bill eventually passed. None other than her neighbor wrote the op-ed.

If you provide journalists with a steady stream of usable tips and information that are accurate and pertinent and respond in a timely fashion to their needs and questions, at least some of your issues and concerns will be reported on. You won't like everything journalists report. Journalists and their news outlets may not totally support your issue. But you will be a participant in the public discussion, which means you will have some power to influence events.

The First Step: Deciding Whom You Want to Reach

It is very important that you define whom you are trying to communicate with so that you can determine how you will communicate. For example, there are audiences or "publics" that you can reach without the news media. If you are trying to explain a new protocol to the clinical personnel in your hospital, you might distribute a memo or send it to recipients via e-mail. If patients with a particular illness need to know some specifics about self care, you might participate in preparing a brochure or sheet of instructions they can take home or a videotape that they may watch when they come in for treatment. Similarly, you might do a mailing to people in your neighborhood or community to advertise new services at your health care facility. You might also purchase newspaper ad space or commercial time on local television.

At the same time, you might want to tell the public about some of these things via the news media. This means that you will have to convince intermediaries—journalists and television and radio producers—that your information is newsworthy, so that they, in turn, will make it into a story that reaches the public.

Before you pick up the phone or send out a news release, you need to decide the audience you are trying to reach and which media outlets would be most effective. Perhaps you would like people in your community to know about a nursing program that can serve them. In that case your best vehicle for communication might be weekly community newspapers. A feature story on the program could be loaded onto your institution's Web site.

Perhaps you will be rallying in front of your state or provincial/territorial capital to support new legislation or regulations. You'll want as much publicity as possible across the state or province so that citizens throughout the area will urge their political representatives to support your cause. Therefore, you won't want to limit your efforts to the media in the state or provincial/territorial capital. You'll want to get advance press releases to newspapers, television and radio throughout the region. If you're working with a public relations professional, he or she should know whom to contact and how to distribute information. You can find out yourself by contacting the capital news bureau and/or pressroom.

Whether you are seeking a national audience or a more limited one, one of your tools will be an up-to-date media list.

Experienced public relations specialists who work with nurses have contacts with the press. We discuss the role of public relations practitioners more fully in the next chapter. But whether you employ a PR person or not, nurses must establish and tend relationships with reporters who can be helpful to them.

Introducing Yourself

You introduce yourself to the media by bringing them something that's newsworthy. A letter, press release or phone call describing a newsworthy event or project can be your introduction. Since nurses are not usually regular sources for reporters, nurses will have to do personal outreach to journalists to establish a connection. Journalists need to know that the people behind the news release are credible.

A good story is the vehicle for establishing a relationship. But how do you know if what you are doing is a story? Stand back and look at your work with some objectivity. Have you seen articles or television reports on similar topics? Does your activity have some of the news values outlined in chapter five? Is your issue relevant to the kind of broader audience that a media outlet would reach? Can you present your work in a way that makes its value and relevance obvious? If your work is narrowly focused, ask yourself if it can be generalized. Is it poignant, dramatic, quirky, offbeat? Does it challenge conventional wisdom?

Considering the newsworthiness of all sorts of activities and issues is a constructive activity for nurses inasmuch as the goal is to fully integrate nursing into health care coverage. Reaching out with a variety of events and activities will make a broad range of nursing expertise more visible. It will open the door for nurses to become regular news sources on health matters far beyond those related to hospital working conditions. Professional organizations can broaden the public view of nursing by becoming as vigorous in promoting stories about nursing practice as collective bargaining groups have been in exposing threats to nursing and patient care.

Any research study or program that enhances patient care is a possibility for a nursing angle. When a study reported in the *New England Journal of Medicine*, for example, discusses parental reluctance to stop futile aggressive treatment of children with advanced cancer, nurses have an opportunity to show how they help parents make difficult decisions. Another good patient care story is nurses' involvement in understanding why heart attack patients delay going to emergency rooms and their efforts to teach patients the symptoms that call for immediate treatment.

Opportunities

Be alert to your particular issues surfacing in the media. When the media focus on a dramatic or even sensational event, be prepared to jump in. In both Canada and the US, the care of the dying is a subject of continuing debate. Periodically an event—a tragedy, a new study, a court decree, a new law—catapults the issue to the top of the news agenda where it receives intense coverage for a while. Nurses must take advantage of these openings even though some may be created by controversial or unpleasant events.

Each time Dr. Jack Kevorkian killed another patient, that was a story. In Canada, after Robert Lattimer killed his 12-year-old severely disabled daughter to "put her out of her pain," the story resurfaced with every new development in the case. Although these events provided opportunities for nurses in hospice and palliative care to present their views, some told us they were reluctant to enter the discussion because they feared that palliative care would suffer from guilt-by-association with euthanasia. This fact alone gives nurses an unprecedented opportunity to educate the public about palliative care and argue for expanded use in the care of the terminally and chronically ill.

In such a case, the press is looking for credible sources to present various sides of the issue. If you want your side to be represented, you need to be ready with appropriate spokespeople. This is how Gerri Frager, a former nurse who is now a pediatrician and palliative care physician in Halifax, Nova Scotia, became a national spokesperson for pediatric palliative care in Canada. When the Lattimer tragedy occurred, she spoke eloquently about the fact that seriously ill children need palliative care. "It's terrible what the child and family went through," Frager said. "But what we need now is a public discussion about what can be done to relieve pain and suffering rather than a call for euthanasia and physician-assisted suicide. It's important for the public and health care professionals to know that pain can be relieved in the overwhelming majority of cases."[2]

In many instances, the kind of events that will propel an issue are predictable. If a blue-ribbon panel has been considering a particular problem or policy, most likely the media will cover its findings. Such groups make a point of packaging their reports in a media friendly way. Journalists will report on a high court's decision in a controversial case. They usually know in advance when the court will hear the case. The agendas of legislative, policy-making and regulatory bodies can be monitored to predict when newsmaking developments will occur. Journalists often get advance notice of new research findings. As a profession concerned with health care issues, nurses can stay abreast of these processes and be ready with their stories when the issue is about to crest again.

Focusing the Story

Pretend that you are the reporter trying to tell the story. You'll have to come up with something that can serve as a "peg."

Say you are a geriatric nurse practitioner who has initiated a program to release nursing home residents from physical and chemical restraints. Your work could be a timely and relevant story. One peg for a story could be how the health of the residents improved at a particular nursing home when this program was implemented. A research study showing how this approach prevents suffering and saves money could also be a peg for a story.

For nursing, the point of outreach is to show, in a newsworthy way, how *nurses* understand patient needs, prevent problems, enhance public health, offer alternative policies, and meet contemporary health needs. It is not to get free publicity for your institution. Reporters will resist that kind of overture.

Unless you are working with a journalist who has demonstrated his or her knowledge about nursing, assume ignorance. The natural tendency of many journalists is to credit physicians with any improvement in health care delivery. That's why you'll have to highlight the *nursing* component of the story.

Assembling Written Materials

Reporters generally expect to see something written on the story you are trying to pitch. It makes their job easier and more efficient if they have something to read that gives the gist of the story.

Most of the time this is a brief letter, a news release, or both. Sometimes a news release will be more effective if it is backed up by research studies or news clippings. Reporters may pay more attention if they see that other journalists have found the topic newsworthy. However, they will be looking for their own "peg" in the form of a new development or angle.

If you are mounting a campaign like one of those described in chapter eight, you will want to assemble a media kit for distribution to journalists and influence makers. A kit is often just a two-sided pocket folder containing pertinent materials. If your organization has sufficient resources, the cover can be specially designed and printed. If you have fewer resources, you can buy folders at a local office supply store and print labels on your computer. The kit might contain some or all of the following:

- A press release or letter that piques the interest of the reader, briefly gives the facts, conveys a sense of immediacy, explains the relevance of the event or issue, and tells how to contact the people involved.
- A simple fact sheet that lists important points or background events or developments.
- A fact sheet or brochure describing the organization or organizations sponsoring the event or involved in the issue.

- A "backgrounder" or briefing paper that gives in-depth information. If the backgrounder includes statistics or research data the sources must be listed in a bibliography.
- Biographical sketches of the important players including information on how to contact them.
- Copies of articles that have appeared in the press and brief descriptions of television reports and features on this or a similar topic. You could include a videotape on the subject. However, in general, it is more efficient for a journalist to sift through papers than to view a tape.
- Copies of pertinent research articles.
- A question-and-answer sheet that suggests and anticipates key questions and provides the answers.

Don't make your press kit confusing by putting in too much material.

Initial Contacts: News Releases

News releases are often belittled by journalists. Many claim they barely look at the scores of handouts that cross their desks or their computer screens. The reason journalists toss or delete the great majority of the news releases they receive is because the form is greatly abused by corporations peddling products and by organizations that indiscriminately crank out statements containing nothing remotely newsworthy. According to a public relations researcher, news releases are usually poorly written, have no local angle to interest news outlets in a given area, and have no news elements. This means that the information in the release is not particularly interesting or timely, is not of consequence, and lacks impact, oddity, conflict, known principals, or proximity.[3]

But companies, organizations, and public relations firms continue to put out news releases because a good one can be effective. When a release is informative and targeted properly, it can be put to use in various ways.

A weekly newspaper, for example, might run an excerpt from or even an entire news release on programs of interest to the public or on people in the community. Most of the health service announcements in such publications— a blood drive will be held, flu shots will be administered, a blood pressure screening clinic is operating—originate in news releases. So do many ideas that can be developed into good stories.

Larger newspapers and radio and television news organizations use news releases in a number of ways. They might use the information for an immediate story. They might cover an event because of a release. A reporter might hold on to a release for use in a future story. She might add the cited expert sources to her Rolodex™. Since journalists receive so many news releases, they scan them very rapidly, usually reading only the headline and the first paragraph.

Neil Rosenberg, the health editor for the *Milwaukee Journal-Sentinel*, describes his modus operandi this way: "I don't know what other reporters do—I'm sure some see Eli Lilly on the envelope and throw it out—but I open every piece of mail. Ninety-nine percent of it is cast aside. I'm like a fisherman, I'm looking for an idea that I can make into a very good story. Some days I get skunk and some days I get muskie."[4]

If journalists don't see a "peg" for a story right at the beginning, you can be sure they won't spend their time wading around in your verbiage. Like the newspaper reader or the television viewer, they want to know what the story is right away. Then they can decide if they're interested.

Format

A news release must be typed or printed from a computer—never hand written—on standard 8 1/2 x 11-inch white paper. Use a standard business typeface, not script or a peculiar font. Put a 1 to 1 1/2-inch margin around the page. Double space the lines, or, if you are trying to save paper, at least the first couple of paragraphs. Single-spaced paragraphs should have double spacing between them. It's best to use only one side of the page. Limit the release to one to three pages. One to two pages are preferable.

Note the reprinted news release (page 135) by the Canadian Nurses Association on an abrupt shift in nursing education policy announced in Saskatchewan. That release didn't need to be long because it's purpose was to respond to an important, unforeseen event. But it does make clear within its five paragraphs that the CNA has a major stake in nursing education and will be heard from again.

Background material can be included separately, or a note can be added about additional material and where to get it.

Components of a News Release

1. Letterhead. Your news release should have a letterhead with your name or the name of your organization, mailing address, phone number, and perhaps e-mail and Web site addresses. You can create this yourself on a computer if you don't have a printed letterhead.
2. Contact information goes at the top of the release. After "Contact:" put the name(s) of the person or persons a journalist can contact to verify the information in the release and to learn more. Be sure to give their day and nighttime phone numbers and/or pager numbers, and e-mail addresses.
3. The standard news release identifies itself with the word NEWS or NEWS RELEASE written in very large type at the top of the page.

FOR IMMEDIATE RELEASE   <u>en français</u>

CNA BAFFLED BY SASKATCHEWAN GOVERNMENT BACKTRACK ON EDUCATION

(24 January 2000 - Ottawa)

The Canadian Nurses Association (CNA), the professional voice of nursing in Canada, is baffled by the sudden changes announced Friday related to entry to practice requirements for registered nurses in the province of Saskatchewan.

"Targeting education, and ultimately, the level of care patients have a right to expect across the country, is not the way to get at the root cause of a growing, national nursing shortage," says CNA President Lynda Kushnir Pekrul, adding, "It simply doesn't add up. Reducing education requirements to offset the nursing shortage is a knee-jerk reaction to a long-standing challenge. What we must do is move quickly to address the recruitment, integration and retention of nurses into the system nationally."

In the early 1990s, the challenges of health care delivery including advances in technology combined with greater patient acuity as the population ages, led CNA to spearhead the movement to provide registered nurses with an entry level of education that is in line with the needs of the public. "For CNA, says Kushnir Pekrul, the issue of entry to practice requirements was, and is, about nursing professionals providing the best patient care. Canadians deserve no less. With Friday's announcement, the Saskatchewan government is downgrading the importance of nursing."

Governments in the provinces of Newfoundland, PEI, Nova Scotia, New Brunswick, Manitoba and Ontario have formally moved towards baccalaureate education for registered nurses.

CNA is the professional voice of nursing in Canada. It is a federation of 11 provincial/territorial nurses' associations.

For information contact:

Carole Saindon
CNA Media Relations
Tel: (613) 237-2159, ext. 310
Fax: (613) 237-3520
E-mail: <u>csaindon@cna-nurses.ca</u>

---

4. Next a release time is given at the top of the page. Usually the release time is FOR IMMEDIATE RELEASE, which means the news organization can use the material as soon as it comes in or any other time. The date the release is being issued should be provided. Some releases, reports and studies will have an "embargo" date on them. Journalists will be given an advance copy so that they will have time to prepare their stories, but they must wait to publish or broadcast them until the specified time and date.

5. A headline, or tag line, goes at the top to catch the interest of the recipient. This is not the headline that the news organization will use. They will write a headline that fits their own format.

Note the headline on the news release that follows on the next page from the University of California at San Francisco: FEDERAL ENFORCEMENT OF NURSING HOMES MAY BE INADEQUATE, SAY UCSF RESEARCHERS. Like an actual news headline, it captures the point of the news release. It uses a present-tense verb ("say") to convey timeliness. Try to make your headline dynamic. Employ active verbs when possible. Like the "UCSF Researchers," in the headline, make as strong an assertion as you accurately can. This is not the time to fudge the issue. The UCSF release uses the qualifying word "may." Nevertheless, the researchers are alerting journalists to a major societal problem.

The Lead of the News Release

Like a news reporter, never save the best stuff for last. Construct your news release like a news story—inverted pyramid style with the foundation for the story at the top. The first paragraph of a news story or news release is called the "lead." Like the headline that preceded it, a good lead is a small story all by itself.

A summary lead is the most common type. It usually contains several of the five Ws—who, what, where, when, why (and sometimes how). It does it in one or two sentences. Look at the first sentence of the UCSF release:

"The deteriorating quality of health care in US nursing homes may be due, in part, to poor enforcement of federal regulations, according to researchers at the University of California, San Francisco."

The "what" of the lead is the problem: the deteriorating quality of health care in nursing homes.

The "why" in this case is the nub of the story: poor enforcement of federal regulations.

The "who" refers to researchers at UCSF.

The "where" is nursing homes in the United States, but the location of the researchers is also important to the local media.

University of California
San Francisco

News Services

UNIVERSITY OF CALIFORNIA, SAN FRANCISCO

3333 California Street
Suite 103, Box 0462
San Francisco, CA
94143-0462
tel: 415/476-2557
fax: 415/476-3541

Alice Trinkl, News Director
Source: Rebecca Sladek Nowlis, (415) 476-2557
E-mail: RSNowlis@pubaff.ucsf.edu

FOR IMMEDIATE RELEASE
December 6, 1999

**FEDERAL ENFORCEMENT OF NURSING HOMES MAY BE INADEQUATE,
SAY UCSF RESEARCHERS**

The deteriorating quality of health care in US nursing homes may be due, in part, to poor enforcement of federal regulations, according to researchers at the University of California, San Francisco.

The average number of deficiencies issued to US nursing homes for various violations of federal standards declined nearly 50 percent during a seven year period, say the researchers. Although this could suggest that nursing homes are improving their overall quality of care, a more likely explanation is a gradual weakening of the federal enforcement process, they said.

"We don't know why the number of deficiencies are going down, but we definitely don't see an improvement in quality of care," said Charlene Harrington, RN, PhD, UCSF professor of social and behavioral sciences and principal author of the study. "There's clear evidence that the quality of nursing home care nationwide is substandard."

The authors' evaluation of federal nursing home standards between 1991 and 1997, the first since passage of the Nursing Home Reform Act of 1987, appears in the December 1999 issue of *Medical Care Research and Review.*

The researchers examined Health Care Financing Administration (HCFA) records from the On-Line Survey, Certification, and Reporting System (OSCAR), the only source of comprehensive and uniform data about nursing home resident conditions and deficiencies for the United States. OSCAR compiles data from site evaluations done by state survey agencies every nine to fifteen months. If a facility fails to meet federal standards of care, surveyors hand out deficiencies or citations. The most frequently cited violations included inadequate food sanitation, improper resident assessments and care plans, and failure to prevent accidents and pressure sores.

Using a subset of the OSCAR data set, the researchers report a 44 percent decline in the average number of deficiencies given to nursing facilities, falling from 8.8 per facility in 1991 to 4.9 per facility in 1997. The researchers also report a 100 percent increase in the number of facilities with no deficiencies, from 10.8 percent in 1991 to 21.6 percent in 1997.

In light of numerous reports documenting the poor quality of care found in the roughly 16,000 nursing homes nationwide, the decline in deficiencies is suspect, said Harrington. Earlier this year, the US General Accounting Office (USGAO) issued reports

(more)

Federal Enforcement of Nursing Homes May Be Inadequate, Say UCSF Researchers-- Page 2

that found widespread health and safety violations in more than one-fourth of nursing homes.

"If nursing home quality continues to be problematic, a reasonable explanation for the decline in deficiencies is inadequate enforcement by HCFA and the states," said Harrington. "There is evidence that deficiencies may be unreported by the HCFA survey process. The whole survey process is pretty weak."

In 1998, the USGAO found that surveyors were unable to detect serious quality of care problems and concluded that HCFA enforcement policies have not been effective in ensuring that deficiencies are identified and corrected. There is also documented variation in the deficiency rates across states, said Harrington, suggesting that the survey process and the process of issuing deficiencies are inconsistent.

The researchers report that the average number of deficiencies in 1997 varied substantially across states, from 1.8 per facility in Vermont and New Mexico to 14.3 in Nevada. Forty-five states and the District of Columbia showed a decline in the average number of deficiencies cited per facility from the 1991 to 1997 period, with Colorado and New Mexico having a more than an 80 percent decline.

In addition to the overall decline in deficiencies, the authors examined the data for six conditions commonly used to assess quality of care in nursing homes. Two conditions, being bedridden and the use of contractures to immobilize joints, increased significantly. Over the seven year study period, the average number of bedridden residents increased 125 percent, from 3.5 to 7.2. Most residents should not be in bed except when there is a serious medical condition, so a high percentage of bedridden residents is considered a potential indicator of poor care, said Harrington.

The percent of residents with contractures, or immobilized joints, also increased significantly, up by 45 percent. Contractures can be a sign that residents are not receiving appropriate joint exercise and adequate care, said Harrington.

Only one condition, the use of physical restraints, improved significantly between 1991 and 1997. Physical restraints restrict freedom of movement or normal access to one's body and are viewed as negative indicators of quality, said Harrington. Their use decreased by 30 percent. Bladder incontinence and pressure sores increased slightly, and urinary catheter use decreased slightly.

In addition to Harrington, Helen Carrillo, MS, UCSF statistician in the department of social and behavioral sciences, co-authored the paper.

This research was funded by the Agency for Health Care Policy and Research and the Health Care Financing Administration.

###

(RSN Harrington)

The "when" is not a big factor in the UCSF release, but it is crucial in the news release below put out by the Massachusetts Nurses Association announcing a demonstration by nurses "today."

When writing the lead (and the rest of the news release) don't be melodramatic or flowery. Write the way reporters do—in simple declarative sentences in the active voice.

MASSACHUSETTS NURSES ASSOCIATION

NEWS RELEASE

FOR IMMEDIATE RELEASE
November 8, 1999

Contacts:	David Schildmeier	781-821-4625 x717 or 508-426-1655 (pager)
	Barry Adams, RN	617-437-0550
	S. Stephen Rosenfeld (Adams' Attorney)	617-723-7470
	Denise Garlick, RN (Protest Organizer)	(781) 449-7338

Nurses To Demonstrate Outside Headquarters of Nursing Board on Nov. 10th
Await Decision on Complaint Filed by Nurse Whistle Blower Barry Adams Against His Former Nurse Executive

Nursing Board Has Come Under Fire by Nurses From Across the Nation
For Its Handling of Adams' Concerns and the Board's Efforts to Protect Executives While Punishing Frontline Care Givers Working Under Dangerous Conditions

Board Begins its Deliberations at 9 a.m. Nurses to Demonstrate outside BORN Headquarters at 239 Causeway Street from 10:30 a.m. to 12:30 p.m.

Boston, MA – Outraged nurses from across the Commonwealth as well as the nation have called for a demonstration outside the headquarters of the Massachusetts Board of Registration (BORN) in Nursing on Nov. 10, 1999 to protest the BORN's failure to hold all nurses equally accountable for the care they deliver. *Call the MNA for names of nurses attending from your coverage area.*

The demonstration coincides with the day the BORN has announced it will issue its final determination to pursue a complaint filed by nationally recognized nurse whistle blower Barry Adams against his former nurses executives. Adams has filed a complaint of unethical conduct, unprofessional conduct and patient neglect against his former nursing administrators at Youville Health Care of Cambridge, who illegally fired Adams for blowing the whistle on deplorable staffing conditions that led to a patient's death and harm to other patients at the facility.

At the heart of Adams' complaint is the issue of accountability of all licensed nurses, including nurse executives, for decisions they make which adversely affect patient care. The case comes at a time when nurses across the nation have been voicing their concerns about the deterioration of patient care in light of chronic understaffing in America's hospitals.

The BORN will begin its deliberations on complaints and other issues beginning at 9 a.m. Nurses will be demonstrating outside the BORN headquarters on 239 Causeway St. from 10:30 a.m. to 12:30 p.m.

The demonstration is part of a "Campaign for BORN Reform" begun by the Massachusetts
-MORE-

340 TURNPIKE STREET ■ CANTON, MASSACHUSETTS 02021-2711
781.821.4625 ■ FAX 781.821.4445

®—◆—19

NURSES TO DEMONSTRATE OUTSIDE NURSING BOARD ON NOV. 10TH/2 . . .

Nurses Association and other concerned nurses following the BORN's actions at an investigative hearing held on September 22, 1999 when Adams was invited to submit information to the BORN's Complaint Committee and to provide witnesses in support of his complaint.

With the media and a number of nursing leaders in attendance, the BORN announced that it had dismissed the most salient components of Adams' complaint and redrafted his complaint to mitigate the impact on the nurse executive. According to observers, the BORN was disorganized, disrespectful and inconsistent in their handling of the issues, which are of great concern to a growing audience of nurses from throughout the state (and the nation).

The MNA's Committee for BORN Reform has been working with nurses from across the state and the nation since the Sep. 22nd hearing to raise awareness within the Executive Branch of their concerns for the Board of Registration's ability to fairly and effectively carry out its mandate to protect the public. A letter writing campaign has been initiated to request that the Governor's administration conduct an immediate investigation into the policies and practices of the agency. It also seeks a mandate that the BORN hold all nurses (executives and staff nurses) equally accountable, and it asks for the Governor's support for whistleblower language, which is expected to be passed as part of the state budget.

Adams, with the support of nurses from throughout the nation, has also retained Rosenfeld & Associates, a prominent health care law firm that specializes in consumer protection, to assist in seeking justice, not just for himself but for all nurses and patients cared for by nurses in the Commonwealth. "The need for this legal action speaks loudly to the gauntlet nurses must face when making well substantiated assessments in the patients' interest and safety, "Adams said. "The system in place to protect patients failed for me and for the patients in this case, from the hospital to the BORN I was blocked at every juncture."

Adams' attorneys have submitted a "bill of particulars," to the BORN, which is a legal document providing evidence and arguments as to why the BORN should reverse the decision of the complaint committee to dismiss his complaints regarding patient neglect, unprofessional conduct, and unethical conduct. In failing to do so, the attorneys argue that the BORN would be in "violation of the principles it is charged with upholding.... in violation of its public mandate... and in violation of Massachusetts law."

It concludes that the BORN's handling of the case "...leads to the inescapable conclusion that the BORN is capriciously selective in the complaints it wishes to hear, and that it categorically favors complaints made by superiors against staff nurses and disfavors complaints by staff nurses against superiors. Such a pattern is an abuse of the BORN's discretion and would be enjoined by a court of competent jurisdiction if proved."

Editors and Reporters Note: For a fax or email copy of Adams' complaint, his attorney's "bill of particulars," additional background on the issue, or the names of other sources, including nurses attending from your coverage area, contact David Schildmeier at 781-830-5717. You may also find additional information on the MNA web site at www.massnurses.org.
###

Body of the News Release

Stick to the facts. Use direct quotations to introduce subjective material, opinions, or allegations. Get in a pithy quote as soon as possible. Quotations are essential to your news release because they allow you to inject "voice," opinion, vigor, and, sometimes, colorful language.

A direct quotation is a good way to make a strong point as experts did in the second paragraph of the CNA release and the third paragraph of the UCSF release.

Direct quotations for news releases are anything but spontaneous. The speaker herself might construct one or a public relations person might write it with her or for her. But the quote is carefully tailored to deliver maximum impact and still sound like something the person would say. It should also be conversational and sound as though it was spoken rather than written.

Direct quotations must be attributed to the speaker. Inexperienced writers tend to put the name and the title of the speaker before the quotation. But unless the name is the most important element, advance attribution slows down the eye and lessens the impact of a dramatic or colorful quote. Look at the quotations in this book and at those in newspapers. You will see that the sentence often begins with the quote and finishes with the attribution. Also note the punctuation. Quotation marks go *after* the punctuation at the end of a quote.

The Elements of Style, by William Strunk, Jr. and E. B. White, is an excellent and inexpensive source of information on quotation and other matters of style and content.[5] This slim volume is a classic reference guide used by tens of thousands of students and writers.

A speaker is credible in a news release (or a news story) because he or she has expertise or authority. Credibility is established by the person's title, position, work, and experience. Nurses often worry that being "just a nurse" is insufficient. For the working nurse, doing the work of nursing is precisely the credential that matters.

Note how Charlene Harrington is identified in the UCSF press release. She has many credentials. She is a PhD, a professor, a researcher, an RN. By using the RN credential first, she is emphasizing its importance to the subject matter. She is a *nurse*, who is an authority on *nursing* homes, which are places that are supposed to provide *nursing* care.

Be sure to emphasize your nursing credentials in your news release. In some instances PhDs let their institutions send out news releases with no explicit mention of their connection to nursing. Their name appears as Mary Smith, PhD, or as Dr. Mary Smith. This not only contributes to the invisibility of nursing, it actually risks giving medicine credit for nurses' accomplishments.

Although PhD nurses may feel strongly that they have earned their "Dr." title, in this society they will generally be mistaken for physicians unless they make an extra effort to identify themselves as nurses.

When you are writing your news release, plan to spend about half of your time on the headline, the lead, and the first direct quote. These are the most important elements and it's reasonable to rewrite them until you have reduced them to the essentials. This is also true for e-mail releases and media alerts. The rest of the release elaborates upon the main points. For an inverted pyramid-style release, you don't need a snappy ending. Just end before you start belaboring the points. Remember the release is designed to be a quick read.

Organizations often end their releases with a "boilerplate" paragraph that describes the function of the organization. The Canadian Nurses Association ended its release with just two short sentences: "CNA is the professional voice of nursing in Canada. It is a federation of 11 provincial/territorial nurses' associations."

Accuracy

Make sure your news release is accurate. Check and recheck all of the names and other proper nouns for correct spelling. Then have someone else proofread your release. It is astonishing how easily errors can creep in and not get caught. Your credibility could suffer if there are errors in your release. It is a maxim in journalism that if a name is spelled incorrectly, then nothing else is believable.

A release must be honest as well as accurate. You are expected to present information from your point of view. However, you must not mislead, exaggerate or distort the truth to build your case.

Broadcast Releases

Radio and television stations can use information in a standard news release to create a report, but they cannot broadcast it as is. If they are interested in doing a report based on the release, they will convert its essential information into a short, broadcast-style piece. When you are trying to get media attention for timely events—such as a major nursing demonstration at a state or provincial/territorial capital—it might make sense to fax a 200-word (one-minute-long) broadcast release to radio and television stations around the state or province. Small radio stations might use it, although they will probably tighten it further. You would want to include an extra sheet with exact information on where and when the event will take place, and the names of participants who will be available for interviews.

For broadcast writing simplify the issues. Write for the ear, not the eye. Use short sentences. Use colloquial language. Avoid hard-to-pronounce words. Don't use abbreviations. Follow a difficult name with a phonetic spelling in parenthesis so that the reader will know how to pronounce it. Spell out numbers. By all means use participants as sources of information, but in most cases, paraphrase instead of quoting directly, e.g., "Stella Smith is among the registered nurses who say a safe staffing law will improve the care of patients in area hospitals."

Distribution

There are times when you will want to distribute broadly a news release to news organizations. You might fax your release to all the news organizations in the area or, for a fee, get it onto a PR newswire that goes to news organizations. Even with widespread distribution, targeting is important. You will want to make sure that appropriate reporters get their own copy.

In some instances, it's better to contact just a few reporters. If you have a story that you think would be of particular interest to a certain feature writer, a columnist, or a writer who focuses on health policy issues, or would fit the format of a television newsmagazine show, put your efforts into making a good match. Tailor your presentation to that reporter or media outlet.

Write a short letter to accompany your materials explaining who you are and why your project might make a good story. If you are pitching to television, make sure you can provide good visuals, an interesting setting, and people who will appear on air to tell their stories. National television newsmagazine shows specialize in what Lawrence K. Grossman, former president of NBC News and PBS, calls "nonfiction entertainment," and thus require drama or even melodrama.

If you are seeking attention for new research or for your participation in a health care campaign, don't make the mistake of thinking that a journalist will read your release just because it is on your Web site. Some journalists may check your Web site for news. But nursing organizations and institutions can't assume that journalists will routinely monitor them, as they do the sites of some medical associations. Even journalists who pay attention to nursing advise nursing groups not to use materials posted on their Web sites as substitutes for assertive outreach to journalists.

"I go immediately to the *New York Times* homepage on the Internet each day," Madge Kaplan, senior health desk editor for the public radio program "Marketplace," says describing her routine. "I check a number of sites either daily or weekly. But no journalist can monitor all the Web sites they have bookmarked, nor can they afford the time to search the Web for interesting health news. I have 35 nursing sites bookmarked. If I devoted time each day to those sites—plus all the other health care sites—I would spend my whole day scouring the Web."

Kaplan and other journalists depend on organizations to send them e-mail alerts advising them of breaking, interesting or significant stories. "I receive e-mail alerts from *JAMA* and the AMA and from a lot of other health care sources, but almost none from nursing organizations," Kaplan says. "I don't want to be swamped with e-mails, but an alert signals something you may need to know about. It's a good device since most journalists can't resist glancing at their e-mails."

Journalists can be directed to a well-designed, substantive Web site. An infrequently updated Web page, though, with little newsworthy material, won't be useful for media coverage.

Phone Calls

When you send a letter containing the elements of a news release, or a conventional news release, follow up with a phone call. You can't be sure the reporter has read his or her mail, paid attention to the specific piece or even received it. That phone conversation will allow you to elaborate on the initial communication, or present it if the release hasn't been read or has gotten lost. Don't call to ask if the reporter received it. Use the opportunity to sell the story.

If you've made phone contact with the reporter before sending the release or letter, it is wise to have a written version before you so that you can make your points without getting flustered.

Getting through to a reporter is not always easy. Many news organizations have voice mail systems that act as fortresses. Try to get the direct extension for the person you want to reach. You may encounter difficulty in getting a person on the phone. But keep trying.

Just as patients need advocates in the hospital, nurses need advocates in media institutions as the following story illustrates.

A freelancer who writes for major media outlets received a press release and a follow-up phone call about a nursing program at a hospital she had written about in the past. Intrigued by the program, she called an editor at the city newspaper offering to do a story on the program. The editor confessed she had received the same press release, but because she didn't know much about nursing, the release went into the waste paper basket. She did, however, respond to the call from a journalist she trusted, and assigned her to do the story.

Arranging Meetings with Editorial Boards

One of the best ways of establishing relationships and stimulating interest in nursing stories is to meet with the editorial board of a newspaper. Editorial boards—the people who write the editorials and the section editor—schedule frequent meetings with experts and community members to discuss current issues. Sometimes the reporters who cover the subject participate in the meeting as well.

"For coverage of the news, we depend on our reporters. But in terms of argument on public policy, we depend on advocates to present all sides of an issue," says Judy Dugan, assistant editorial page editor of the *Los Angeles Times*. "When we hear the arguments and nuances of the debate, we are more able to form a solid public policy position. The lifeblood of editorial pages consists of frequent meetings with advocates."

Dugan says that those involved in the issues usually call the editorial board. "If advocates have an issue that's on the front burner—or that should be on the front burner—we want to talk to them. PR operators all know this and know how to arrange meetings. We try hard to get non-profits and people who don't realize they can come and talk to us to come forward.

"But don't call just to come in and say, 'Howdy,'" she advises. "Be prepared to discuss your issue in depth and to respond to hard questions."

Not every call you make to an editorial board will produce a meeting, and not every meeting will produce favorable editorials.

For example, in 1999, when the California Nurses Association was fighting for new legislation to establish safe nurse-to-patient staff ratios, they met with editorial page editors and writers at all the major California newspapers. As a result, several newspapers ran editorials supporting safe staffing legislation.

The California Nurses Association wanted the *Los Angeles Times*, the biggest newspaper in the state, to come out for the staffing bill while it was being debated in the state legislature. But the *Times* didn't run an editorial at all on this subject. The op-ed page, however, published a piece by a nurse from Massachusetts on what nurses and patients confront in understaffed hospitals throughout the US. Thus, the point was made, and the op-ed was distributed to other news organizations on the *L.A. Times* wire. Later, when it looked like California governor Gray Davis would veto the bill if it passed the legislature, the *L.A. Times* ran an editorial sympathetic to mandated staffing minimums.[6] Davis, in fact, signed the bill into law.

If a newspaper has provided good coverage of your issue, by all means compliment them during an editorial board meeting. Poor coverage or no coverage at all, however, can be the reason for arranging a meeting with the editorial board of a newspaper or with producers at a television or radio station.

One such meeting more than a decade ago helped attract attention to nursing at the *Boston Globe*. Under the aegis of the Nurses of America campaign, four nurses—Claire Fagin, then dean of the University of Pennsylvania school of nursing and president-elect of the National League for Nursing (NLN); Pamela Maraldo, then executive director of the NLN; Joyce Clifford, then nurse-in-chief of Boston's Beth Israel Hospital; and Nancy Valentine, then vice-president for nursing of McLean Hospital—arranged a meeting with *Boston Globe* editors and reporters. They were concerned about the *Globe*'s failure to depict accurately the crucial roles nurses play in health care. They talked about what nurses do and suggested avenues for coverage. The journalists challenged the nurses to explain why nursing was newsworthy, and the nurses told them.

As the nurses spoke, one editor recalled that he had been hospitalized when he was a teenager. Like many people, he had had a positive experience being cared for by nurses, but had no broader conceptual framework about nursing. But when he told his story about his nursing care, it was, Fagin recalls, "like a light going on. The tenor of the meeting immediately improved."

That meeting and continuing overtures from the public relations professionals at the Beth Israel Hospital, the Massachusetts Nurses Association and others, helped to establish a relationship between nurses and the paper. The *Boston Globe* became more inclusive of nursing in its health care coverage and now covers nursing more seriously than most newspapers in the US.

"If more nurses reached out to editorial boards," Fagin says, "they'd be surprised at how responsive journalists can be. The only negative that can happen is that journalists might say no. But they also might say yes."

Inviting Reporters to Visit You

Another way you can forge relationships with the press is to invite journalists to your institution to look at a project or an example of innovative practice. You could invite them to seminars or meetings that illuminate current practice. Imagine that a hospital has just opened a palliative care unit in which nursing plays a prominent role. The nursing staff can work through the nursing department or through the hospital's public relation office to inform journalists about this development and show them how it works.

Invite a reporter to follow a nurse for a day. This could make an excellent television or radio report as well as a print story. In the early 1990s, Joyce Clifford and Antony Schwartz-Lloyd, the hospital's media director, launched Boston Beth Israel's Nurse-for-a-Day program. It encouraged journalists and others to spend a day with a particular staff nurse and even act as an assistant. Journalists used this experience to inform their coverage of health care.

To spotlight the newsworthiness of what nurses do, the Nurses of America campaign in 1990 invited newspaper reporters, magazine writers and editors, and television producers to a media luncheon in New York City at which three nurses in various areas of practice did presentations. Jane Brody, health columnist for the *New York Times*, was the moderator for the event and later wrote an article on nursing for her newspaper. A similar luncheon was organized in Philadelphia the next year.

There are many other opportunities to get the media to come to you. When hospital shows like *ER*, *Chicago Hope* or *Side Effects* burst out of the fevered imagination of a television writer, it is time to pick up the phone and invite reporters to see the real ERs, as the Emergency Nurses Association did.

You can also ask journalists to come to your group to describe how they work and what they need to cover nursing adequately. After Sigma Theta Tau released its report on the status of nursing coverage,[7] it scheduled seven regional meetings at which journalists spoke to nurses about how to improve "nursing's voice in the media." According to Nancy Dickenson-Hazard, Sigma's executive officer, journalists explained how they work, the stresses they are under, and what they consider to be news. Nurses told the press "about the uniqueness and diversity of nursing," Dickenson-Hazard said. Journalists and nurses discussed ways to change coverage.

Other organizations have invited journalists to meetings and conferences to talk about coverage of nursing. The American Academy of Nursing asked radio editor Madge Kaplan to speak at one of its meetings. The University of Pennsylvania featured a *Philadelphia Inquirer* reporter at a conference it sponsored for nurse executives.

Presentations to Journalists

Nurses can do presentations to journalists about nursing issues in settings other than editorial boardrooms. They can ask to appear at chapter meetings of journalistic associations such as the American Medical Writers Association. There are networks of journalists that cover health and aging. Ask journalists you know about these and see if nurses can make a presentation either at a meeting or through an on-line listserve.

Journalism school courses on health and science writing welcome guest experts who can tell them what is new in these areas. It's a safe bet that few ever invite nurses, but you can ask to visit. Nurse researchers should definitely alert such classes and conferences to their important work. Nurses can even write articles for publications for journalists telling them what they need to know to cover nursing. This is exactly what Bernice Buresh and Nurse Jean Chaisson did in articles for *Nieman Reports*, a quarterly publication for journalists published by the Nieman Foundation at Harvard University.[8,9]

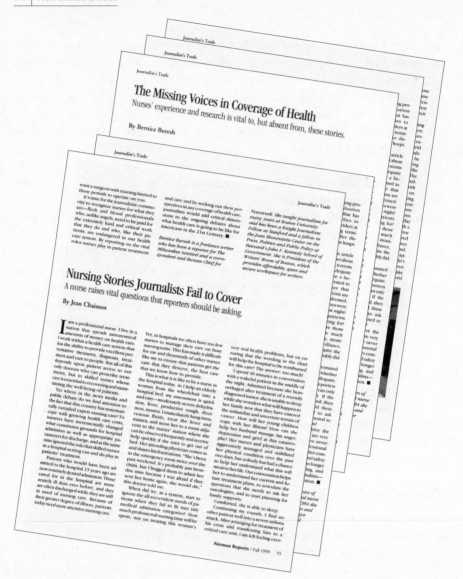

Organizational Meetings as a Form of Outreach

Professional meetings and conventions can be outreach tools by providing a focus for coverage. However, don't expect journalists to pay registration fees. They are there as observers not participants; their fees should, therefore, be waived.

One reason journalists will come to your conference is to cover a speech by a prominent person. The simple appearance of a celebrity speaker, however, will not be enough to draw attention. The speaker will have to talk about newsworthy issues.

If a political candidate is using a conference to advocate a policy change, for example, the media may come, particularly if the speaker holds or is running for high political office. The appearance of entertainers or celebrities known for their social advocacy may also draw coverage if they are speaking about an issue or event that is in the news. Unless your conference is showcasing original research or presenting new information, reporters won't treat your organizational meeting as anything other than a setting for the appearance of celebrity keynoters. They will cover the speech and leave. Only if you make the link between the keynote and the experiences or research of your members, will a reporter remain to talk with other participants. If that link is made, they may interview people at the conference about their views. Your conference may then be the launching point for continued coverage of these issues (see the Hawaii Nurses Association example in chapter seven).

Speakers can help you significantly with outreach to the public if they do more than use your organization to advance their platform or popularity. All too often organizations provide a platform for prominent speakers without asking anything in return. If speakers are well briefed in advance, they can refer to problems in the delivery of nursing/patient care, practice innovations and important policy proposals that will improve patient care or health care delivery. This will help direct coverage to your organization and concerns, not just to the speakers' agenda.

This is, however, a delicate negotiation. Speakers will not respond well if they believe you're trying to write their speeches. On the other hand, speakers like to appear to be knowledgeable about the group they're addressing. So when you're preparing speakers or their representatives, brief them on the critical issues and suggest certain points or research they could highlight that would make the audience more receptive and responsive. Unless the speaker specifically requests such help, it's not a good idea to present speakers with "talking points" or written material that they should insert into their remarks. However, speakers may be grateful if you provide them with background information and the talking points "we give to our members."

If a reporter, producer or editor, or politician or health policy expert—or any other prominent individual—is speaking at your conference, woo them to your cause. Invite them to a luncheon or reception following their presentation. If they are staying overnight—which is often the case—invite them to dinner. Ask a select group of your members to meet with the speaker. This group might include researchers on health policy or nursing practice, nurses who give direct care, or managers, academics or administrators who can explain what nurses do and why their work is important.

Prominent keynoters or panelists may decline your invitation. They may be too tired or too busy to attend such a gathering, or they may have other plans. But often they will be delighted to have the opportunity to converse with members of your organization. The point is, give them the opportunity to say yes, and give yourselves the opportunity to take advantage of yet another educational opening.

News Conferences

Because people see news conferences so often on television, they may think that the news conference is the first choice for disseminating information. In reality, it is the last. It is another device that has been so abused by publicity-seeking people or organizations that journalists tend to be wary of them. A full-blown news conference requires a great deal of labor-intensive organizing and should be used only for carefully defined purposes.

A news conference would be warranted, for example, if several nursing organizations in the US or Canada formed a coalition to fight for national safe staffing standards. They could use a news conference to present the various issues involved from the point of view of nurses and patients. Pre-conference organizing would include the preparation of media kits, rehearsing the speakers' presentations, checking audio-visual equipment, and doing extensive outreach to encourage journalists to attend.

A press briefing, on the other hand, can be an efficient way to update journalists. Hospitals often hold news briefings on their premises to keep journalists informed about the condition and treatment of a government official, a movie star, or some other highly visible personage. They use the same forum to update reporters when many people are injured in a massive accident or when an extremely unusual or experimental procedure, such as the separation of conjoined twins, occurs.

An impromptu press briefing can be held at the site of an action. A few nurses, for example, could be pulled aside to talk to journalists covering their demonstration or strike.

Broadening the Story's Impact

The news media are interested in stories that may represent a trend. A trend—something that is occurring in more than one place—has currency because it affects a lot of people. Newsmagazines, because they circulate nationally and internationally, seem to specialize in trends, particularly those that have major economic, cultural or political impact. National publications and TV news organizations cover trends by having their bureaus contribute information on what is going on in various geographical areas. Correspondents look for particular and dramatic examples to illustrate the phenomenon. The illustrating example requires spokespeople who are willing to talk as well as occasional appealing visual elements.

To convince a reporter that you have a good story, you might want to brief her on how the program/event/phenomenon is happening elsewhere and thus is part of a national or international trend. Good nursing trend stories will be unrealized if organizations and institutions promote only what is going on within their walls or among their members. Being unique may work in some instances, but backfire when a broader appeal is called for.

For example, a nursing department, eager to promote an experiment that allows family members to be present when a loved one is undergoing intense and invasive emergency treatment, may resist telling the media that this program is being tried at another hospital in the same city or in other facilities around the country. Similarly, a nursing union on strike in one area may want to talk only about the local issues involved. But the story could gain an appeal it would not otherwise have if it is presented as part of a trend. If journalists know that nurses all over the world—in Ireland, Poland, Canada, and the US—are striking over similar issues, they might be more attracted to writing about a strike in a local area.

Pitch Your Story in a Variety of Ways

When you're trying to get media attention, be aware that there are many ways of presenting a set of facts, a program, an activity, or event. When talking about a potential story, an editor will ask a reporter, "What's the angle?" The editor is not seeking just a set of facts. She wants the reporter to explain why the story is appealing enough to displace other competitors for time on the nightly news or space in the morning paper.

To convince his editor, the journalist will have to come up with an angle that indicates clear news value. Because many stories are multi-faceted, you must also consider which angles to highlight when you are trying to attract coverage.

Consider the latest nursing shortage. It was just beginning to surface as a story in 1999. The *New York Times* and other newspapers got into the subject by concentrating on the aging-of-the-nursing-workforce angle. Others, such as the Canadian magazine, *Elm Street*, and the *Boston Globe* Focus Section, ran pieces suggesting that the mistreatment that is driving nurses into more militant actions does not portend well for the future of the profession. But there are other angles to the story.

First and foremost, it is a public health story and should be pitched as an invisible public health crisis. The message is simple: Without nurses, hospitals—which are, after all, nursing institutions—will not be able to provide patient care. Credence was given to this point in the winter of 1999–2000 when hospital closings and reduced nursing staffs left US and Canadian hospitals in flu-ravaged cities unable to provide needed patient care.

The nursing shortage also has a women's angle. Nursing is the largest female profession. Writers and editors who cover women's issues, or who are sensitive to gender, may be attracted to a subject that concerns millions of women as health care professionals and patients. Women are the people most often pressed into service to provide care to sick family members in the hospital and the home when professional nurses are not available.

The nursing shortage also provides fodder for business coverage. Nurses can point out that a chain of undesirable business and economic consequences are attached to this issue. Some hospitals will try to raid nursing staffs elsewhere by throwing monetary incentives at nurses with expertise in certain areas. They and others may also try to compensate by hiring more unlicensed aides to fill RN vacancies. Many hospitals will increase their demands for mandatory overtime. Nursing organizations and unions will protest. Stopgap responses to a shortage of nurses will lay the groundwork for labor unrest and perhaps nursing strikes. With conditions deteriorating and nurses being poorly treated, more of them will leave the profession thus exacerbating the problem. This is a realistic scenario that nurses should spell out for journalists.

The nursing shortage also has an educational and policy component that must be brought to the attention of reporters who cover those areas. It is a serious matter when policy makers may try to circumvent university education, as they did in Quebec and Saskatchewan, to speed up the production of nurses. Although lip service is constantly paid to the extensive education and training required for contemporary nursing, efforts to produce nurses more quickly and cheaply undercut quality patient care. The gender and educational angles mingle nicely in this story, as Suzanne Gordon's op-ed on nursing education in Quebec (see chapter nine) demonstrated.

Journalists should be encouraged to compare how physician population fluxes are handled. No one would dare implement policies that shave a couple of years off medical training so that doctors can enter the workforce more quickly. The supply of doctors is manipulated by regulating how many people are accepted and graduated from medical school, not by reducing the time they spend there or by reconfiguring their curriculum.

Keeping a Story Going

In some cases, a major goal will be to get one good story on your program or practice. It could mean more visibility for nursing and the beginning of a journalistic relationship you may be able to return to at another time. If, however, you are working on an on-going issue, one good story does not mean it is time to sit back and relax. It means it is time for more action so that the story does not fade from the news.

Stories can have either a long and robust life span, or they can suffer sudden cardiac arrest and die. For stories to remain vital, they must be fed with "new" material and activity.

You need a plan to create new developments and take advantage of those that come along. Start a pipeline to journalists with new studies, surveys and reports on your issue. Engage in research or analysis yourself and issue reports. Participate in forums organized by allies. Testify at hearings and distribute written copies of your testimony to journalists. Even if you are not called upon to testify, you can bring your own documentation to the hearing and distribute it to the press corps. You can use other people's testimony in your reports and analyses as well. Plan "media events" around the issue.

These are the kinds of things that people involved in the nursing home reform movement do to keep the story alive. Among many others, nursing researchers Charlene Harrington and Jeannie Kaiser Jones at the University of California, San Francisco, regard public education as crucial to improving nursing home care, given the industry's reluctance to provide adequate resources. As authorities on the subject, they help to keep these issues public by providing expert testimony at all kinds of legislative and government hearings, by continuing their research into pertinent areas, and by making sure their findings are widely disseminated to groups that can use them in their push for nursing home improvement. The Service Employees International Union (SEIU), senior citizens groups, and consumer activists have all used these research studies as they worked for reform.

Negative Coverage

Having an active relationship with the news media not only increases the chances of favorable coverage, it is an asset when stories come along that are not kind to nursing.

In recent years there have been a number of stories that questioned the qualifications of nurses. One was an ABC-TV "Day One" program on anesthesiologist fraud broadcast in January 1995.

The program was focused on anesthesiologists "who violate Medicare laws and their own professional rules, who supervise many more operations than they are permitted, are not present at critical moments during surgery, and even fraudulently bill for services they never provide." These renegade anesthesiologists—greedy, incompetent and negligent as they may be—were not shown to be injuring and killing patients directly. That sort of thing occurred, the program asserted, when the anesthesiologist was out of the room and the patient was under the care of a nurse anesthetist, also referred to in the program as an "assistant."

The report had a subtext that has often plagued nursing: Although there are individual physicians not worthy of the title, physicians as a class provide safe medical care when they are present. Nurses, on the other hand, are not competent either as individuals or as a profession to deal with patients without close physician supervision.

The program cited four cases in which severe patient injury or death was attributed to the lack of an anesthesiologist in the operating room. The most bizarre involved a nurse anesthetist who, left to her own devices, warmed a bag of blood in a microwave oven. The patient who received the blood died.

Bad press like this understandably terrifies many nurses. They may think that if this is what they are going to get in the media, no coverage at all is preferable. There are things you can do, however, to avoid or soften bad coverage and to respond if it does occur.

1.   Anticipate. When you hear that a story is being developed on an area of nursing that concerns you, contacting the producer or the reporter and offering to provide pertinent information will usually serve your interests better than waiting to see what will happen. You can anticipate that difficult questions about nursing might be raised. Journalists have a legitimate interest in probing incidences of patient suffering, medical errors, fraud, denial of treatment, and withdrawal of care. Their job is to expose flaws in the system and to question the way things are done. In today's world, every profession has to justify its existence. Conflicts and competition among health care professions can be intense and may color news stories. Nurses must plan to use the media effectively to communicate how and why their work is beneficial to the public health.

If it appears that the story will present nursing negatively, try to find out what the issues are and try to help the reporter understand their complexities. Many, if not most, reporters who do serious coverage want to be accurate. They might be influenced in their approach if they are made aware of aspects they didn't know about.

If a producer or reporter is insistent upon forcing the story in a direction that makes you very nervous and refuses to listen to you, you don't have to deal with him. But you should weigh this carefully. Opting out of a game you fear you can't control might not get a better result.

The American Association of Nurse Anesthetists (AANA) was confronted with this sort of choice when it learned what "Day One" had in the works.[10] The organization's board decided not to provide on-camera interviews out of concern that cooperating with a report implying widespread anesthesiologist fraud would be detrimental to certified registered nurse anesthetists (CRNAs). As a courtesy, the AANA notified the American Society of Anesthesiologists of its decision.

Later, however, when the AANA thought the program's focus had changed, it sought to put nurse anesthetists on camera as patients' advocates, but producers resisted the overture.

"Day One" found nurse anesthetists on its own. It interviewed two in shadows to hide their identities. These nurse anesthetists said that to make more money, anesthesiologists regularly violate practice regulations and that nurse anesthetists cover up for them. The program also had no trouble finding a credentialed physician to slam the whole nursing specialty. Dr. Wilson Wilhite, the past president of the American Society of Anesthesiologists, the organization that the AANA treated so courteously, implied, on the air, that medically directed anesthesiology delivered by nurse anesthetists is dangerous.

Nurses can anticipate that things are going to get tough in this sort of situation, and that doctor groups under attack are not going to treat them with kid gloves. They may even make nurses the scapegoat. Knowing that you cannot possibly control the content of such a television program relieves you from trying to do the impossible. Then you are free to try to have at least some influence.

2. Act. It is impossible to duck scrutiny. If nurses are to have professional credibility and access to the media when they need it, they have to get involved and stay involved.

By doing interviews and taking a tough stance with the "Day One" producers, AANA might have been able to cast nurse anesthetists in a better light. Maybe it would have made no difference. But the overriding urge that nurses sometimes exhibit to protect the welfare and reputation of another profession can limit nurses from acting on their own behalf. Other professions are capable of looking out for their own welfare. When nurses act in their own interest, it does not mean they are being disrespectful of others.

Acknowledging a problem within the profession does not invalidate nursing. Not every nurse is a great nurse; not every nurse gives high quality care, but of what profession is that not true? Unless you are willing to admit this fact, it is very hard to defend nursing. Indeed, rather than defending nursing or a nursing specialty in the abstract, concretely describe the problems nursing has delivering quality care in the context of the issues being probed. If the subject involves practices that jeopardize patients, this can be an opportunity for nurses to advocate for patients and come out against practices not under their control.

3. React and respond. Don't get tempted into thinking that a strong response will merely fan the flames of criticism. Don't believe for a moment that if you are quiet, it will all blow over. Media reports are powerful because they can leave a lasting impression.

Although AANA limited its ability to shape the story, it did respond assertively. Before "Day One" aired, the AANA sent its members survey forms for recording their responses to the program. They included fact sheets on CRNAs and anesthesia to help nurse anesthetists answer questions from patients or others in their workplace. This groundwork produced a virtuoso response.

Nurse anesthetists were outraged by the show and refused to let it stand. The day after it aired, Mary DePaolis-Lutzo, president of the American Association of Nurse Anesthetists, sent a letter to the president of ABC, other network executives, principals on "Day One," and managers of ABC-owned stations stating that the program had misled the public and unfairly attacked nurse anesthetists. Accompanying the letter was a six-page point-by-point rebuttal to 19 distortions she said occurred in the report. She strongly refuted the assertion that "patients' lives are at risk" if an anesthesiologist isn't in the room by pointing out that Certified Registered Nurse Anesthetists (CRNAs) administer more than 65 percent of the 26 million anesthetics given to patients in the US each year. She explained that CNRAs are permitted to practice in every state, and that "they work with surgeons independently of an anesthesiologist, or collaboratively with anesthesiologists."

DePaolis-Lutzo put a message on the AANA's president's hotline advising callers where to send protests. Some 2,000 persons called ABC and 1,500 of those who wrote letters sent copies to the AANA.

Two weeks later, "Day One" acknowledged the "huge response" to the program. For the first time in its history, it quoted on air letters it had received.

Nurses must respond to serious inaccuracies and misinformation. This means talking to and writing to journalists, editors and producers. It may mean taking out advertisements.

In the end, even a negative report can help organizations discern what issues they need to address publicly. It can be an opportunity to go forward with new communication activities that will benefit both the public and nursing.

Establishing the Rules of the Game

People inexperienced in dealing with the media may fear they will be at the mercy of reporters. Of course you cannot control everything, but you should expect an honest working relationship with reporters. You should inquire about what information is being sought, why it is being asked for and how it will be used. You should do all you can to assure accuracy and clarity. But don't ask for or expect to see an advance copy of the story.

The late Edward L. Bernays, who was a legend in the public relations field, said he always told his clients that there was only one rule in talking with reporters: "If you don't want it printed, don't say it." Always assume that you are speaking on the record to a journalist even if the conversation has an informal tone. Journalists are in the business of conveying information, not in keeping it to themselves. It is in nurses' interest to speak clearly and directly about their work and not shrink from that role.

If, however, there is an instance when you do not want your name or information that you give used, you must make that agreement up front, not after the fact. Here are some ways in which reporters temper information.

- **Not for attribution**: There may be times when you want a journalist to report on something that has happened, but you fear the personal consequences if it is attributed to you. You can work out an agreement with a reporter that the facts can be used but not attributed to you by name. You should discuss with the reporter how general the attribution should be, such as "a clinical nurse specialist in oncology said Tuesday," or "a nurse at the hospital said Tuesday." The more sources a reporter has who can confirm and expand on the information, the more you are off the hook.

- **Off the record**: Contrary to what you see in the movies, these agreements are very rare. "Off the record" really means that neither the information nor the source can be used. A person might seek this agreement if he or she was the only person who could have possibly been the leak for something that was explosive or possibly criminal. By making an off-the-record agreement, the journalist is saying that he or she will not use the information unless it can be found from another source without identifying the original source.

To take advantage of the media opportunities that occur and craft strategies that will amplify nurses' voices it makes sense to work with public relations professionals. How they work and how to work with them is the subject of the next chapter.

Endnotes

1. T. Hunt and J.E. Grunig, *Public Relations Techniques* (Fort Worth: Harcourt Brace College Publishers, 1994).

2. B. Buresh, *Profile of Gerri Frager, MD, RN* (Project on Death in America media packet, 1999).

3. L. Morton, "Researcher Finds Complaints against Press Releases are Justified," *Editor & Publisher*, 8 May 1993: pp. 52, 42.

4. B. Buresh, "Extra! Healthcare Forms New Media Partnership—Nursing Must Participate," *Revolution: The Journal of Nurse Empowerment,* 1998 (spring): pp. 68–75.

5. W. Strunk, Jr. *et al., The Elements of Style* (Allyn & Bacon, 1999).

6. Editorial, "HMO Reform Far From Done," *Los Angeles Times,* 8 September 1999: Editorial Page.

7. *The Woodhull Study on Nursing and the Media: Health Care's Invisible Partner* (Sigma Theta Tau International, 1998).

8. B. Buresh, "The Missing Voices in Coverage of Health." *Nieman Reports,* 1999 (fall): pp. 52–55.

9. J. Chaisson, "Nursing Stories Journalists Fail to Cover," *Nieman Reports,* 1999 (fall): pp. 55–56.

10. B. Buresh and S. Gordon, "Fighting Scapegoat Journalism," *American Journal of Nursing,* July 1995.

Chapter 7

WORKING WITH
PUBLIC RELATIONS
PROFESSIONALS

As nurses seek to expand their relationships with the public, they can be greatly assisted by public relations experts. Public relations often refers to planned or managed communication with the public. Public relations is not an end in itself, but a means to achieving important goals. This chapter describes what public relations professionals do and how they approach their work with nurses.

While effective public communication depends upon the participation of large numbers of individual nurses, it is unrealistic to expect nurses to know all the ins and outs of media work. Nurses go to nursing school to learn how to be nurses not public relations or media specialists. Yet, sometimes nurses who are inexperienced with PR find themselves talking solely with other nurses about how to devise media strategies for their organizations or media research projects for their nursing schools.

Just because the media are familiar, it doesn't mean that the process of working with the media is self-evident. The better part of wisdom is knowing when outside help is needed. If nurses don't get expert communication assistance when they need it, they risk spinning their wheels on fruitless activity and growing demoralized when results are lacking. This may discourage them from engaging in more productive activities in the future.

Public relations experts have a lot to offer nurses.

"One reason to hire a public relations specialist is to get someone who is not inundated in your reality but is sensitive to the issue," says Scott Foster, a communication consultant who has worked with the Hawaii Nurses Association. "A little bit of distance may be needed to shape the information and focus it."

PR experts can help nurses develop a media strategy and enlist allies to achieve certain goals. "I don't operate in a vacuum," Foster explains. "When I work with a group, I bring in other people—say political consultants—who can provide an important perspective and important contacts."

Many of the problems that nursing groups face are more political than they are technical. Therefore, it is essential that nurses find public relations consultants or political organizers who are well-versed in public outreach and grassroots organizing. "Instead of hiring a traditional adman or PR hack, nurses usually will be better off finding a PR person who is experienced in community activism and coalition building and who will do it from a nursing perspective," says David Schildmeier, communication director for the Massachusetts Nurses Association (MNA).

Not only should a PR person know how to reach the mainstream media, she should be able to access patient groups, other health care workers, unions, doctors, other clinicians, consumer advocacy and patient groups, and seniors, among others.

When it comes to nursing, one of the most important things a PR person can do is encourage nurses to end their silence and talk about their practice. A good PR person will help nurses feel comfortable doing this by showing them how to shape information and talk about their work in a way that captures public attention.

An effective public relations professional will be well versed in the mores and culture of the group or individuals he is working with and will know what obstacles come with their territory.

For example, gaining access to the media is usually much easier in a small or medium-sized city than it is in a Toronto, Chicago or New York where there is heavy competition for media attention. Nurses in smaller communities might find little difficulty in placing a story on something they are doing. For them, however, an inhibiting factor might be "what people will say" if nurses are doing something unconventional or "stepping out of character" by pursuing a more visible and feisty role. If nurses, for example, suddenly decide to wage a campaign over hospital staffing, they may fear that they will lose whatever public support they have won in the past by adhering to more "professional" or caring behaviors. A skilled PR professional can help nurses weigh these concerns and work them through.

In a big city, nurses might be quite assertive and still not capture media interest. The challenge in an overheated media market may be to determine the right moment to take on a particular issue, what tactics to use and whom to contact. A good PR person can make all this easier.

A public relations specialist should have access to the latest information and studies in the field. She should make these materials reader friendly and available to nurses so that they can prepare themselves for discussions with journalists and legislators. A PR staff member should bolster nurses' communication efforts and save them time and energy by disseminating relevant materials to journalists.

Most PR specialists can help nurses craft letters to the editor and op-ed essays. If the news demands a nursing response, a PR person may want to generate an outpouring of letters from nurses by sending an alert through communication channels established for this purpose. Some issues might require op-eds or letters from nurses with specific expertise. The PR person should be able to contact just the right nurse and, if needed, help her construct her argument. When an organization is waging a campaign, the PR person will work with members to produce communication materials such as news releases, slogans, banners, posters, videos, advertisements, and media kits.

Expert public relations practitioners not only shape information, they know to whom to take it. They must know the phone and fax numbers and e-mail and snail mail addresses of journalists and have good working relationships with many of them. The PR person cannot guarantee that the story he pitches will be picked up, but in most instances, he should be at least well enough established with key media outlets to get his phone calls returned. That's because a good PR person, as Foster says, will have established credibility with journalists who recognize that he is, in turn, bringing them credible clients and information.

In nursing, the job isn't only to convince journalists to talk to nurses, it is to convince nurses to talk to journalists. PR experts will have to encourage nurses to take first steps—and then giant leaps—forward. They may have to conduct media training sessions with leaders and members of the group, and do a lot of handholding to help nurses negotiate this new public arena.

If you want to promote a particular issue or program, and you do not have in-house expertise, you can get it from the outside. Many PR professionals will work on a consultancy basis to help you develop a communication strategy or help you publicize a particular project.

If your group has little or no budget for PR, you may be able to get help from public relations students in schools or departments of communication in colleges and universities. There are student groups that take on non-profit organizations as "clients." Some public relations and advertising firms do *pro bono* work. National and international organizations of PR specialists— like the Public Relations Society of America—will send speakers to advise you on how to set up a PR program.

When you work with public relations specialists who have little or no knowledge of nursing, you must be clear about what you want to convey. These people, like so many others in our culture, may harbor misperceptions about nursing that could lead you in the wrong direction. It is up to you to instruct them even as they instruct you.

Do not go along with a plan that can sabotage the strengths of nursing, diminish nursing practice, or imply that one group of nurses is superior to another.

"Internal" and "External" Communications

On the surface, nursing seems to be awash in public communication specialists. Many nursing organizations, nursing schools, and hospitals and other health care institutions have PR specialists working for them. Therefore, some nurses might find it mysterious that nursing still ranks as the least visible health care profession. The mystery can be solved, however, by looking at what many of these PR practitioners are actually assigned to do.

A major goal of any organization is to serve and retain its members and to recruit more. Most nursing organizations expect their PR people to do more "internal" than "external" communication. In other words, their primary mission is to communicate with members, and enhance the image of the organization with members as well as with others in the profession.

In a nursing school, for example, a communication specialist might spend most of her time putting out promotional materials for prospective students and alumni and promoting the nursing school *within* the university. Or, in a subspecialty organization, a PR staffer might put out an organizational newsletter, supervise the publication of clinical journals and books, and help plan annual conventions. She might hire speech and media trainers to teach officers how to make speeches, do interviews with journalists, and appear on television and radio. She might even invite journalists to speak about the how-tos of health care coverage—with a focus on nursing coverage, or the lack of it—at nursing meetings or conventions.

While internal communication activities are critical to organizational functioning and survival and may improve the communication skills of nurses, they are not the same as a viable "external" communication strategy. Internal communication activities do not get nursing into the news, nor do they necessarily raise the public profile of the profession, even though they are both equally critical to nursing and organizational viability.

"If people don't see nurses playing important roles, then the public and policy makers don't really give nursing what it is due in terms of money and a significant place at the policy table," says Dan Mezibov, director of public affairs for the American Association of Colleges of Nursing. "As a result, nursing research doesn't get funded to the level needed. This affects nursing school budgets and the number of faculty that can be hired, which in turn affects the number of nursing students, which then affects the future availability of nurses."

This calculus is pertinent to every nursing organization. However, the reality is that the vast majority of nursing organizations, subspecialty groups and professional associations do very little "external" communication. One unintended consequence of *not* having an external communication plan is that it reinforces the silence of nurses. When nurses don't see members of their profession in the news, they might conclude that the media simply aren't interested in their stories and that nothing can be done to change that.

That's why it is important for members to inquire about their organization's definition of its public relations mission. What are its stated public relations goals? What are its major priorities? What are staff members doing to advance stated goals? What will it take to achieve them? How long will it take? What resources will be needed?

If your organization has PR people on staff, they should be taking an active role in promoting nursing beyond the organization and the profession. Members can push their organizations to create, fund and implement an explicit external communications program.

Making Your Workplace Work for You

It's critical for nurses to address how the PR staff in their institutions work—or do not work—for nursing. Many of the health care institutions in which nurses work do not promote nursing and won't unless nurses intervene.

The media officers who work for hospitals and medical centers usually do an excellent job of promoting doctors and medicine. If a journalist needs an expert to bring him up to speed on urinary incontinence, he can phone the media relations department at a medical center and ask them to arrange an interview with an expert on staff. Almost invariably—even if the subject is one in which nurses have particular expertise—that authority will be a physician. In pitching stories and responding to requests from journalists, PR people are practically on automatic pilot at the institutions where most nurses work. The flight instruction is: Find a doctor.

"Why is this?" we asked the director of public relations at a major medical center.

His analysis was that since the medical staff is considered the core of a hospital or medical center, the fortunes of the institution are viewed as being synonymous with those of the medical staff. The *raison d'être of* the public relations staff, then, is to promote the medical staff.

Whether they agree with this perspective or not, PR officers quickly get the message that doctors think anything interesting in their institution revolves around them. The PR representatives are also influenced by the attitudes that some physicians have about nurses. "Because medicine is a 'male' field," this public relations expert asserts, "doctors don't like nurses who see themselves as being equal to doctors and, worse, who can go about proving it."

The physician pecking order also leads to disputes among doctors. "Surgeons complain if there's a story about dermatologists," he explains. "So if it's this bad between medical disciplines, it's even worse if you pay attention to other areas that doctors regard as marginal. If PR people get a reputation for promoting what doctors consider to be frivolous—meaning stories that aren't about 'real' medicine—they lose physician support."

Without institutional support, communication specialists at medical centers and hospitals might be wary of promoting nursing even if they would like to. They might worry about how far they can go. A public relations officer at the Massachusetts General Hospital once told us she could help promote the nurses in the hospital by arranging interviews with a physician and nurse together for some stories.

We suggested that nurses were also capable of speaking to the press unescorted and sometimes know more than physicians about certain health problems. She was startled. "Oh, we could never promote that idea," she retorted.

The failure of PR staff to promote nursing creates a self-reinforcing cycle. Nursing doesn't appear in the media because the PR professionals don't send releases or pitch stories about nursing. They also don't educate journalists by talking with them about developments in nursing. With no one initiating the conversation, PR people don't get journalistic inquiries about nursing. They thus conclude that nursing won't "sell" because journalists aren't—and never will be—interested in nursing stories. Because nursing is not sold, they're convinced it's not salable, and therefore may discourage nurses who approach them with good stories.

The premise that nursing is not salable has certainly been tested and found wanting.

In the 1980s, the Beth Israel Hospital in Boston successfully placed a succession of stories on nursing in the local and national media. "It took five years to sell primary nursing, which Beth Israel was developing and implementing, but eventually we did it," says Antony Swartz-Lloyd, the former PR director of the hospital. According to Lloyd, Mitchell Rabkin and Joyce Clifford, then the hospital CEO and Nurse-in-Chief respectively, encouraged the PR staff to learn about nursing and promote it. This high-level administrative commitment gave the PR staff the resources and authority to go in a new direction, and shielded the staff from medical sniping. Time and again, through print and television stories, the BI proved that the nursing story is salable.

This is why, in spite of the difficulties, it's essential for nurses to try to work with their PR departments.

Just as relationships are key to patient care, they are critical to getting the PR staff to work for you. Get to know the PR people so that you can bring them up to date on what is going on in nursing. Suggest potential stories based on nursing activities and events that contain some of the news values outlined in chapter five.

Think about inviting a PR staff member to follow an RN for a day. Suggest that she invite journalists to do the same. Compile a list of nurses who are doing interesting work in the institution and ask the PR staff to pitch stories on them. Include a brief description of the relevance of their work to the public. Ask the PR staff to refer reporters to nursing sources for expert comment. Furnish a list of the appropriate names with areas of expertise and contact information.

If the PR staff insists that journalists want to talk only to doctors, persist. You can explain that you're not in competition with doctors or trying to displace them, but by giving visibility to nurses, the hospital raises its public profile. To buttress your case, collect news stories about nurses from elsewhere.

If the PR people remain cool, nurses have other avenues for getting their stories out. Let's say that the critical care nurses at a certain hospital develop a new protocol for working with cardiac patients, but the hospital doesn't pick up the ball by putting out news releases or talking with health care reporters about it. There is no need to let the story die. The nurses' professional organization or union can pitch it to the news media. The nurses involved can then speak to journalists as representatives of their professional organization or union.

Unions that represent nurses can and should do more to promote the professional work of their members. The PR professionals who work for nursing unions or collective bargaining associations are generally very experienced and active in external communication. They could expand their outreach beyond workplace conflicts by making the practice of their members visible.

No matter where you work or what organization you belong to, public relations outreach about nursing should be central to its mission and activities. PR people who understand how to communicate to external audiences will institutionalize outreach activities and make them part of the organization's standard operating procedures.

There are many books that will teach you how to pick a good public relations staffer or consultant. We offer some guidelines of our own.

- Choose someone who understands nursing or is willing to learn about nursing.
- Pick someone who respects the core of nursing and is not trying to turn nurses into something they consider more respectable or legitimate. A communication specialist who advises you to ditch the word nurse in "nurse practitioner," who wants to sell NPs as junior or cheaper doctors, who uses the term "medical news" when referring to nursing or broader health care news, or who views sick, vulnerable human beings as "customers" may not be a good candidate.
- Beware of specialists who suggest advertising slogans or communication that belittles or effaces, rather than builds upon, the profession's reputation for caring and compassion. Similarly, be wary of practitioners who downplay patient care to create what they believe to be a more "professional" image of nurses. Find a practitioner who can grasp that caring is highly skilled work.
- Be wary of someone who unknowingly reflects societal stereotypes of nursing.
- Make sure the candidate is willing to learn not only the facts about nursing and health care but also the nuances of nursing culture so that they can effectively work with nurses. No matter how highly paid, or how extensive his client list, a media-trainer who frames issues in sports and battle metaphors will probably fail to win the confidence of nurses or inspire them to speak out. Similarly, a media trainer who shows nurses videotapes of politicians who have ruined their campaigns with a mistaken response, will terrorize rather than embolden nurses.
- Hire someone who will respectfully make demands upon nurses by pushing them to be more assertive, more willing to speak, and more able to take on controversial issues.
- Hire a person who understands that promoting positive images of nursing and taking assertive stands on health care issues is as much political work as it is communication technique.
- Don't have unrealistic expectations of what a PR expert can do for you. In some cases, he or she may get you good press in the *New York Times* or *Globe and Mail*, but only if you give them newsworthy material and spokespeople who will talk to the press. He or she can talk *with* you but not *for* you and can make contacts that will *facilitate* your work but not be a *substitute* for it.

Public Relations Specialists Talk about Their Work

The following texts are from public relations specialists who work with nursing organizations.

1. Joan Meehan-Hurwitz is director of communications for the American Nurses Association, which has 180,000 members in its 53 constituent state and territorial associations.

The primary purpose of my job is to develop and maintain a positive, highly visible, public profile of the American Nurses Association and nursing in general to help achieve strategic goals and objectives. This "reputation management" function includes responsibility for internal and external communications as well as for special events and "crisis" communication.

Public opinion is critical in waging a political battle or winning a policy victory. Given increasing competition and unprecedented changes in health care—including who makes decisions about how a shrinking economic pie is divided—nursing must be aggressively promoted.

Interestingly, the current institutional devaluation of nursing has motivated nursing and individual nurses to articulate publicly the value of nursing. This makes my job as liaison between the ANA and the media, and between the media and nurses, easier. I always try to find the right match—who is the best spokesperson for this reporter on this issue at this moment. I have to deal with constant deadlines. That's why developing relationships is so critical. It's hard to be a good matchmaker if you don't know who you're fixing up.

Successful media relations are based on preparation, preparation, preparation. I brief spokespeople by providing talking points, sound bites and anecdotes. I review possible tough questions, and remind spokespeople of their rights in an interview. I constantly remind them to stay "on message" so the interview will be successful.

I'm thrilled to help a nurse frame a letter to the editor or write an op-ed. I am, conversely, dismayed when a nurse calls the ANA outraged about something in the media and demands that we "do something to fix it," yet resists my suggestion that he or she join the chorus and channel his or her energy into a personal letter.

I understand why some nurses are reluctant to do this. I believe nursing—like any group that historically has been oppressed or disenfranchised—must acknowledge how this legacy affects confidence and self-esteem. In my view, a fundamental building block for self-esteem is promotion that builds pride in nurses.

Nurses need a fundamental understanding of the relationship between politics and policy and practice, as well as how public opinion plays into this equation. This must be incorporated into nursing education to ensure that future generations of nurses understand that it is appropriate, professional and pragmatic to advocate for themselves and for their profession.

Once that foundation is laid, nurses must be groomed and organized to take on media relations work and to commit to building on-going relationships with reporters.

2.   Carole Presseault is manager of health policy for the Canadian Nurses Association, which has more than 110,000 members across Canada.

I don't view media relations as an end in itself. It's a means to an end. Having a front-page story is not a goal in itself. It is a means of influencing the public and decision-makers to see an issue from your perspective. For example, if you want government to act on recruitment of nurses, one strategy is to go public.

If we want to influence decision-makers, one way to do that is to influence public opinion, which means you need a media strategy. This is where a PR professional can help you. They can help you do the important work of framing stories. The PR expert is the middle person who helps translate issues in a way that highlights their public salience.

Creating press releases is only one thing a PR person does. I give workshops all the time and tell people that the outcome of this workshop is not just a press release. In any political action strategy, a news release is one tool among many. In fact, issuing a press release is a tactic that should be carefully weighed. The CNA once issued a press release that was very critical of a government decision. In this case, it would have been better to talk to the minister in question first. It's not always good to be publicly critical.

When you are looking for a public relations person, the motto should be "buyer beware." You need to interview candidates carefully. You need someone who understands your issues, but obviously, they don't know the issues as well as you do, so they should be willing to do background work on them. If someone is interested in having your group as a client, they should prepare a presentation that's pitched to your organizational needs and concerns.

Our staff has done some training in media relations, but we always like to get independent advice to validate what we know and to keep us current. When we are choosing PR help, we don't want to be dazzled by the bright lights. We prefer someone who is willing to find out more about us to someone who has a lot of big-name clients.

Media relations is not something you do overnight. It takes time and investment.

3. Anne Schott is director of communications for the New York State Nurses Association, which has more than 33,000 members, the majority of whom are in collective bargaining units.

In the early 1990s, pressure to cut costs began to squeeze the health care system in New York state. Managers concerned chiefly about their hospital's bottom line targeted the nursing staff for restructuring and layoffs. Many facilities outlined plans to use unlicensed assistive personnel (UAP) to "help" registered nurses deliver care. In theory, UAP were supposed to do only a limited number of simple tasks under the supervision of RNs.

In fact, hospitals attempted to expand the duties of UAP, and sometimes included tasks that were illegal under the state's Nurse Practice Act. Nurses who were already carrying heavy patient loads could not adequately supervise these minimally trained workers.

To make matters worse, in something of a stealth campaign, hospitals dressed UAP in white uniforms with identification badges that said "nursing department." It was almost impossible for a typical patient to recognize that these workers were not RNs.

The New York State Nurses Association (NYSNA) recognized that this inappropriate use of unlicensed workers was a danger to patients and a threat to the nursing profession. The public relations challenge was to alert the public to the danger and explain why it was important to receive skilled nursing care from a registered nurse.

To meet that challenge, NYSNA hired a New York City ad agency and launched a four-year advertising and public relations campaign that cost $2.5 million. It was built around the message, "Ask for a Real Nurse, Ask for an RN." The campaign used radio, TV, newspaper, and magazine ads as well as subway and bus posters to tell the public: "You have a right to know who's caring for you when you're in the hospital." The ads warned: "A lot of the people you think are nurses, may not be nurses at all."

Every ad carried a toll-free number people could call for more information. The first year, those who responded received a postcard advising them to ask a series of basic questions about their hospital care, such as, "Will I be cared for by a registered nurses? How often will I see my RN? How many patients will be assigned to the RN caring for me?"

In subsequent years, we expanded the information and sent callers a free hospital evaluation kit that explained why patients should ask for a real nurse.

It included a button patients could wear to the hospital that read: "Excuse me, are you a Real Nurse?" It also provided the telephone numbers of local hospitals so people could easily call and ask the questions. In the final year of the campaign, we sent out a "Consumer Guide to Being a Confident Patient," that included information on both home care and long-term care.

We received tens of thousands of calls and sent out more than 50,000 pieces of literature to patients and their families. Reporters began to call and ask, in disbelief, if the information in the ads was true. Hospital patients began to ask nurses who came to the bedside, "Are you a real nurse?"

The campaign generated many news stories and significantly raised public awareness of the issue. In many hospitals where we represented the nurses, plans to replace RNs with UAP were curtailed or scrapped. Perhaps the clearest evidence of success was an advertisement placed in the *New York Times* by a hospital that adopted our basic message at their expense. It read:

"Maybe She Just Looks like a Real Nurse. Don't assume your nurse is a real nurse unless you're at White Plains Hospital Center. Here, 92 percent of our nursing staff are Registered Nurses."

The unlicensed personnel issue has faded in New York. Now the key issue is short staffing, which we are addressing in labor negotiations and through legislative initiatives. Public relations supports both efforts by explaining to the public how short-staffing affects the quality of care patients receive.

Individual staff nurses play a key role here. We help them describe in simple, concrete language what happens when they are trying to take care of 15 seriously ill patients. We also help them deal with the kind of troubling questions reporters often ask, like, "Has anybody died as a result of short-staffing? Has any patient been maimed?"

Often a nurse's first impulse is to say, "Well, no."

We encourage the nurse to go further, to use the opportunity to educate the reporter. Nurses know that poor care isn't confined to those instances that result in tragedy. If a patient has gone without pain medication for six hours or is lying in urine or feces, that's unacceptable.

Nurses understand what patients need and how the current system often fails them. Fortunately, the media want to hear from nurses who are close to patients and who can provide the insight and anecdotes that make health care stories come alive. What nurses need is the confidence to speak from the heart about what they know. The real job of a public relations expert who works with nurses is to help them gain that confidence.

4. Dan Mezibov is the director of public affairs for the American Association of Colleges of Nursing (AACN).

Until about fifteen years ago, nurses were only talking to themselves. The culture of nursing is so other-oriented—do for the patient—that nursing has never paid enough attention to self-promotion. Nurses tend to think of self-promotion as being selfish. But there's nothing necessarily selfish about it. In fact, self-promotion is intimately tied to the health and well being of the profession.

Much of what I do goes beyond broadening the awareness of the general public and the news media about what nursing is and what nurses really do. A large part of my job is to help nurses themselves make sure that when they're talking to the news media, they get their message out and that nursing is given full credit for its achievements and its work.

At the AACN, an organization of more than 540 nursing schools that have bachelor's and graduate-degree programs, we do this in a number of ways. We hold media training sessions for our deans and for school PR officers. A minority of nursing schools have their own PR officer. Most schools, though, have a PR or communications officer who is assigned to the nursing school by the college or university press office. This can lead to tensions particularly if there is a school of medicine or a psychology department at the university. In that event, the nursing school will have to encourage the press officer to spend enough time to get to know and promote the nursing school. The medical school, or even a psychology department, often is seen by university press officers as the source of "more sexy" news material. In contrast, there isn't enough attention given to equally interesting and important news stories developing at the nursing school, which is why it's more effective for a school to have its own PR person.

However, if that's not possible, we suggest ways that the nursing school can work more actively with the university press office. There are simple things a school can do such as inviting the university press officer to attend nursing school staff meetings on a regular basis. That way when interesting developments are discussed, the PR officer may recognize their newsworthiness even if the dean or faculty does not.

We also try to teach them to think in unconventional ways when placing a story that's newsworthy. For example, one state university we worked with has a joint-degree program in nursing and law. They have similar tracks combining nursing with economics and management. They wanted to push the story but didn't know what kind of media to take it to. So I suggested they think of it not as a health care story, but view it as a workplace or business story

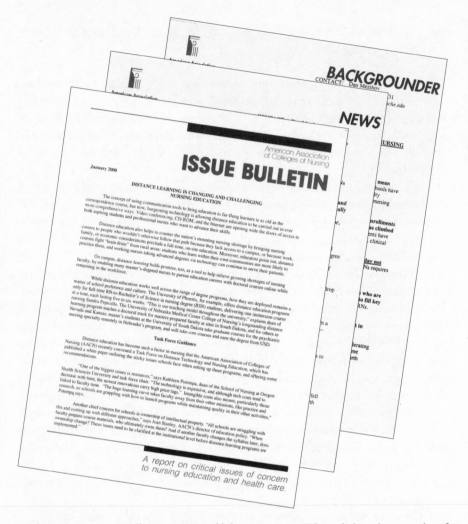

American Association of Colleges of Nursing

ISSUE BULLETIN

January 2000

DISTANCE LEARNING IS CHANGING AND CHALLENGING NURSING EDUCATION

The concept of using communication tools to bring education to far-flung learners is as old as the correspondence course, but now, burgeoning technology is allowing distance education to be carried out in ever more comprehensive ways. Video conferencing, CD-ROM, and the Internet are opening wide the doors of access to both aspiring students and professional nurses who want to advance their skills.

Distance education also helps to counter the nation's mounting nursing shortage by bringing nursing careers to people who wouldn't otherwise follow that path because they lack access to a campus, or because work, family, or economic considerations preclude a full-time, on-site education. Moreover, educators point out, distance courses fight "brain drain" from rural areas: students who learn within their own communities are more likely to practice there, and working nurses taking advanced degrees via technology can continue to serve their patients.

On campus, distance learning holds promise, too, as a tool to help relieve growing shortages of nursing faculty, by enabling many master's-degreed nurses to pursue education careers with doctoral courses online while remaining in the workforce.

While distance education works well across the range of degree programs, how they are deployed remains a matter of school preference and culture. The University of Phoenix, for example, offers distance education programs only for full-time RN-to-Bachelor's of Science in nursing degree (BSN) students, delivering one immersion course at a time, each lasting five to six weeks. "This is our teaching model throughout the university," explains dean of nursing Sandra Pepicello. The University of Nebraska Medical Center College of Nursing's longstanding distance learning program teaches a doctoral track for masters-prepared faculty at sites in South Dakota, and for others in Nevada and Kansas; master's students at the University of South Dakota take graduate courses for the psychiatric nursing specialty remotely in Nebraska's program, and will take core courses and earn the degree from USD.

Task Force Guidance

Distance education has become such a factor in nursing that the American Association of Colleges of Nursing (AACN) recently convened a Task Force on Distance Technology and Nursing Education, which has published a white paper outlining the sticky issues schools face when setting up these programs, and offering some recommendations.

"One of the biggest issues is resources," says Kathleen Potempa, dean of the School of Nursing at Oregon Health Sciences University and task force chair. "The technology is expensive, and although tech costs tend to decrease with time, the newest innovations carry high price tags." Intangible costs also mount, particularly those linked to faculty time. "The huge learning curve takes faculty away from their other missions, like practice and research, so schools are grappling with how to launch programs while maintaining quality in their other activities," Potempa says.

Another chief concern for schools is ownership of intellectual property. "All schools are struggling with this and coming up with different approaches," says Joan Stanley, AACN's director of education policy. "When faculty prepare course materials, who ultimately owns them? And if another faculty changes the syllabus later, does ownership change? These issues need to be clarified at the institutional level before distance learning programs are implemented."

A report on critical issues of concern to nursing education and health care.

and pitch it to a *Wall Street Journal* labor reporter. They did and a couple of weeks later it was in the "Work Week" column on the front page of the *Wall Street Journal*.

One important thing that we do at the AACN is produce media backgrounders on breaking issues within nursing education. In March 1999, we did a backgrounder on nursing school enrollments, why they are declining, and the major factors driving the growing nursing shortage. We did another backgrounder that month on the expanding use of nurse practitioners in the health system. In that, I also described NPs' educational programs. In February 2000, we sent out a news release on our latest annual enrollment survey that provided updated information on declining enrollments and the nursing shortage.

We do backgrounders as issues warrant, perhaps two a year. These backgrounders are usually six to eight pages long or about 1500 to 2000 words, and are accompanied by a cover memo. One version goes to about 400 people in the mainstream news media; another 250 go to the nursing, health care and higher education trade press. A duplicate version will also be sent to deans and to press officers at each of our member schools of nursing, and, when we have their addresses, to press officers shared with the college or university. We also send backgrounders to approximately 250 executives of nursing, higher education, and health care organizations and foundations, as well as to the chief staff members of key congressional leaders and to the heads of federal agencies involved in nursing education and research.

In addition, we've established a media referral service to provide the names of nurse researchers who are experts in various areas of health care. Print and broadcast journalists looking for expert sources are put in touch with leading researchers who have agreed, in advance, to respond to media inquiries.

The nursing community often thinks of media relations as an afterthought. It's the last thing on the list, if it's on the list at all. The goal of nursing education shouldn't be only to help nurses enhance their communication with patients, but to help nursing as a profession communicate with the public through the media. When people talk about health care, they tend to think in terms of medicine. Reporters who cover health care are often called "medical" reporters and tend to see their job as searching out the latest "medical' breakthroughs. It ought to be the goal of nurses to promote the profession as the largest in health care —not simply in terms of numbers, but in terms of its impact on patients' lives.

5. Rand Wilson is campaign support coordinator for the Service Employees International Union. SEIU represents 650,000 nurses, physicians, technicians, aides, and other professional, administrative, and service employees in the US.

The biggest difficulty is to convey the links that exist between union collective action, the long-term interests of the institution, and the good of patients. This flies in the face of almost everything that the public—and even many nurses—believe. The public believes that management is running the institution—the hospital, clinic, home care agency—and that, therefore, they always give top priority to the patient care mission of that institution. In fact, there are times when management is forced—say by managed care or government cutbacks—to make the financial bottom line its highest priority.

Another problem is unique to caregivers, especially women. Although the public holds nurses in very high esteem, many people believe that nurses should not be motivated by financial considerations. There is an expectation that nurses should be willing to sacrifice their health and financial well being to take care of their patients.

Some nurses reinforce these perceptions by arguing that their union colleagues shouldn't engage in any militant action to protect themselves and their patients because it is unprofessional or un-nurselike.

So that's the challenge: union members must illustrate how their bargaining objectives will advance both the mission of the hospital or health care institution and the well being of the public. If that's not done well in advance of any contract deadline or collective action, then union activities will appear blatantly opportunistic.

You have to do a lot of work up front to get satisfied patients who've had a good experience with nursing to speak out for you. You have to encourage patients who've had a bad experience because of short staffing or lack of time with nurses to speak out too.

It's important to use academic research to support your case. Recruit experts to speak—in a more objective fashion—about the problems and pressures within the health care industry. You also need to reach others in the profession—like doctors or other clinicians who can link their concerns to yours.

It's also important to connect workplace conditions, such as mandatory overtime or such high patient loads that prohibit nurses from taking a lunch break, with issues of concern to patients and the public. You need to explain why a nurse who walks 20 miles a day on a hospital floor needs to fuel up with a sandwich. Or why a nurse who's burnt-out and exhausted after working a ten-hour shift, cannot safely care for patients when she's forced to work another ten-hour shift.

It's also useful to link these issues to the problems of women in the workplace, the fact that many nurses are single parents and sole breadwinners in their families, or that, as women, they bear the lion's share of care-giving responsibilities in the home. When you add a second eight-hour shift to the "shift" women work at home, they're really working a 24-hour day.

If you do a good job up front to rally public support, it's less likely that you will have to go on strike. However, if you do have to go on strike—which is rare—you have to be even more aggressive in reaching the public. Increasingly, contract issues aren't settled at the bargaining table, they're settled in the court of public opinion. That's why an effective communication strategy is essential.

6. Art Moses is the coordinator of communications and campaigns for the British Columbia Nurses Union. The BCNU has 26,000 members.

Our fundamental challenge is to explain to the public what nurses do, and to win the public over to the idea that registered nurses are undervalued and should receive recognition for their critical work. They should receive much higher compensation and better benefits. Nursing care and other services should be organized in a way that contributes to patient care and nurses' satisfaction with their work. We also want nurses to play a greater role in primary health care.

Like all the Canadian nurses' unions, the BCNU runs public education campaigns that spotlight what RNs do. We use conventional advertising and try to get RNs to speak on television and radio and to the print media. Our campaign tools are designed for members' use in their lobbying, in working with fellow nurses, and in reaching out to members of their communities.

In 1997, for example, we needed to alert the public to the fact that employers were considering or actually replacing RNs with less-expert personnel. Rather than viewing RNs as expert clinicians giving direct care, they increasingly saw the registered nurses' role as supervising practical nurses and unlicensed staff. We launched a campaign that used two 30-second television ads highlighting the assessment skills bedside nurses bring to their work.

In newspaper ads, we depicted a nurse talking to a hospital patient who's just had a meal tray delivered to his room. The ad copy read: "He thinks he's having a conversation about the hospital Jell-O. She's actually mid-way through about 100 assessments." It continued with the explanation: "In the seconds it takes to reach the bedside of a patient to ask how they feel, a registered nurse will have made over 100 assessments—any one of which could mean the difference between recovery and tragedy."

In l998, the thrust of our bargaining was to increase staffing in long-term care facilities. Our video on the issue ran on the local community cable television network. We also circulated the video to members so they could show it at bargaining meetings and use it to lobby politicians and health employers.

We developed a television ad that showed an old man in a nursing home not as a stereotype, but as a human being who had had a rich full life. Older people deserve the highest quality care, but, as the ad said, there could be one RN per 100 residents on a night shift. "Tonight," the ad warned, "that might not be enough."

In long-term care and in other settings where nurses work, the issue today is increased workloads. Through a poll of our members, the BCNU documented that increased RN workloads have led to great disaffection on the part of nurses for the profession. In this poll, many nurses said they would quit nursing if they could and would not recommend it as a career choice to others.

Because of the nursing shortage, some health employers are training LPNs to do registered nurses' work. To help the public understand that this is not the answer, and to explain why higher wages and better working conditions are needed to keep RNs in the profession, we've done two things. We have initiated a campaign at workplaces and through the media to relieve RNs of their non-nursing duties like delivering meal trays, mopping floors, answering phones, cleaning, and filing. We want employers to hire more service staff to do that work. Our question to employers is: Why are you spending money to train LPNs to do RN work and wasting money by asking RNs to transport patients and deliver meal trays?

We're working on an innovative communication approach—a humorous musical theatrical production that will dramatize the content of nursing work. We've hired an experienced theater producer to write and stage the play. It will tour British Columbia.

The producer held focus groups to collect stories from nurses who work in various settings throughout the province. The nurses gave us great stories. Originally, we anticipated that we would have three professional actors and two nurses in the production. However, as the meetings between nurses and the producer unfolded, we saw that we could easily find working nurses capable of acting in the production. Thirty nurses responded to the casting call out of which we chose five. So we have an entirely RN cast. The play opened in Vancouver in April 2000.

Like everything else we do, this theatrical production uses public communication techniques to encourage nurses to speak out for themselves. Our campaigns are successful with the public because they stem from the actual experiences of real nurses and involve them as actors rather than spectators.

7. David Schildmeier is the director of communications for the Massachusetts Nurses Association. The association has 20,000 members, 17,000 of whom are in its collective bargaining unit.

My job is not only to solicit media interest in nursing issues, but also to encourage nurses, wherever they practice, to solicit media coverage of themselves. I try to help them develop an understanding of the importance of the media to their practice. I liken that job to the work of a lobbyist who needs to know legislators, educate them and stay in contact with them. If professional issues are to be heard, you have to know who reporters are, what they like to hear and what motivates them. You have to watch for openings to talk to them. You also have to watch out for problems with coverage and respond immediately so that there is a direct cause and effect.

Several years ago, nurses at the Brigham and Women's Hospitals were trying to get contract language giving them more power over delegating nursing activities to unlicensed assistive personnel. The nurses had contacted the *Boston Globe* about an upcoming strike authorization vote over this issue, and took great pains to explain to the *Globe* how this issue of unlicensed personnel might affect the quality of patient care. A *Boston Globe* labor reporter did a story on the strike authorization vote. But she turned it into a labor dispute about wages and benefits, not a patient care story.

I had told the nurses at the Brigham to be on the lookout for the story and to write or call if they didn't like it. The nurses flooded the reporter with phone calls complaining that she had missed the story's real significance. The next day I got a call from the reporter asking why the nurses were so upset. I told her. The reporter did another story on the patient care issues and later did a story on the nurse who was the main MNA leader at the hospital. Those calls were a turning point of that coverage at the *Globe*.

Nurses in Massachusetts have become valuable, cooperative sources for reporters. I tell nurses to be patient if a reporter doesn't know about the issue. You don't get mad at a family member because they don't understand what's wrong with a patient. You educate them.

Many nurses worry that reporters will misquote them. They will. About 70 percent of the time they won't get it exactly right. But that's close enough to be effective.

Part of my job is to find nurses who will talk to reporters, who will follow the first rule—return reporters' phone calls. I never work with a nurse if reporters say, "I tried to call her and she said she was busy." The whole key to media work is answering a journalist's call.

I do a lot to make reporter's jobs easier. Like nurses, reporters are spread thin today. In many instances, reporters want to do a story but don't have time to chase everything down. This means that I have to get them a lot of material and help them conceptualize the story. The easier I make that reporter's job, the more likely that reporter is going to trust my information.

I think PR directors like me should also focus on promoting more positive stories about nursing. There is a lot that nurses can take to the PR people in their institutions and organizations to show what they are doing. Our association, and organizations like ours, gives awards to nurses for expert and innovative practice, but we need to take those accomplishments beyond the walls of nursing. This is particularly important today.

The public has to know that the house of health care is burning down. Today it is rare to find a nurse who can say that things are wonderful in her institution. We have to promote what nurses do so nurses can get back to doing it.

The Hawaii PR Story

In 1999, the state of Hawaii was experiencing an all-too-familiar problem: its hospitals had cut nursing positions or not filled those left vacant. Patient lengths of stay were reduced. Queens Medical Center, the largest hospital in Honolulu, announced it would implement work role redesign. The Hawaii Nurses Association (HNA) feared the three other Honolulu hospitals would follow suit.

The HNA, which represents 3,800 RNs statewide (2,500 for collective bargaining), wanted to include staffing and patient safety in contract negotiations with the four Honolulu hospitals before their current contracts expired in December 1999. The hospitals refused to bargain over this issue.

"We were at our wit's end. Everything we said to them about staffing and patient safety was falling on deaf ears," says Nancy McGuckin, executive director of the HNA. "To change the employers' position, we knew we needed to get the support of the broader community. To do that we needed to get nurses to talk about the significance of these issues. Our members were telling us, 'Go out and tell the public they're in danger,' but we had no idea how to deal with the media. We worried that we would not be able to get our message across in a way that would encourage public support."

The Honolulu hospitals also tried to discourage nurses from taking assertive action. "The hospitals had told us they would respond to anything we did, tit for tat," McGuckin continues. "We had to get past that. We needed a comfortable way to take a leap off the cliff into this kind of public communication."

The HNA knew that the Massachusetts Nurses Association had gotten a lot of press attention and public support through its Safe Care Campaign and had integrated staffing into its contract negotiations. They invited David Schildmeier, MNA's communication director, to come to Hawaii to advise them.

Schildmeier spent a week listening to HNA staff explain the situation. His advice? Get professional communications help. He cautioned them not to hire someone who only knows traditional public relations. The job the HNA had to accomplish demanded political organizing too. Schildmeier's precise words were: "You need someone like Ralph Nader."

The HNA searched for the right candidate and selected Scott Foster— who had in fact worked with Ralph Nader—as a part-time consultant. When Foster first met with HNA leaders and members he was very impressed. "I told them they had an *embarras de richesses*," Foster recalls. "Here were people who knew the health care scene inside and out, who were articulate, passionate and angry about what was happening to patient care, and who were prepared to do something about it. What more could you ask for when you're about to launch a media/political campaign?"

With Foster's help, the HNA created an internal and external public communication campaign that turned a traditional labor dispute into a highly visible public health issue.

To apply pressure on the hospitals, Foster had to find a way to get into the media well before the contracts expired. However, he couldn't approach the media or other public forums without nurses who would describe articulately their working conditions and link them to patient safety. The HNA also needed an outside expert on health care policy and nursing who could frame the issue as a major, nationwide public health problem. The association asked Suzanne Gordon to speak at its annual convention in late October. There the HNA hoped to rally nurses to the cause and bring the issue to the press.

Foster and the HNA leadership wanted Hawaiian policy makers and consumer advocates to learn what was at stake when hospitals cut nursing staff. They set up a breakfast meeting for Gordon to talk to nursing and health plan executives, state government officials, health policy academics, and patient and consumer activists. They wanted her to present a national perspective by explaining the impact of cuts in nursing staff on patient care and health care costs on the mainland.

Before the meeting and the convention, Foster and the HNA staff did an enormous amount of preparatory work. "People make the mistake of believing that if they publicize an event, people will come," Foster says. "A lot of work has to be done to get them to come."

Foster assembled media kits. He wrote 16 separate letters to his press contacts announcing Gordon's visit. Each letter was tailored to the interests of the particular journalist. He hand delivered the letters and media kits to his contacts at newspapers and radio and television stations.

"One editor was a feminist, so in her release I focused on the women's issues," Foster explains. "Another, to a business magazine writer, emphasized business and cost issues. For press contacts one size doesn't necessarily fit all. If you are doing this for the first time, it sounds like a lot of work. But once you know the people involved, it's not so daunting."

Foster followed up with phone calls to make sure his contacts had received the press kit and to focus their attention on it. As the date of the conference approached, he was on the phone constantly getting commitments for press, television and radio interviews with Gordon. During her visit, Gordon met with editors at the major Honolulu paper and was interviewed on TV and radio. The day before the HNA convention, a TV interview that was shot in a Honolulu hospital and presented a strong case against restructuring and staff cuts was carried without rebuttal on the evening news.

Nurses who saw the television interview were very receptive to Gordon's message the next day at the convention. It was: "It's up to you to tell the world what you do. You're the ones who will win this campaign."

The tactic of bringing in an "outside expert" was the bridge into the public arena. Nurses saw that they could have their concerns presented in a positive way through the media. Over the next month, Foster and the HNA staff worked on a press strategy and coached nurses on speaking to the media. When contract talks stalled, and management refused to put staffing and work redesign on the table, the HNA was able to be proactive not just reactive.

Between November 25 and December 29, as nurses took strike votes at the four Honolulu hospitals, the HNA sent out daily news releases. "This made the media's job easier," says McGuckin. "The press was very appreciative that we were constantly providing them with concise, usable information. I kept my cell phone on 24 hours a day. I even slept with it," McGuckin recalls. She says that Foster instructed her to call the three evening news shows each day—fifteen minutes before they went on air—to let them know the status of the strike votes and/or how contract talks were going.

When the hospitals released a report titled "Hospitals' Bleeding Budgets," that insisted the state's hospitals didn't have money to maintain or enlarge their nursing staffs, the nurses assertively reframed the issue. They argued that the dispute was not primarily about wages, but about patient safety.

Throughout the campaign, Foster had a line up of nurses giving interviews to various media. When the nurses were at the HNA offices painting picket signs, TV reporters and camera crews were there too. "The office was constantly filled with reporters with their cameras rolling recording nurses who simply spoke from the heart," McGuckin says. "We had 137 hits on TV for that 30-day period."

The nurses won their campaign. "Queens Medical Center completely capitulated," McGuckin reports. "They withdrew their work role redesign scheme. They agreed to include the American Nurses Association staffing principles and nursing-sensitive quality indicators. They said there would be no further staff cuts. Period. They would negotiate over staffing. We got the best contract language in the country. And the other hospitals were a variation on the theme. The bleeding stopped."

McGuckin believes it is essential for nurses to make their work and their concerns visible and to get the right kind of professional help to do it. "It didn't break the bank," McGuckin says of the HNA's contract with Foster. "It was highly affordable. Nursing organizations can afford to do this. In fact, they can't afford not to. If you lose jobs, you lose members. And if you lose enough members, then you have no organization at all."

According to McGuckin, after the settlement, people approached nurses on the street to thank them. "Our collective bargaining director and chief negotiator had her car broken into and so she called the police," McGuckin recalls. "When the officers came to take her report, they recognized her name from all the media attention. They thanked her for what the nurses did to protect the public.

"We found out the public really supports nurses. We'd all heard that. We'd read the polls that say the public respects us and thinks we're honest and ethical. But it wasn't real to us. We'd never really tested the extent of our public support. And then for two months, we tested it and people were there for us. It was a wonderful experience."

For that the nurses are immensely grateful. To express their thanks, in January 2000, the nurses picketed in front of the state capital at rush hour. Only this time, their signs read, "Mahalo," Hawaiian for "Thank you."

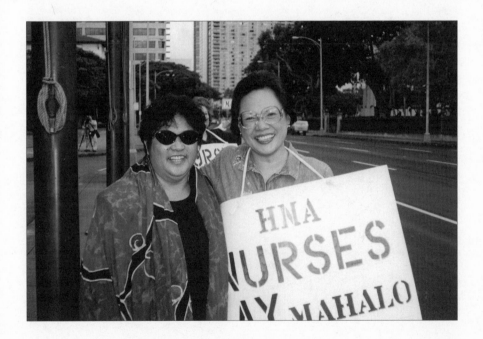

Nurses Joey Ibarra and Aggie Pigao Cadiz say "Mahalo."

Chapter 8

CONSTRUCTING CAMPAIGNS THAT WORK

This chapter examines six advocacy "campaigns" nurses have conducted to achieve specific goals. In all these campaigns, nurses "went public" to secure a remedy for a serious problem. They employed extensive internal and external organizing and communication strategies. They achieved their goals.

In 1999, two historic events occurred in North American nursing.

In the United States, California became the first state to mandate safe nurse–patient staffing ratios despite opposition from its powerful health care industry.

In Canada, the federal government earmarked C\$25 million of new health care funding for research specifically on nursing's contribution to patient care and the impact of restructuring on nursing and nursing care, factors that affect the health of the profession.

These watershed commitments to nursing and patient care didn't just happen. They were the hard-won victories of thousands of nurses who engaged in strategic planning, collective advocacy, and extensive public communication to reverse the erosion of nursing care brought about by relentless budget cutting. Their determined activism on behalf of their profession and patients was far from novel. Indeed they were acting in the finest tradition of nursing, which, throughout its history, has waged campaigns to win practice and patient-care advances.

Although many don't think of Florence Nightingale as a whistleblower or lobbyist, she was both.

It was the press that first drew Nightingale's attention to the poor treatment of British soldiers in the Crimean war. William Howard Russell, the first British war correspondent to file dispatches from the front, reported in the *Times* that cholera and other enteric diseases—not artillery fire—were responsible for hospitalizing 20 percent of the expeditionary force. Because of abominable hospital conditions, these soldiers were more likely to die than survive. Moreover, while France provided nurses to care for its sick and wounded soldiers, Great Britain did not.

When Nightingale learned of this, she contacted her friend Lord Sidney Herbert, then Secretary at War and the person in charge of finances and supplies. After much negotiating, in November 1854, Florence Nightingale embarked for the Crimea with a force of 38 nurses. During her stay in the Crimea, Nightingale used the popularity she gained through newspaper reports on her activities to lobby for money to finance her efforts. When she encountered military, physician and bureaucratic recalcitrance, she threatened to go to the press to advance her cause.

After she returned to England, Nightingale used every means to improve military and civilian hospitals, to provide home care to the sick poor, and to give respectable women paid work outside of the confines of the Victorian household. One of the first health care statisticians, she used research findings to bolster her arguments. Nightingale also collaborated with a notable female political writer, Harriet Martineau, who was then a columnist for the *Daily News*.

As Lois Monteiro writes: "Nightingale contacted Martineau when her attempts to pressure reform in the Army in 1857–58 were going too slowly; she turned to public opinion as the pressure source."[1] In 1858, Nightingale sent Martineau a "private reading" copy of a report she had produced on army reform. Over the years, Nightingale continued to feed Martineau information that later appeared in the journalist's columns. Martineau's book, *England and Her Soldiers*, grew out of the two women's working association.

The significant advances in nursing have come about through nurses' individual and collective advocacy. Their earliest struggle "was the effort to distinguish trained nurses from everyone else who purported to care for the sick," says nursing historian Joan Lynaugh. "It involved the insistence that nursing work required education and standards." This campaign took from roughly 1860 to 1915. But, finally, according to Lynaugh, the idea that "there is a distinct thing called nursing" requiring a distinct education achieved worldwide acknowledgment.

"Efforts to bring about significant change require coalitions that have a purpose, leaders who won't give up, and public activity," Lynaugh asserts. "They grow out of the awareness that the only way you can achieve anything is to connect your own little world to other worlds in which people share your views, at least about one particular issue."[2]

More recently, nurses who specialize—nurse midwives, nurse practitioners, and critical care nurses, among others—have won acknowledgment for their distinct work. Nurses have also succeeded in winning reimbursement and prescriptive authority for nurse practitioners, instituting PhD programs in nursing schools, developing the National Institute of Nursing Research in the US, adopting baccalaureate education as the standard entry into practice in the majority of Canadian provinces, and adding nursing as a visible clinical category to the Canada Health Act. These achievements came about by mobilizing coalitions within and beyond the nursing profession.

The nuts and bolts of advocacy campaigns are described in the following six case studies. Campaigns are created to deal with a pressing issue or problem. They are grounded in a convincing analysis connecting the issue to larger public concerns. They are aimed at winning sufficient backing to bring about the desired solution to the problem. A campaign is not a one-shot event. It has a beginning and continues over time until the issue is decided. A campaign for a specified remedy, however, is almost always part of a larger, long-term program.[3]

The campaigns described in the following case studies are characterized by the creativity, persistence, and assertiveness the nurses involved brought to them.

Case Study Number One:
The Fight for Safe Hospital Staffing Legislation in California

With a stroke of his pen, on Saturday, October 10, 1999, governor Gray Davis made California the first state in the US to require hospitals to meet fixed nurse-to-patient ratios in an effort to force hospitals to provide high quality patient care.

It was a day of celebration for the 30,000 members of the California Nurses Association. They had spent years contending with the pervasive cost cutting that left nursing staffs in the nation's most populous state at dangerously low levels. Two years previously, a similar remedy had made it through the California legislature, but was vetoed by governor Davis's Republican predecessor, Pete Wilson.

But now a new law required the California Department of Health Services to set standards for nurse-to-patient ratios for all hospitals and mandated hospitals to assign additional nursing staff on the basis of patient acuity and need. The law, which covered all licensed registered and practical nurses, restricted hospitals from assigning certain nursing functions—such as invasive procedures, patient assessment, administration of medication, and patient education—to unlicensed assistive personnel (UAP). It also addressed the issue of floating by prohibiting hospitals "from shifting nurses trained in one unit to duty in another without adequate preparation."[4]

"This is one of the most significant days in the history of nursing," California Nurses Association president Kay VcVay said after the signing. "This law will save the lives of countless numbers of patients needlessly endangered by unsafe hospital conditions."

For nurse activists, the safe staffing law was the most significant victory in an ambitious and on-going union program to "reclaim the health care agenda" in the state where managed care was born. A month before, the Democratic governor had signed bills that expanded patients' access to mental health care and their rights to sue health insurers for punitive damages and seek outside reviews of decisions denying coverage.

Once seen as an innovative and economical means of expanding access to health care, by the mid-90s, it had become abundantly clear that market-driven managed care was making it increasingly difficult for clinicians to provide high quality care to patients. Rather than trying to adapt to a bad situation, rank-and-file nurses took their concerns to the union.

They reported that to save money, hospitals were laying off registered nurses and replacing them with UAP that lacked the training or experience necessary for proper patient care. They complained about enormously expanded RN workloads, understaffing, and the assembly-line treatment of patients forced out of hospitals by length-of-stay reductions imposed by their health maintenance organizations. As it turned out, it would not be long before managed care would bring the same problems to other states.

The California Nurses Association argued that nothing short of mandated nursing care levels would stem the tide. However, the campaign to gain legislation for this solution took six years.

In 1994, the association proposed its first staffing bill. With a Republican majority in the assembly, it never got out of committee. But the California Nurses Association was mobilizing for the long haul. One of its most innovative tactics was to find patients who had suffered from short staffing by advertising for them.

"It's 3 a.m. Who will come when you need help?" asked ads that ran in California newspapers and the *New York Times*. The ads asserted that "hospitals and HMOs are cutting care to make record profits. Patients are paying the price." They explained that nursing staffs were being cut and that "unlicensed staff, often with no clinical background or experience, are being forced to make decisions about your health."

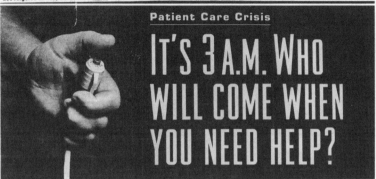

Patient Care Crisis

IT'S 3 A.M. WHO WILL COME WHEN YOU NEED HELP?

Hospitals and HMOs are cutting care to make record profits. Patients are paying the price. Just ask any registered nurse who provides direct care.

We're the health professionals patients call on most. And we see dangerous changes that can put you at risk at a time when patients in hospitals are more critically ill than ever.

Untested, experimental work redesign schemes are reducing the standard of care and cutting skilled care givers by up to 50%. But with staff cuts of just 8%, mortality rates can jump as much as 400%.

Registered nurses and other skilled health care professionals are being removed from directly caring for patients. Unlicensed staff, often with no clinical background or experience, are being forced to make decisions about your health.

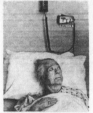

✖ Dangerous short staffing leads to death and injuries due to omissions and accidents.

✖ Nurses and other health care professionals are threatened with termination when they speak out on behalf of patients.

✖ Doctors are prevented from making necessary referrals and treatments.

Yet health care is the number one profit industry in the country. What's wrong with this picture?

When hospital corporations like Alta Bates in Berkeley talk about "patient focused care" and "cost efficiency," what they really mean is higher profits and cut-rate care.

This is the real health care crisis. The kind that happens at three in the morning when you reach for the buzzer and there's no one there.

At the California Nurses Association we are very concerned about your safety. We are asking Congress to take action against this threat to patient safety. But we need your help. Please write our "Patient Watch" program and tell us if your care or the care of your loved ones has suffered because of short staffing or inadequate care. Join the California Nurses Association in the fight for quality care.

 CALIFORNIA NURSES ASSOCIATION

Write to: "PATIENT WATCH"
California Nurses Association
1145 Market Street, Suite 1100
San Francisco, CA 94103

A HEALTH CARE BULLETIN FROM THE CALIFORNIA NURSES ASSOCIATION

The ads asked people to write to "Patient Watch," a program of the California Nurses Association, "if your care or the care of your loved ones has suffered because of short staffing or inadequate care."

The Association received many responses. Some told tragic stories. "Our family has suffered from the death of our daughter because of short staff and/or inadequate care in a local hospital," one parent wrote. "At about 3 a.m., Tuesday, June 7, she vomited and aspirated the vomit, causing cardiac arrest and then seizures. She then went into a coma and was in the coma until she died."

The mother of an infant born prematurely wrote: "I can't count the number of times I saved my son's life and the life of the child in the neighboring room. The nursing was five [patients] to one [nurse], at least that is what they told us. We had things happen [like] being told to pay for a baby-sitter to watch our son if we wanted to leave...We would go for eight hours without seeing a nurse."

For the most part, the patients and family members who wrote in did not blame individual nurses for the terrible neglect they had experienced. They saw it as a system problem. "Nurses do a terrific job, but more nurses are needed to nurse the patients in the hospitals, not just to hook up patients and take the vitals," said a San Francisco respondent.

In 1994, activists were pursuing every avenue to halt the decimation of nursing care, including national legislation. But the news media were treating managed care largely as a business story. Reporters had trouble finding working nurses who would talk to them about the human costs. Gag orders, threats and employer retaliation against nurses made it difficult for RNs to come forward. Some did, but only if reporters cloaked their identity. One nurse interviewed by NBC News was shown only in silhouette behind a screen.

In this atmosphere, the "Patient Watch" stories were an invaluable tool even when they were used without the names of patients and hospitals to avoid lawsuits. To encourage coverage, the Association faxed a new patient horror story to journalists each night (when the phone rates were the lowest).

With support from unions and other organizations working for health care reform, the Democrats regained control of the California assembly in 1996. A new, safe staffing bill finally made it through the legislature in 1998 only to be vetoed by governor Pete Wilson. That fall, Californians elected a Democrat, Gray Davis, to the governorship. Davis had told the California Nurses Association he would favor the legislation.

The union knew that even with a friendlier governor and Democratic majority in the legislature, a staffing bill would face intense industry opposition. Only thousands of nurses—working with other health care workers and patient groups—could overcome this opposition.

To mobilize nurses, the Association built a statewide campaign network. Articles in its publication, *California Nurse*, explained why hospitals were so short staffed and why legislation was necessary to insure better patient care. Activists distributed leaflets on the issue in both unionized and non-union hospitals. In their workplaces, RNs signed petitions to unit managers and administrators asking them to support the bill. Although Association members recognized that few of these administrators would actually support the bill, for some nurses, the action of signing a petition was the first step toward greater involvement in the campaign.

The Association distributed educational material to all California nursing schools. It used its own as well as other nursing Web sites and listserves to post and distribute a continuous stream of information.

Association members and other supporters were asked to write letters to state senators and assemblymen and assemblywomen. Model letters were made available, but nurses were encouraged to tell their own stories in their own words. A torrent of heartfelt letters—sometimes five or ten pages long—flowed to legislators and the news media, often followed by personal phone calls presenting the case for legislation.

Nurses spoke at hearings on the bill, before church and consumer groups, and on television and radio shows. Patients and the families of patients who had suffered were encouraged to join the lobbying effort. They also testified at hearings, wrote letters to the editor, and contacted legislators.

Nurses organized press conferences. They met with the editorial boards of all the major newspapers in California and won a number of supportive editorials. Individual nurses also wrote letters to the editor and op-eds.

One of the campaign's most persuasive documents was a study by the Institute for Health and Socio-Economic Policy commissioned by the Association. The study analyzed 18.2 million California patient discharge records and other hospital and government data. It found an 8.8 percent increase in the average number of patients cared for by each full-time RN, and a 7.2 percent decrease in the number of full-time RNs employed in the period from 1994 to 1997. Between 1995 and 1998, the number of patients per staffed bed increased 7.7 percent.

The study indicated that California had the second lowest ratio of registered nurses to patients in the nation. When the California Nurses Association commissioned a poll to assess public attitudes toward a safe staffing bill, support was overwhelming.

After the California assembly passed the staffing bill in the summer of 1999, the California Nurses Association organized large rallies to encourage the more reluctant Senate to follow suit. When the senators were set to vote on the question, 2,400 RNs gathered at the state capital building in Sacramento. Hundreds more from 50 different hospitals—union and non-union alike— rallied in Los Angeles. The outpouring of grassroots support pushed a sufficient number of fence sitters to cast pivotal votes for the bill.

But the governor's signature was still needed to turn the bill into a law. Although Gray Davis had signed other pro-patient measures, he complained that the legislature was sending him too many bills on health care. He hesitated to sign the staffing bill. He refused to sign another bill—a major nursing home reform measure that he worried would place too great a burden on the state budget.

Eleventh-hour lobbying by hospitals and HMOs was intense. Nurses feared that Davis would be swayed by the industry's argument that the bill was too rigid. Campaigners turned up the heat with more letters, faxes and phone calls, trying to make it politically unacceptable for Davis to refuse to sign. To get the governor's signature, assemblywoman Sheila James Kuehl, the sponsor of the bill, agreed to offer a follow-up bill the next year postponing implementation of staff rations from 2001 to 2002 to give the state time to work out the correct ratios.

The California Nurses Association is now working to make sure the new law will be effectively implemented.

Case Study Number Two:
Saving Baccalaureate Nursing Education in Quebec

Given the complexity of contemporary patient care, the trend in both Canada and the United States is toward making the baccalaureate degree the educational threshold for entry into the nursing profession. Reports by commissions and health care policy groups emphasize the need for education that will prepare nurses to care for increasing numbers of patients with complicated needs and to function effectively in dynamic health care settings that call for more independent decision making. In both countries, nurses most in demand are those with baccalaureate and graduate degrees. In fact, in Quebec, the government had previously announced *Virage ambulatoire* (Turn to the Ambulatory Setting), a policy that would move more patient care into the community through "community health centers" or CLSCs that mainly hired nurses with university degrees.

Therefore, it was a shock to nursing educators in 1998 when Quebec's education minister, Pauline Marois, announced a plan to limit access to university nursing programs in the province to students who first complete a three-year community college nursing program. This technical program awards a nursing diploma. The rationale for the government's proposal was that funneling all nursing students through the three-year CEGEP (Collège d'enseignement général et professionel) technical program would standardize Quebec's two-pronged nursing education system.

Quebec has an unusual system of post-high-school education. All higher education students must first attend a community college for at least one year. In the CEGEP, nursing students choose either a three-year technical track leading to a diploma, or a two-year pre-university science track. The latter is followed by a three-year university nursing program that awards a BSN degree. The government's view was that the CEGEP program would be sufficient for most nurses. Under the government proposal, post-CEGEP university education was conceived as *perfectionnement* or continuing education for those who wanted to specialize or teach, or go into administration. This proposal would have constituted significant barriers for students who wanted a broader university education.

The government claimed it was concerned about duplication of educational programs in nursing. However, policy changes of this nature are rarely non-political. Quebec, Canada's only French-speaking province, has long formulated its own policies independently, some of which differ markedly from those of other provinces. Critics suggested that the proposal was a parochial attempt to deal with the Quebec nursing shortage by churning out nurses more quickly and cheaply. Harsher critics went so far as to argue that a mandated technical program was a government ploy to make sure that nurses stay in Quebec by making them unemployable in other provinces requiring more education. The move would have also limited the professional mobility of nurses in Quebec itself. A technical diploma limits access to supervisory jobs and those in the community.

When the deans of the major nursing schools in Quebec learned of this proposal, they immediately and publicly opposed it. Laurie Gottlieb, director of the School of Nursing at McGill University, called the Canadian Association of University Schools of Nursing (CAUSN) to alert deans throughout Canada.

Leading Quebec nursing educators including Gottlieb, Suzanne Kérouac, dean of the faculty of nursing at the Université de Montréal and president of the Quebec region of the Canadian Association of University Schools of Nursing (RQ-CAUSN); Edith Côté, dean of the faculty of nursing at Université Laval, Quebec City; Louise Chartier, director of the School of Nursing at the University of Sherbrooke, and other nursing department heads throughout Quebec, mobilized a protest.

A key element of their strategy was to enlist interdisciplinary and national and international allies to help convince the government that its approach would not only shortchange potential nurses and patients in Quebec, but would put the province uncomfortably out of synch with nursing in the rest of Canada, the US, and other countries throughout the world. Within hours of the announcement, the appalled deans and directors began a letter writing campaign directed at critical Quebec government ministers.

Gottlieb also called the Canadian Nurses Association executive director, Mary Ellen Jeans, who had been her predecessor at the McGill nursing school, and asked for CNA's support. Quebec does not belong to the CNA and the CNA does not usually intervene in provincial/territorial matters. But, the association, which supports university education for nurses, knew that there were national implications to this Quebec development. If Quebec rolled back the clock, other provinces could do the same.

"We wrote letters providing a national perspective. What the provincial government was doing was contrary to international trends, going against what good sense and good research tells us," said Carole Presseault, CNA's manager of health policy.

Wendy McBride, executive director of CAUSN, said that such a policy would deter would-be nurses from getting a baccalaureate degree because it would take too long. It would also cut off access to RN certification for students in the province's nine university nursing programs.

Andrea R. Lindell, the president of the American Association of Colleges of Nursing told Marois in a letter that her proposal had "ramifications that can cross international boundaries." Lindell said that the US also is experiencing a nursing shortage similar to the one in the mid-1980s, but "the need is not merely for higher numbers of RNs to meet increasing demand, but rather, for more nurses of the right educational *mix* to handle the more complex requirements of today's health care environment." The AACN encourages direct entry into baccalaureate and higher-degree nursing tracks. Lindell noted that employers seeking nurses were recruiting across the border (an activity likely to increase as the nursing shortage worsens). She pointed out that it is in the interest of both the US and Canada "to ensure that educational programs produce sufficient numbers of nurses who have the requisite knowledge and skills to provide high-quality, cost-efficient care in a rapidly changing health environment."

The Quebec media quickly picked up the educators' arguments. "We're going backward here," McBride said of the Marois proposal. "Elsewhere, diploma schools of nursing are closing or moving toward collaborative programs with universities ... Nursing is a profession and as a profession it requires basic education at the baccalaureate level. We need the sciences and theories of nursing. It's not a task-oriented profession."

McBride was quoted in an article in the *Canadian Medical Association Journal* headlined: "'Dumbing down' of Quebec RN education irks nurses, MDs."[5] The article cited physicians' objections. "This is clearly wrong," Patrick Vinay, the dean of medicine at the University of Montreal, said of the proposal. "We need well-trained nurses who can collaborate with us. Without university education this bond is extremely difficult."

Educators gathered information about the international trend toward university education for nurses. They reached out to colleagues in other disciplines (including medicine), to those in hospitals and other health care institutions, to a wide sweep of organizations and to individuals with influential relationships with government ministers. In short, they mustered all of the clout they could find. Their contacts included the president of the Ordre des Infirmiers et Infirmières de Québec (the Quebec nurse licensing association), the Council of Nurses of the McGill University Health Centre, and the Quebec Federation of Nurses, the nurses union. The campaigners set up an e-mail network to keep participants abreast of the latest developments.

The deans of nursing had been told that the government was basing its decision on a 1980 report by a committee on the formation of nursing science headed by Ginette Lemire Rodger, a former director of nursing at one of Quebec's major hospitals. Gottlieb contacted Rodger, who had moved to Alberta, and informed her of the situation. Rodger was stunned that her report was being used as a justification for limiting access to university education in Quebec. She wrote to Pauline Marois explaining that her report had been misinterpreted—in fact, it recommended an end of diploma programs in favor of university nursing education. She told the education minister that the plan would "put Quebec nurses at a dead-end and keep them from playing their role as leaders of the science of nursing in the francophone world."

("Madame La Ministre, je joins mes commentaires à tous ceux qui, j'en suis sûre, vous ont fait part de l'erreur que serait l'implantation de cette orientation. Les conséquences seraient de mettre dans un cul de sac les infirmières du Québec et de les empêcher de jouer leur role à titre de leader du monde francophone dans le domaine des sciences infirmières.")

Gottlieb contacted Nicolas Steinmetz, the physician in charge of a plan to unite the five McGill University teaching hospitals into a health center network. Steinmetz, who had an excellent working relationship with the provincial ministry of health and social services, expressed his concerns about inadequate preparation of nurses to health minister Jean Rochon. Gottlieb spoke to the board of governors of the McGill University Health Centres to enlist support from the whole university hospital community.

Bernard Shapiro, the principal (equivalent to provost in the US) of McGill University, and president of the Conférence des Recteurs et des Principaux des Universités du Québec (CREPUQ), the organization representing the principals of all Quebec universities, organized a CREPUQ teleconference on the government's proposal. In a letter to Marois, Shapiro expressed CREPUQ's support for community college nursing education, but insisted that university nursing programs must continue, especially given the government's intention to use more nurses in ambulatory settings.

Nursing dean Suzanne Kérouac garnered support from the Université de Montréal. In fact, the university senate passed a motion against the government's intended action. Kérouac, Côté, Gottlieb, and Ghislaine des Rosiers, of the Ordre des Infirmiers et Infirmières de Québec met with representatives from the government ministries.

When the academics met with Quebec business people and members of the Association des Hopitaux du Québec, they highlighted the contradiction in the government's new direction. Why, they asked, would the government want to produce nurses that these employers would not hire?

This was the point the president of the Association des Hopitaux du Québec made in her letter to ministers Marois and Rochon. "We have difficulty understanding how this decision can fit in with the context of the evolution of the health care system in Quebec," wrote Marie-Claire Daigneault-Bourdeau.

Early on, the campaigners held a major press conference featuring a broad spectrum of educational and health care experts all opposed to the move. They provided press kits of material that explained the issues, and copies of all the participants' statements. The conference attracted local and national radio, television, and newspaper coverage. Nursing students from across the province held their own well-covered press conference. Local press conferences and briefings were held outside of Montreal.

Throughout their campaign, the educators appeared on radio and television and kept in close contact with journalists, some of whom had a field day with this story. To give them background on contemporary nursing, the group gave copies of the book, *Life Support: Three Nurses on the Front Lines*, which describes the day-to-day work of three American nurses, to journalists, physicians, and politicians. The book's author, Suzanne Gordon, provided an international perspective in an op-ed for the *Montreal Gazette*.[6]

Faced with so much intense lobbying, the government set up a committee to consider the future of nursing education in the province; it included university, union, and health care representatives. "This was the government's way of recognizing that the issue was far more complex than they had originally understood," says Gottlieb. "They began to understand that nursing wasn't just a set of technical tasks, and that the solution they proposed wouldn't work."

This committee met for more than a year. Although its members have still not resolved the thorny issue of multiple routes to nursing practice, they abandoned the idea of closing direct access to university nursing programs. The educators, realizing that their campaign was only a phase of a long-term effort, established a committee to monitor the issue. With contributions from the Quebec universities, they hired a public relations company to continue public education around an issue they knew would become more acute as the nursing shortage worsens.

Indeed, in both Manitoba and Saskatchewan, overtures have been made to reopen diploma schools of nursing. "The campaign waged by Quebec nurses in 1998 is a useful model for nurses who want to maintain university education," says McBride.

Gottlieb feels the campaign demonstrated the importance of creating internal and external alliances. "Nursing has a great deal of power when nurses activate their own networks, communicate the issues clearly and passionately, and reach beyond themselves to educate and involve other interested parties such as physician colleagues, and, when the issue permits, employers.

"During this campaign, we heard that the Bouchard government was overwhelmed with faxes, letters, phone calls, and e-mails from a wide variety of constituencies. During one meeting, a deputy minister told me with surprise, 'You are so well organized. First, I hear from schools of nursing across the country. Then I hear from the Americans. Then I hear from the doctors.'"

Gottlieb says she replied, "Actually, we haven't organized yet. Just wait to see what happens when we do."

Case Study Number Three:
Massachusetts Whistleblower Legislation

In the 1990s, as staffing conditions in many health care institutions deteriorated, many nurses found themselves taking on a role they had neither sought nor trained for—that of whistleblower. Nurses in this category followed a similar path. First, they went through channels to rectify problems. When this was unsuccessful and patient care became even worse, they took some action that either intentionally, or as an after effect, made public the problems within their institutions.

Their "blowing the whistle" on institutional problems was one of the things that eventually caused the press to turn a critical eye on the growth of managed care in the United States. Whistleblowers risked their jobs to protect the public from hidden health care risks. But one whistleblower, Nurse Barry Adams, of Cambridge, Massachusetts, became a symbol for the need for legislation that would protect caregivers from retaliation wherever they worked.

The Massachusetts Nurses Association (MNA) had lobbied for whistleblower protection in 1996. MNA leaders understood that passage of such a bill would require public support. But few members of the public were then aware of what was happening to patient care in hospitals and other institutions. Nor did they understand the risks of retaliatory dismissal of those caregivers who revealed unsafe conditions to the public or to governmental agencies.

Members of the MNA had tried to raise public consciousness about this problem. When Barry Adams was fired and the story hit the press, the public was given a vivid illustration of the restraints on caregivers who try to protect their patients.

Four years previously, Nurse Adams had gone to work at the Youville Health Care Center, a rehabilitation hospital in Cambridge. As the facility experienced mounting pressure to cut costs, Adams witnessed a dangerous erosion in patient care standards. He documented cases of poor wound management and mistakes that occurred because newly graduated nurses were not adequately supervised.

Adams tried to address these problems in-house. He talked with his immediate supervisor and two other managers who were also alarmed by the eroding quality of care. But when Adams tried to discuss his concerns with Youville's director of nursing, she refused to meet with him. So he sent a memo to the director of nursing and to the chief hospital administrator, who was also a nurse. Both dismissed his reports. As the risks to patients mounted, Adams persisted. The director of nursing threatened to fire him for documenting his concerns. Suddenly his supervisors claimed he was having "time management" problems.

On October 15, 1996, Adams went to the Massachusetts Board of Registration in Nursing (BORN) and filed a complaint of "unprofessional conduct," "unethical conduct," and "patient neglect" against the director of nursing and the administrator of the Youville Center. He asked for clarification of nurses' responsibilities under the state Nurse Practice Act, specifically, whether nurses who were in charge of institutional finances were responsible for the safety of care given under their administration.

Three days later, the hospital dismissed Adams. Two other nurses who had protested were forced to work rotating shifts and resigned soon after.

Although Youville was not unionized and Adams was not an MNA member, the first thing he did was contact the association. "I'd never been involved in any political or union activity," he said. "But I knew they were the professional organization for nursing in the state, so I called them and said, 'I just got set up and fired.' They talked to me, told me they would help and said that the first thing I needed was an attorney."

The MNA put Adams in touch with Marie Snyder, an attorney who had been a nurse. She filed a wrongful dismissal suit in state court. She contended that it was a violation of the public trust to fire a nurse for speaking out on behalf of patient care.

Adams and the other two nurses filed a complaint of unfair labor practices against Youville with the National Labor Relations Board (NLRB), the enforcer of federal labor law in the US.

While these cases were pending, Adams went to work for the Visiting Nurse Association of Boston, whose members are represented by the collective bargaining arm of the MNA. The MNA asked Adams if he'd be willing to talk publicly about his experience. "You bet your boots I would," he responded.

After Adams completed his six-month probationary period at his new job, MNA's director of communications, David Schildmeier approached the *Boston Globe* with an offer of an exclusive on the Adams story. Coincidentally, *Globe* reporters had been digging through Massachusetts department of public health records and discovered that a Youville patient had died from an accidental drug overdose. They learned that the health department had cited Youville for eight deficiencies in patient care. Two were specifically for "patient-care neglect" and two were for "lack of professional and technical services" in the department of nursing.

The *Globe*'s story incorporated this information into the saga of Adams as a health care whistleblower. The story generated widespread media coverage. Adams became a symbol for all of the health care whistleblowers who had been penalized for trying to protect their patients. The MNA recognized that Adams was a focal point for the issue and helped him hone his media skills.

Soon after the *Globe* story appeared the American Nurses Association (ANA) unveiled its Patient Safety Act, a proposed federal bill to provide whistleblower protection throughout the country. Adams was a featured speaker at an ANA press conference on the legislation held in the National Press Club in Washington, DC.

In May 1997, the NLRB held a two-day hearing on the complaint of Adams and his two colleagues. Six months later federal administrative law judge Arthur Amchan ruled that his firing was an "illegal attempt to silence [Adams] and retaliate against him." Amchan found that Youville's disciplinary actions against the three nurses were discriminatory, punitive and carried out with "animus." He dismissed testimony by the hospital nursing director and ordered the RNs reinstated with back pay. The judge also ordered the hospital to post a notice reassuring employees that they would not be harassed, fired or disciplined for joining together for mutual aid or protection.

While Adams won this case, he lost the one in state court. Adams and the MNA saw the state court verdict as a demonstration of the need for statutory protection. One reason Adams fared well with the NLRB was that he could show that he had acted in concert with two other nurses. Under US labor law, workers—even non-union ones—cannot be legally fired or disciplined if they engage in "group" activities related to wages, hours and working conditions. They have protection if they can act as a "group." Many nurses, however, are unaware of this and act alone, sometimes because their colleagues are afraid of what will happen if they speak out with them. While NLRB rules do not discriminate between union and non-union workplaces in this regard, state courts usually offer no protection to "employees at will" in non-union workplaces, unless there is a specific statutory ban against recriminations.

In March 1998, a measure to provide such a statutory ban was again introduced into the Massachusetts legislature. Adams appeared on radio and television as a spokesperson for the bill. Over the next year, he testified several times at legislative hearings. This time, he was joined by another health care whistleblower, Cathleen Kyle, a cardiac critical care nurse, who had received excellent performance reviews of her work at the Massachusetts General Hospital until she began to file incident reports on understaffing and unsafe conditions on her CCU. Management suddenly insisted she was compromising the nursing teamwork on her unit and fired her.

To keep the whistleblower story alive and draw national attention to legislative activity in the state, in December, Schildmeier contacted a reporter at NBC "Nightly News." After extensive discussion, NBC carried a piece on the Adams case.

PROTECTING OUR PATIENTS

Nurses should be free to speak out against dangerous practices—it could save your life

BY BARRY ADAMS

NOBODY REALLY LIKES GOING TO A HOSPITAL OR nursing home. But all of us will probably need to at some point in our lives, either for a loved one or for ourselves. The unfamiliar environment of a health-care facility can be frightening, and the realization that we are at the mercy of our doctors and nurses can make us feel even more vulnerable.

I am a registered nurse who has worked on the front lines of patient care for the last seven years. We are the only licensed health-care professionals at a patient's bedside 24 hours a day. Nurses today are in charge of patients who cannot be cared for either at home or in outpatient clinics. With managed care's emphasis on cost-cutting, only the most seriously ill are permitted an overnight stay in a hospital, and that stay is as brief as possible. As a result, most hospital floors resemble the intensive-care units of the past, with patients' conditions changing rapidly from moment to moment. Nurses are in the best position to know when they are stretched too far to provide good care. Unfortunately, in most states we are not protected against retribution if we report short staffing or other dangerous circumstances that put patients in harm's way.

I know, because I stood up for my patients and paid a painful price. I reported dangerous staffing levels in my hospital. At first my complaints were brushed off, and when I persisted I was fired. Eventually I was legally vindicated, and the state board of health found the hospital in violation of eight standards of care including "patient neglect." Now I am supporting federal legislation to protect health-care professionals when they speak up about patients in danger.

My difficulties began two years ago when the hospital trimmed costs by reducing the nursing staff. The number of patients assigned to my care doubled, from six to 12. This meant I couldn't even look after basic hygiene, let alone assess patients for subtle changes in their conditions, give them medication on schedule or monitor them for possible side effects—nursing skills that keep patients safe and comfortable. I found a 92-year-old stroke victim soaking in her own urine, unable to reach her call button to alert nurses. I saw patients who, tired of waiting for someone to help them to the bathroom, had tried to make the trip themselves, only to slip in their own urine and feces.

What's more, newly graduated nurses were frequently left alone to perform complicated procedures without training or supervision. One day I found an inexperienced nurse rushing to administer a man's medication. She was preparing 50 times the prescribed dosage to inject into the unsuspecting patient's central venous line. Had I not caught the error, the man would have died.

Along with other nurses, I expressed my concerns to the direc-

tor of nursing and the administrator in written memos. Three months before I was fired, my personnel review stated that I was "an excellent role model ... conducts himself in a professional manner ... is an advocate for his patients ... and channels his concerns appropriately." After I spoke up, my supervisors began to find fault with my performance. I was wrongfully charged with having "time-management problems" and fired for being "unprofessional" when I refused to sign the disciplinary notice. In November 1997, after I filed a complaint with the National Labor Relations Board, a federal judge ruled that my termination was unlawful and motivated by "the [institution's] desire to silence [me] and retaliate against [me]." The judge ordered the hospital to reinstate me, pay all back wages with interest and expunge all record of my illegal termination.

In October 1996, the same month I was fired, my worst fears came true. A nurse who had never been trained by the hospital to administer intravenous medication accidentally gave a woman an overdose of morphine, and the woman died. Within one year after I was fired, a second patient was given the wrong medication but survived, and yet another unattended patient fractured his skull when he fell down two flights of stairs while strapped to his wheelchair.

I wish I could say the situation is better in other states. But a recent survey by the American Journal of Nursing found that more than two thirds of nurses don't have time for basic nursing care, like teaching patients how to tend to wounds or inject themselves with insulin. More than half are too busy to consult with other members of the patient's health-care team. A full one third would not recommend that their family members receive care at the facility where they work. State boards of nursing and the nurses-association code call on us to safeguard our patients. Where is the legal protection we need to truly uphold this charge?

There is some progress. Just this year Kentucky passed legislation to protect nurses who speak out. Similar measures are pending in seven states. But will they pass soon enough to protect you or someone you know?

Many health professionals, like me, are willing to speak out and take the risk of being fired. But forcing us to choose between keeping our jobs and meeting our obligations to ensure safe care can put patients in jeopardy.

A new Patients' Bill of Rights contains whistle-blower language that would allow nurses to uphold the trust people place in us during their time of need. We could report patient-safety concerns without fear of termination. Every American should understand that "ungagging" health-care professionals is one of the best ways to guarantee that life-threatening conditions are brought to light. As a Louisville Courier-Journal editorial stated, "Americans rightly expect their doctors and nurses to be vigorous advocates for the care they need, not silent partners in settling for less."

You really don't want to go to the hospital. But if you have to go, and you are lying in that awkward bed in a paper-thin gown, worried, helpless in a sea of intimidating equipment, unfamiliar sights and smells, wouldn't you want to be looking at a nurse who is free to speak on your behalf? It's time to stop settling for less.

ADAMS *is an IV infusion nurse.*

Joan Meehan-Hurwitz, the ANA's communications director, then suggested that Adams submit an article to *Newsweek's* "My Turn," a premier forum for personal experiences that have national implications. With the ANA's help, Adams wrote the article and submitted it. *Newsweek* published it on November 16, 1998.[7]

The *Newsweek* column produced national reaction. Thanks to Adams, and all the nurses who had spoken out, whistleblower legislation was passed in Massachusetts in 1999 and signed by Republican governor Paul Cellucci.

However, the fate of Adams's complaint to the Massachusetts Board of Registration in Nursing proved to be a different story. In spite of nurses' insistence that the board had been protecting nurse managers while holding staff nurses accountable for lapses in patient care, in March 2000 the board dismissed Adams's complaint against his nurse manager and administrator.

"Being a public speaker and a spokesperson for an issue has been very intimidating to me," Adams says. "But I can cope with this kind of scrutiny because no matter what kind of legal wizardry or spin is placed on what I say, it's still the truth. Getting the support of other nurses and learning that I can deal with even the toughest questions has been very rewarding to me because it has helped nurses improve their working lives. If I had to do it all again, I would."

Case Study Number Four:
Protecting the Public from Medical Errors

What are nurses to do when they know that patients are being harmed by medical errors or negligence yet the authorities in their institutions will not listen to them or act on their reports?

This was the challenge that Carol Youngson and her nurse colleagues in Winnipeg, Manitoba, faced when they saw 12 infants and young children die, and others suffer serious injury, at the hands of a surgeon they considered to be incompetent. It is a challenge that nurses everywhere face when they are given responsibility for patient safety without the authority to correct conditions that jeopardize patient care. For all of the public attention being paid to medical errors, one of the least visible aspects of this crisis in North America is the failure of physicians and health care institutions to value and use the expertise of nurses.

In Canada, it took the nation's longest running coroner's inquest to demonstrate finally the critical role that nurses play in patient safety and the cavalier way that many institutions disregard nurses' expert judgments.

Carol Youngson—a nurse with 23 years of surgical experience—was the RN in charge of the cardiac operating room at Winnipeg's Health Sciences

Centre Children's Hospital when the hospital's veteran pediatric cardiac surgeon left in 1993. The unit was shut down for a few months until a replacement, Jonah Odim, arrived in February 1994. He was an American surgeon with impressive credentials—Yale education, University of Chicago medical training and a fellow at the Harvard-affiliated Boston Children's Hospital when he was recruited.

He was soon functioning as the sole pediatric cardiac surgeon in the province of Manitoba without back up or on-site supervision from experienced surgeons. As became evident later, he had little experience performing cardiac surgery in general and none in the kind of pediatric surgeries the program was designed for.

Nurse Youngson, who assisted Odim in the OR, quickly became concerned about the doctor's surgical technique. She had worked with 150 surgeons and realized that Odim's work was far below par. Within a month, three young patients were dead. The surgeries on these children had been considered low to medium risk, but all had bled to death because of failed repairs.

Youngson discussed the situation with two other nurses—Carol Bower, who also worked in the OR, and Irene Hinam, a high-risk anesthesia nurse who worked in the neo-natal ICU. Youngson reported the concerns of her group to the nursing supervisor and the director of nursing. The nurses also approached their medical colleagues about the quality of Odim's surgery. There was no response. Desperate, Youngson begged Nathan Wiseman, the hospital's director of surgery, to attend one of Odim's operations. Although Youngson had considered him a friend, he refused. He told her bluntly that he didn't take orders from nurses.

In May with the death of the fifth patient, the program's mortality rate reached 50 percent, and other infants experienced serious complications. Although it had been unwilling to act on the earlier alerts from experienced nurses, the hospital abruptly suspended the surgical program when cardiac anesthetists threatened to withdraw their services unless the pediatric cardiac surgery program was evaluated.

At that point, the hospital administration formed a committee, with Youngson as its only RN member, to review the program. Interestingly, Youngson notes, none of the concerns of nurses that she voiced at the meetings were mentioned in chairman Nathan Wiseman's minutes. The committee decided that, at least temporarily, Odim should only perform low- and medium-risk surgeries.

However, within a short time, he was again performing a full range of pediatric open-heart procedures. Again, nursing's concerns were ignored and unrecorded. And, again, babies started dying.

"In December, we lost three neonates, bang, bang, bang," Youngson recalls. "One bled to death, another had a canula in and Odim knocked it out and destroyed the repair. The repair on this three-day-old baby's heart was complete and things were looking pretty hopeful. As I briefly looked away, I heard a gasp. I looked at the heart and saw that the aortic canula, the tube that returns oxygenated blood from the by-pass machine, had been knocked out. In his efforts to restore it, Odim destroyed his repair. The baby died on the table."

This 13-hour case finished on a Sunday night. The next day Youngson went directly to the medical director and to the director of nursing. Finally, responding to the concerns of Youngson, other nurses, and doctors, the hospital required Odim to have a cardiac surgeon present when operating on complicated cases. Nevertheless, three weeks later he did another open-heart surgery on a neonate without requesting help. The baby bled to death in the OR.

This 12th death was Odim's last case—ICU physicians said they would no longer refer patients to him.

Surgeons from Toronto were called in to conduct an independent review of the program. They documented the same serious problems delineated by the nurses and pronounced the program's pediatric mortality rate to be "unacceptable." But rather than seeing the nurses as acting on behalf of patients, the two physician reviewers seemed to think the nurses just held a grudge against the surgeon. The report said they were "concerned" with "the degree of animosity that existed between the surgeon [Odim] and the anesthetists and the surgeon and virtually all of the nurses."

As a result of the review, however, Winnipeg Children's Hospital sent out a news release announcing the program's suspension. Parents, whose children had died under Odim's care, were stunned when they read the news. They soon discovered that this was Odim's first job as surgeon, that he had no experience with complicated surgery, and that the anesthetists had threatened to withdraw their services. "They went wild," Youngson said. They brought their complaints to the provincial/territorial government, which demanded an inquest into the functioning of the program since its founding in 1981.

Youngson was soon notified that she and other nurses would be represented by the hospital's attorney during the proceeding. She and Irene Hinam, Carol Bower and the unit manager Karin Dixon met with the hospital's lawyer, director of nursing and a senior administrator. At this meeting Youngson revealed that she had made copious notes about those operations that had gone wrong. So did Carol Bower. The nurses presented their notes and opinions to the hospital. "Here," Youngson said," you should take a look at this."

Several days later, the hospital told Youngson and her fellow RNs that the hospital's attorney could not represent the nurses because a of conflict of interest. The nurses were told to seek their own legal representation.

Youngson and her colleagues were taken aback. They knew they couldn't pay for attorneys on their own. So they called the Manitoba Association of Registered Nurses (MARN) and asked for help.

Diana Davidson-Dick, executive director of MARN, had already asked her board to seek standing in the inquest. "This was consistent with MARN's legislative mandate, which is to protect the public from harm," Davidson-Dick recounts. "If the system in which the public is cared for and in which nurses work prevents nurses from protecting patients and the public, then it's the obligation of regulatory boards to try to intervene."

Davidson-Dick realized that the RNs' testimony in the inquest could "provide insights into how the hospital system was preventing nurses from acting for patients. The nurses could provide evidence that might be used to prevent this from happening again."

When MARN's board okayed the request, Davidson-Dick hired counsel to represent the association and the nurses involved.

Before the inquest began, Davidson-Dick organized meetings to plan the group's media strategy. She worked with Marion McGee, a researcher on nursing who helped MARN and the attorneys, "develop the kinds of messages we thought were important for the public." Davidson-Dick also feared that if the association didn't employ its own means of communication, the nurses could be scapegoated for their inability to stop Odim in time.

The inquest into the Health Science Centre program began in March 1996. In September, Carol Youngson took the stand as the first person from the operating room to testify. For 13 days, she was examined and cross-examined about what she saw. She spent two of the days being questioned by lawyers for families that were suing. One observer of the proceedings said he didn't know how the parents could bear to be present. "The nurse's testimony about the babies dying was just horrific," he said.[8]

"In this case, nurses had something to say that had to be said," Youngson insists. "I had been there through 11 of these 12 cases. I was the person most involved in terms of what happened when the surgeries occurred."

Attorney Colleen Suche says that, during the inquest, the nurses had to confront the fact that "no one understands what a nurse knows. The public doesn't understand what nurses *do* in hospitals. They have this idea that nurses sit beside patients' beds and hold their hands—that nurses are a lesser form of being than doctors. We saw this repeatedly with witnesses as well as with the media."

The inquest drew media attention throughout Canada. Everyday that the nurses were on the stand, their testimony made the front-page news in Winnipeg papers. The CBC program, "The Fifth Estate," did a piece on the inquest that prominently featured Youngson. Profiles of the nurses appeared in newspapers throughout Canada. The magazine *Elm Street* did an article entitled "Heartbreak," highlighting the hospital's failure to heed RNs' warnings.[9] At one point, the nurses had even named themselves the "Broken Hearts Club."

At the conclusion of the inquest, judge Murray Sinclair asked all the parties involved to submit their recommendations. The document submitted by MARN made the following points:

"Nurses must be equal partners with physicians in health care. That is not just because of the significance of the role of nursing but to ensure that responsible nursing occurs.

"Participants in health care systems should be held accountable consistent with their authority, power and degree of control. Currently, nurses are accountable, liable and responsible, without the requisite authority, power or influence."

The three-year inquest produced thousands of pages of testimony. Questions were raised about whether there are enough pediatric cardiac surgery cases in Winnipeg to attract a competent surgeon for such a program. It revealed that the program had a troubled history, questionable financial support, and high death rates during previous periods. It raised troubling questions about why a rookie surgeon was given such responsibility and why negative evaluations of his work had not been communicated. It certainly raised issues of double standards—many families who were reassured about the quality of the surgery program were poor, were members of ethic minorities, and did not know how to seek referrals elsewhere. As we wrote this in March 2000, the presiding judge had still not delivered his findings.

In 1995, Odim left Winnipeg for a surgical appointment at Emory University in Atlanta, Georgia. He was less than two months into a five-month appointment when a Canadian reporter called the university and the Georgia medical board to discuss the upcoming inquest. The state board, which had not known about the events in Winnipeg, postponed a hearing to extend Odim's temporary medical license so he couldn't practice in Georgia.

In 1997, Odim obtained a temporary appointment as a clinical instructor at the University of California, Los Angeles Medical Center, and was accepted for a transplantation fellowship. The next year Youngson recounted the story to an American journalist at a nursing conference. Youngson said she was concerned about Odim's patients in California. The journalist agreed that the public had a right to know his background and phoned reporter Julie Marquis at the *Los Angeles Times*.

Marquis interviewed Hillel Laks, the chief of cardiothoracic surgery at UCLA, who told her that "we had an open mind as to causes of problems" in Winnipeg, and that UCLA had hired Odim in a "supervised role."[10] When the *Los Angeles Times* ran a story on Odim, he volunteered to quit treating patients while on a research rotation. During the summer of 1998, he was returned to full privileges and his appointment at UCLA was renewed.[11]

Since the inquest, Youngson and her colleagues have spoken extensively to nurses and others about procedures for preventing and correcting medical errors. In their appearances before nursing organizations, they are encouraging other RNs to challenge institutional barriers that deprive nurses of their proper authority.

As Youngson said in a talk to the Canadian Operating Room Nurses Association, "Yes, we know how to run the complicated pumps, monitors, and other machines at the bedside, but it is our *patient* who is our first and foremost concern...

"Unfortunately, we still work within a patriarchal system. All of us who work on the frontlines know that until nurses are heard, and their concerns taken seriously by the medical profession and hospital administrators, situations like the one [at Winnipeg Children's] will continue to occur."

Case Study Number Five:
The Service Employees International Union (SEIU) Campaign to Prevent Needle Stick Injuries

On Monday, April 13, 1998, readers of the *San Francisco Chronicle* opened their newspapers to find the first installment of a three-day series of articles on "Deadly Needles."[12] *Chronicle* reporters Reynolds Holding and William Carlsen reported that some one million nurses, physicians, nurses aides, hospital housekeepers, lab techs, home care nurses, and other health care workers in the US each year experienced accidental needle sticks that exposed them to the HIV virus, hepatitis B and C, and other diseases. Thousands of health care workers did, in fact, become infected from needle sticks, the reporters wrote. And hundreds eventually died from their illnesses. Most of this, the reporters asserted, was the result of corporate greed, hospital penny pinching, and regulatory agency indifference that had prevented the widespread use of safer syringe needles.

In a total of 12 articles, journalists Holding and Carlsen laid out the "chilling pattern of indifference and neglect within the nation's medical industry" that they had uncovered during six months of investigation.

The reporters found that the hazards posed by conventional needles were widely known by the early 1980s and had stimulated a variety of approaches toward making needles safer. Indeed, the reporters learned that executives at Becton Dickinson, a medical device corporation that has largely controlled the global market in syringes, knew by the 1960s that hepatitis B could be transmitted both by the reuse of contaminated needles and through accidental needle sticks. In the late 1970s, physician Dennis Maki and nurse Rita McCormick at the University of Wisconsin hospital conducted the first systematic study on how disease was transmitted by needle sticks. Their work sounded a more widespread alarm. Ironically, although patients were protected from contamination by the use of disposable needles, health care workers were not.

Safer needle options have existed for almost two decades. But Becton Dickinson, whose revenues reached $2.8 billion in 1997, refused to jeopardize its existing market share by introducing safer needles. Hospitals, in turn, declined to spend any extra money to purchase safer needles from other suppliers. For their part, the US Occupational Safety and Health Administration (OSHA) and Federal Drug Administration (FDA) dawdled and delayed actions that would have protected workers. In 1985, the Centers for Disease Control (CDC), knowing there was a needle stick problem, recommended that health workers wear gowns, gloves and masks to protect against infection, and take the hepatitis B vaccine as a precaution. But the CDC did not recommend the use of safer needles. By then, the reporters pointed out, needle sticks were already spreading a mysterious new disease—AIDS—that was killing with brutal efficiency. In 1988, the *New England Journal of Medicine* published a landmark study that blamed needle sticks on syringe design rather than on the carelessness of health care workers and asserted that needle stick injuries could be reduced by 85 to 90 percent by using safer needles.[13]

Reynolds and Carlsen catalogued the tragic consequences of corporate, institutional and governmental disregard. They profiled health care workers who have suffered terribly, like Ellen Dayton, a nurse practitioner at the San Francisco General Hospital and a University of California drug clinic, who in 1996 was accidentally pierced with an HIV and hepatitis C infected needle. She contracted hepatitis C for which there is no vaccine or cure, and she became ill with AIDS even though she took the prophylactic medications that sometimes stop or slow down the development of the disease after exposure to HIV. Dayton, a member of SEIU local 790, sued Beckton Dickinson, contending that the company made and marketed an unreasonably dangerous product.

The *Chronicle* series was a pivotal event for the hundreds of thousands of nurses, physicians and other health care workers who had been working for years through the SEIU and other unions and health care groups to get safe needles. The series appeared just as SEIU was launching its biggest effort yet— a campaign for safe needle legislation in California and other states.

For almost 15 years, the SEIU had engaged in aggressive and sustained public communication in its pursuit of educational, legal, regulatory, and contractual remedies. Early on, for example, it published educational materials and conducted workshops to teach members how to avoid needle-stick injuries.

Between 1992 and 1994, the union negotiated safe needle requirements in some of its hospital contracts. It filed complaints with California's workplace safety agency, CalOSHA, against the Kaiser Health Plan. This action led to a CalOSHA citation against Kaiser that required the HMO to evaluate and purchase safer needles throughout its California facilities. This was a step forward, but there were still questions about which needles were the safest. Implementation was uneven and health care workers in other facilities were still unprotected. Without strong state laws, there would be no industry-wide implementation to protect all workers.

SEIU and its allies began lobbying hard for such legislation. One of the most active groups in unveiling this hidden menace was the SEIU Nurse Alliance. Communication was especially critical to the legislative campaign. It was central to the organization of a grassroots force powerful enough to be heard by legislators and to elicit public support for a new law.

In January 1998, SEIU's campaign communication department devised a list of "crowd events" and "non-crowd events" that union locals could use to attract media attention.

The categories of crowd events were:

*   Rally—requires a large crowd and could include state legislators and community leaders as speakers in addition to nurses.
*   Speak-out—workers standing on capitol steps taking turns talking about their fears or actual experience of contracting a deadly disease from needle sticks.
*   Candlelight vigil—"even a few dozen people carrying candles at dusk can make a powerful statement," the memo advised.
*   Lobby day—health care workers (in purple scrubs) showing legislators and others how safe needles work by injecting oranges.

Recommended non-crowd events to illuminate the problem included hearings at which health care workers and outside expert witnesses could testify to the dangers of needle sticks; news conferences; donations of a day's worth of safer needles to a hospital; setting up information booths in hospitals and at other health care facilities; informational pickets to distribute leaflets in front of hospitals and regulatory agencies; and "fax-ins" to generate large numbers of fax messages directly to the governor or to a central location from which they can be forwarded.

In 1998, the year of the most intense effort in California, the SEIU readied an arsenal of communication materials to inform and mobilize its own members and allies and the general public, and to encourage reporters to pursue the needle stick story. These included workplace posters, leaflets, model state laws, instructions on how to file complaints with OSHA, and media "tool kits" for union locals.

This tool kit, and another one developed at a later stage of the campaign, was designed to help activists persuasively tell the story of the needle stick epidemic. It featured a list of "talking points," factual statements containing pertinent statistics that spokespeople could use to make their points.

There was a question-and-answer sheet that responded to arguments that might be raised, such as the suggestion that safer needles would be prohibitively expensive.

"They range in cost from 17 cents to 45 cents per unit for safety needles versus 8 cents per conventional needle," the SEIU response sheet stated. "However, these costs are based on demand, which at this time is virtually non-existent because most hospitals are not purchasing them. If manufacturers were to make these devices in large quantities, the unit costs would go down dramatically. And any analysis of cost ought to include liability costs or the cost of sending a health care worker home to their families with hepatitis B or C or HIV."

The tool kits contained prototype op-ed articles that a nurse or a union official could adapt and submit to a newspaper. They provided a draft of a letter that a group could send to a newspaper editorial board to arrange a meeting on the issue. There was a draft pitch to television programs that suggested the guests (nurses who had been stuck by needles) and the peg (pending legislation) that could be used for a TV feature or talk show. It was accompanied by a videotape aptly named "Killer Needles: Our Fight to Stop a Health Care Epidemic."

The SEIU's press work helped pave the way for the *San Francisco Chronicle* series, which was, without a doubt, the most influential media report on the subject. It was spurred by other developments as well. One was a report by the CDC in 1997 that using safer needles could reduce needle stick injuries by 76 percent. Around that time, Retractable Technologies—an upstart firm trying to manufacture and market safe needles—contacted the *Chronicle* because it had a history of covering AIDS and worker safety. During the same period, Ellen Dayton, a nurse member of SEIU, went public about the consequences of her needle stick accident. The situation had the components of a great exposé. The *Chronicle* assigned Holding and Carlsen to investigate. They spent several days in Washington, DC, combing through relevant documents at the SEIU headquarters and speaking to union experts.

"The *Chronicle* series illustrates how newspaper coverage can act as a catalyst on an issue," says Jamie Cohen, an occupational safety and health expert who is the coordinator of the SEIU Nurse Alliance. "Information on the dangers of needle stick injuries had been around for more than a decade before this series came out. But this series brought it all together."

It had an immediate impact. California assemblywoman Carole Migden, a Democrat from San Francisco, worked with the SEIU to draft a bill setting a timetable for study and implementation of safe devices. Union members, particularly the SEIU Nurse Alliance, mobilized to support the bill. The union sent out a full set of campaign materials to activists including sample news releases and other tip sheets and checklists. To lobby legislators personally, nurses went to the state capitol in Sacramento armed with safer needles and oranges.

On September 1, 1998, the California legislature became the first in the nation to pass a bill requiring the state OSHA to enforce the use of safe needles with retractable sheaths and other protections that would prevent accidental needle sticks. But a huge obstacle remained. Earlier that year, Republican governor Pete Wilson vetoed the California Nurses Association nurse staffing bill. He was likely to do the same to the needle stick legislation.

To sway the governor, SEIU members faxed him 1,200 messages. Activists organized candlelight vigils in Los Angeles and San Francisco. Kaiser Permanente, the largest health care insurer in California, and the California Health Care Association (an industry group that had initially opposed the legislation) urged Wilson to sign the bill. He did so on September 30.

Other state legislatures followed California's lead. On April 5, 1999, as 20 states were considering needle stick legislation, the television newsmagazine show, "Dateline NBC," ran a feature on the SEIU's campaign. In January 2000, Republican governor Christine Todd Whitman signed a bill making New Jersey the fifth state to adopt safe needle legislation. As we went to press, campaigns demanding protections from needle sticks had spread to other states in the US and to other countries.

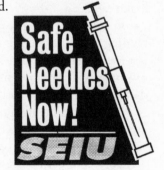

Case Study Number Six:
The Quiet Crisis

In fall 1998, the Web site of the Canadian Nurses Association carried an all-points alert. The CNA was launching a national campaign to pressure the government to vastly increase national funding for health care and to provide specific new support for nursing.

Initiated and led by the CNA and supported by the Canadian Federation of Nurses Unions (CFNU), the Canadian Association of University Schools of Nursing (CAUSN), and student nurses—were seeking a major allotment of C$40 million a year for five years, expressly for nursing.

This move was a response to a decade of federal cutbacks that hit Canadian nursing services especially hard. Over the past several decades, the national government's share of health funding to the provinces and territories had dwindled significantly. Between 1996 and 1999 alone, the federal government cut its annual cash payments to the health care system from C$18.5 billion to C$12.5 billion. As Monique Bégin, a former federal health minister, told CNA members in 1998: "The restructuring of the health care system in our provinces was done—and is still done—on the backs of nurses. In the last few years, it is mainly, almost only nurses who have lost full-time employment and income and worse, in my opinion, who are witnessing the de-professionalization of their occupation."

The success of the CNA "Quiet Crisis" campaign depended on the coalition's ability to convince the Canadian public and its political leaders that, without quick action, Canadians would soon be "deprived of the high quality health care they need, and to which they are entitled."

The reason: A shortage of nurses that is threatening the viability of the nation's health care system.

This effort paid off. A billion dollars was immediately added to the Canadian Health and Social Transfer (CHST) payments to the provinces and territories. A year later the government pledged to restore $15 billion annually for health care.

In the 1999 budget, the nurses' coalition won C$25 million for a new Nursing Research Fund. The fund, administered by the Canadian Health Services Research Foundation, will support some clinical practice research, and will provide a way to examine systematically the contributions of nursing to the health care system and the problems facing the profession.

"This investment signals a fundamental shift in how we value nursing in Canada," says Mary Ellen Jeans, CNA executive director. "This fund acknowledges that quality care begins with nurses, and it will provide the necessary long-term investment in supporting a well-educated and highly qualified nursing workforce."

"The Nursing Research Fund will generate information about the impact of health care reform and management on patient care and nursing," says Judith Shamian, executive director of Nursing Policy for Health Canada. "This research fund is an acknowledgment that changes in the health care system that took place in the '90s had a serious impact on nursing services.

"Traditionally nursing issues were not on the political radar screen. Public appreciation of nursing and nursing activism put it there."

Collaborative action made the "Quiet Crisis" campaign a success. It began two years earlier in a forum organized by the CNA—a historic meeting. Nurses from the CNA, CFNU, and other nurses' unions and professional organizations met to work for common goals.

"This forum represented a huge cultural shift and step forward in the maturation process in nursing," said CFNU president Kathleen Connors. "The tensions that had often divided nursing unions and professional organizations were overcome. We all recognized our common interests in maintaining high professional and ethical standards. We understood that we should all be working together."

Or, as CNA's Mary Ellen Jeans puts it: "We're very privileged to have a relationship with the Canadian Federation of Nurses Unions. We recognize that the organizations are complementary."

The CNA began to develop plans for the "Quiet Crisis" campaign in the summer of 1998. It had previously published *The Ryten Report: A Statistical Picture of the Past, Present and Future of Registered Nurses in Canada.* This report predicted that, without immediate action, Canada would soon face a huge nursing shortage. By the following summer, it had become clear that cuts in the federal health budget were having a significant impact on nurses and patients. Nearly 50 percent of Canadian nurses were employed part time only. Many were holding down several jobs to make ends meet. Others were emigrating to the US. Moreover, Canadians were becoming increasingly dissatisfied with their health care system.

For a number of years, Canadian nursing unions had been similarly trying to draw public attention to the workplace conditions that were driving nurses out of the profession and jeopardizing patient care. For example, the Manitoba Nurses Union had run a campaign called "Standing Up for the Front Lines of Healthcare." A similar effort by the British Columbia Nurses Union was summed up in the slogan "Some Cuts Don't Heal."

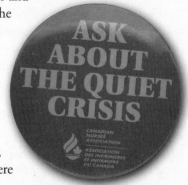

But despite protests and warnings, the 1998 federal budget had no new investment in health care. By later that year, even politicians were acknowledging that there was a nursing crisis. At the 1998 CNA convention, Liberal health minister Allan Rock told participants: "It is time for Canada to care for its nurses."

Now was the time to make Canadian politicians do just that.

The coalition decided upon a single, clear message: The shortage of nurses is threatening the entire health care system. This message directly linked professional issues with larger public concerns. The CNA and other nursing groups were not just fighting for nursing but, through the Health Action Lobby (HEAL), for the integrity of the publicly funded Canadian health care system.

The Quiet Crisis campaign was launched on September 22, 1999, when Mary Ellen Jeans presented CNA's brief to the House of Commons Standing Committee on Finance. At the same session, Kathleen Connors presented a similar brief from the CFNU. "It was really quite amazing," says Connors of that session. "We were quite an effective team. When the heads of the CNA and CFNU spoke forcefully about the crisis facing nurses and the realities of the current work world, that was a very powerful message. And when the executive director of the CNA backed up the unions about the impact of casualization (part-time work) and the importance of maintaining current RNs in the profession as well as bringing new people in, we could not be played one against another." Following this hearing, both Connors and Jeans met with senior government officials, MPs and cabinet ministers.

Participants in the campaign used research to document their analysis of the crisis. Because of cut backs in funding, nurses were unable to get full-time employment. Conditions in the workplace were eroding. Not only were nurses leaving the profession, they were discouraging friends and family members from entering. In addition, some 5,000 Canadian nurses had moved to the US to work. The nurses also explained how the problem arose and why helping to solve it was a federal responsibility.

The CNA gave nurses a road map that helped them take their case to the public. The first step was communicating with the nursing community. In their conversations with other nurses, activists were advised to "analyze how the nursing shortage is negatively affecting your workplace. Examine how patient care is impacted… and discuss how an investment in nursing would improve quality of care for Canadians."

Once enough nurses understood that a political solution was possible, they were able to move the campaign into the broader community by "engaging the media"—writing letters to the editor, working with advocacy and community organizations, churches, and even high schools where they met with parents and guidance counselors to explain the continuing importance of nursing as a career. Tips on how to speak at meetings, sheets of commonly asked questions and their answers, lists of people to contact, talking points, draft letters to politicians, news releases, and sample letters to the editor were all provided.

Individual nurses wrote to their members of parliament, the federal health and finance ministers, and the Prime Minister. They related their own experiences in face-to-face meetings with public officials. Representatives of major schools of nursing and professional organizations also contacted public officials.

The Quiet Crisis was a campaign of very short duration. But there is a continuing effort to encourage provincial governments to alleviate the nursing shortage and improve the conditions of nursing work. So far there has been a flurry of provincial activity to put more money into hiring nurses in hospitals and other institutions, to fund more places for students in nursing schools, and to repatriate nurses back in their home provinces from the US. Interestingly, in promotional brochures, some Canadian hospitals are trying to recruit US nurses by pitching Canada as the only place in North America where profit does not drive treatment and care decisions.

In this campaign, as in the others we have described, nurses weren't just trying to polish their image and increase their status. They were campaigning to secure resources to defend a profession central to the health care delivery system and to protect the health care system itself. In the process, they showed thousands of nurses the power of their collective and individual voices.

Endnotes

1. L. Moneiro, "Nightingale and Her Correspondence: Portrait of the Era," *Florence Nightingale and Her Era: A Collection of New Scholarship*, V.L. Bullough, B. Bullough, and M.P. Stanton, Eds. (New York: Garland Publishing Inc. 1990).

2. J.E. Lynaugh, Interview with the authors, 2000.

3. T. Hunt, and J.E. Grunig, *Public Relations Techniques* (Fort Worth: Harcourt Brace College Publishers,1994), p. 47.

4. T. S. Purdum, "California to Set Level of Staffing for Nursing Care," *New York Times*, 12 October 1999.

5. B. Sibbald, "'Dumbing Down' of Quebec RN Education Irks Nurses, MDs," *Canadian Medical Association Journal*, 158 no. 10 (May 19, 1998): p. 1262.

6. S. Gordon, "Grim Prognosis: Discouraging University-Trained Nurses Threatens Health Care," *Montreal Gazette*, 30 March 1998: p. B3.

7. B. Adams, "My Turn: Protecting our Patients," *Newsweek*, 16 November 1998: p. 17.

8. D. Henton, "Manitoba Haunted by Flurry of Baby Deaths. Inquest Probes 'Excessive' Infant Mortality Rate at Winnipeg Centre," *Toronto Star*, 13 October 1996.

9. H. Robertson, "Heartbreak," *Elm Street*, March 1998.

10. J. Marquis, "Deaths Shadow UCLA Physician," *Los Angeles Times*, 25 June 1998.

11. J. Marquis, "Doctor under Inquiry Gets UCLA Fellowship Extension," *Los Angeles Times*, 29 July 1998.

12. R. Holding and W. Carlsen, "Epidemic Ravages Caregivers: Thousands Die from Diseases Contracted through Needle Sticks," *San Francisco Chronicle*, 13, 14, 15 April 1998.

13. J. Jagger *et al.*, "Rates of Needle-stick Injury Caused by Various Devices in a University Hospital," *New England Journal of Medicine*, 319 no. 5 (1988): pp. 284–88.

Chapter 9

IN YOUR OWN VOICE: WRITING LETTERS TO THE EDITOR AND OP-EDS

Letters to the editor and op-ed sections are places where readers and outside contributors can express their views. These can be powerful forums for nurses. This chapter gives pointers on how to write letters and op-ed articles and how to get them published.

Most news publications provide space for the views of people not affiliated with the publication. The most widely known is the letters-to-the-editor page. Here readers may complain or praise coverage, give their slant on a current issue, set the record straight, or highlight their own or their group's activities in connection with a current issue. The key is to do it briefly.

Letters sections usually receive many more submissions than are published. Newspapers and magazines get a number of letters that are simply unpublishable because they are long-winded diatribes, libelous attacks, or just nonsensical. Publications welcome timely well-written letters and some smaller and medium sized newspapers may publish a good percentage of the acceptable letters they receive. There is much more competition for publication at big-city newspapers and national magazines. Nevertheless, a letter to such a publication may influence coverage even if it is not published.

Today, most news publications and many consumer magazines also provide a place for guest opinion columns. Almost every daily newspaper in North America reserves part of a page or a full page for opinion columns. In journalism jargon, this is known as the op-ed page because it is usually located "opposite" the "editorial" page, hence the contraction op-ed. The actual articles found on these pages are also referred to as "op-eds."

Op-ed pages usually contain a mixture of pieces by regular columnists (on staff or syndicated) and essays or analytical articles by outside contributors. These contributors may be people who are involved in a current issue and have a particular slant or expertise to offer, professional freelance journalists or authors presenting a "take" on a timely topic, or ordinary citizens who have an important insight or experience to relate. Op-ed editors sometimes solicit a piece when they think that certain points of view haven't been represented.

Most op-eds are chosen from the manuscripts that come in "over the transom." Over the last 30 years, the op-ed page or feature has grown in popularity. While some newspapers have very little uncommitted space on their op-ed pages, others, and certainly many magazines, are open to unsolicited submissions.

For nurses, the op-ed offers an opportunity to engage in and influence the national conversation about health care and to convey nursing's expertise to general and select audiences. Whether the op-ed is in a newspaper, business publication, health care publication, news magazine or women's magazine, it provides a singular forum for the writer to put her or his mark on the issue. An op-ed can be like a pebble projecting ripples in a pond. By giving the public a "new" view of the subject, nurses can stimulate wider discussion and media coverage of both an issue and their profession. No other media forum allows the "expert" to direct the discussion in quite this way. This is why many MDs and PhDs use this opportunity so regularly. Nurses can do more of the same.

While the typical op-ed is no more than 750 to 800 words, some publications reserve slots for longer unsolicited analytical pieces. Sunday week-in-review and analysis sections of newspapers may accept pieces up to 1,500 words. Public policy magazines may also accept such submissions. This kind of piece covers more facets of an issue than the typical op-ed. A potential contributor usually talks over a proposed piece with the editor to see if there is any interest and to determine what angle would be most appealing.

Since letters to the editor provide the quickest and easiest route to publication, we'll examine that form first.

Writing Letters to the Editor

The letters page or section is the bridge between the readers and the publication. "It is the one vehicle for regularly publishing citizen comment. It facilitates lively community debate not possible on the news pages. And, it is often the only recourse for those who feel offended or damaged by something they read here," says media critic Mark Jurkowitz.[1]

For nurses, writing a letter to the editor is one of the simplest and most effective ways to:

- Correct an error.
- Affirm and encourage positive news coverage.
- Educate journalists and producers about nursing.
- Educate the public.

- Establish your credentials.
- Change the way a topic is covered and increase public knowledge about that subject.
- Make nursing visible.

Letters to the editor can shape and alter coverage. They do this by providing editors, producers and reporters with feedback on their coverage and sometimes with education on the issues. Radio and television outlets rarely have anything equivalent to a letters page. The way that viewers and listeners get their opinions aired is by calling the talk shows. However, letters directed to producers of news in every medium, including radio and television, assures them that their work is being seen, heard and noted. It shows the media that nurses are out there, that they're paying attention, and that they will respond to what is reported.

If you see coverage that is erroneous and must be corrected, or coverage that deserves praise, by all means respond quickly with a letter and, perhaps, a phone call. When Mark Jurkowitz was ombudsman for the *Boston Globe*, he asked nine editors how readers who want "to connect with a newsroom decision maker and force the paper to rethink its coverage" could do so.[2] The editors suggested that readers should first call the reporter and bring the problem to his or her attention. (We would recommend that such a call be made to commend a reporter as well.) If there is no resolution, or the reporter can't be reached, the caller should try to get through to the editor of the section.

Some of the editors said that they would prefer to receive a letter that succinctly makes the point. Whether the contact is oral, written, or both, "Don't spend a lot of time arguing about what's been printed," said managing editor Gregory L. Moore. "Instead, come in to sell me on what you think should be covered ... with backup information and sources for contacts."

Although journalists pride themselves on not being pressured by organized groups or individuals, positive or negative feedback alerts reporters and their editors to different perspectives and can inform coverage. Reaching out to journalists and editors is particularly important if people are concerned about the treatment of a subject like health care.

A direct but courteous approach works better than a harangue. Maintain an even, reasonable tone in all contacts with the media, oral or written. "No matter how angry you are, avoid conspiracy theories and vicious personal attacks," Jurkowitz advises.[3] A good way to build the bridge is to say you appreciate the reporter's effort and then calmly state your criticism. Give specific examples of what was underplayed, overplayed, or misreported, and suggest what should be handled differently.

Contacting the newspaper ombudsman can be an effective way to call attention to a problem. Bernice Buresh e-mailed *Globe* ombudsman Jack Thomas when she saw an author on science history described in a feature article as "a diminutive woman writer from New York." Buresh suggested that the newspaper apply the same standard to men by referring to John Kenneth Galbraith, for example, as "a tall man writer from Cambridge." Thomas thanked her for sensitizing his antennae to sexist writing, said he would discuss double standards with the reporter and editors, and quoted her remarks in his column.

The aim is to be taken seriously, and that happens when nurses respond in an effective manner. Letters to publications, can, over time, stimulate cultural change. In the 1970s, women wrote thousands of letters to media outlets before reporters put women on their lists of sources, called women for comment, and enlarged their definition of newsworthiness by covering issues of concern to women. Eventually, media stylebooks were rewritten to be less male oriented and more gender neutral. Most style books now point out that professions are not gender specific and, therefore, reporters should not put "woman" or "male" in front of "professor," "writer," "doctor," or "nurse."

One of the most egregious examples of a reportorial double standard toward nursing occurred in a *Washington Post* Health Section article, "Telling the Doctor Where It Hurts." The article was not only oblivious to the contributions of nurses, but demeaned and effaced the nurse who was the initiator of what the reporter described as "a recent revolution in beliefs about children and pain."[4]

"The revolution had an unlikely catalyst," staff reporter Amy Goldstein wrote. "During the late 1970s, a nurse at the University of Iowa Hospital was struck by differences in the way her children and adult patients were treated for pain after operations. In a master's thesis, she concluded that 37 percent of the adults but only 13 percent of the children received narcotics, while 29 percent of the adults and 12 percent of the children received non-narcotic pain treatments.

"In other words, three fourths of the pediatric patients received no relief for pain during their entire hospital stay."

There was no further mention of the nurse researcher in the article. The article did, however, give the names of researchers in other disciplines and quoted them. Nurse Elaine McCann French responded with the letter below.

French constructed a very effective letter.

First, she said that the cited article provided interesting information on children and pain, thus establishing the subject and giving credit for what was conveyed.

Washington Post Health, April 16, 1991

Nurses' Role with Children in Pain

The article on telling the doctor where it hurts [Children's Health, March 26] provided much interesting information on the topic of children and pain. As a nurse, I was concerned by Amy Goldstein's treatment of the nursing profession.

The article states that anesthesiologists, pediatricians, psychologists and "other health care professionals" have made significant contributions in this area. She writes further that the revolution in beliefs about children and pain "had an unlikely catalyst"—research done by a nurse at the University of Iowa.

On the contrary, a nurse is very likely to be at the source of research and health care planning for children in pain, since assessment of pain in children falls very largely in the realm of the nursing profession. Whether in an emergency room or an in-patient unit, a child patient is assessed by a nurse initially as well as on an ongoing basis.

The writer names five health care professionals who have done work on children and pain; however, in describing the pioneering research in this field, she credits it only to "a nurse."

Elaine McCann French
Rockville, Maryland

Then she stated her professional credential ("As a nurse"). It is essential to include this in the body of the letter because some publications cut off the "RN" after a name even though they permit "MD" as an identifier. In the same sentence, French made her general point ("I was concerned by Amy Goldstein's treatment of the nursing profession").

Briefly, French specified the problems:

1. The reporter credits specific professions other than nursing for their contributions to the field.

2. The reporter incorrectly writes that "the revolution" "had an unlikely catalyst" because nurses are likely to be in the forefront both in research and patient care in this area.

We later spoke with the copy editor who handled the children's pain story. She said that, until French's letter arrived, none of the four women (the reporter, editor, copy editor, and section editor) who handled the *Post's* story had even noticed that the name of the nurse researcher wasn't given nor that the tone of the story diminished her accomplishment. She told us this would never happen again.

To us, it could only have happened in the first place because ignorance and prejudice overweighed the journalistic canons of accuracy, balance and fairness. Standard operating procedure would be to name a person who is given such significance in the story. As far as we know, however, despite profuse apologies and the publication of French's letter, the *Post* never did name the researcher. She is Associate Professor Joann Eland, director of the office of information, communication and technology at the University Of Iowa College of Nursing, who continues to do research on children's pain.

New York Times, August 22, 1996

Nurse Layoffs Lower Quality of Health Care

To the Editor:

Your Aug. 19 news article on hospitals' reducing of nursing staffs should alert the public to the dangerous cost-cutting that is expected to accelerate in American hospitals.

The Pew Health Professions Committee, on which I served, recognized that there would be a reduction in the need for nurses in hospitals consonant with the expected reduction in hospital beds in the coming decade. We recommended a reduction in nurses with associate degrees and hospital school programs, in keeping with the need for baccalaureate and advanced-degree nurses to handle the complex problems of patients. We also recognized an oversupply of physicians.

However, the cutbacks you describe have less to do with changes in hospital-bed occupancy and more to do with improving the bottom line of managed-care organizations. They defy thoughtful planning and reflect the views of high-priced consultants or administrators who understand little about the primary aim of the health delivery system—care and cure of people.

Their method is an easy one: to figure out how to replace registered nurses, who represent a paltry 23 percent of hospital wages, with "patient care assistants." In many hospitals these barely trained people now give bedside care to patients who are more acutely ill during their hospital stay than ever before. Not only does this have the potential of doing harm to patients, but it also taxes those RNs who have the responsibility for supervising care.

If the marketplace believes that it can manage care, then care, not profit, is what should be managed. If the marketplace believes that competition is the solution to the health care crisis, then it must create a competitive system that protects quality.

Claire M. Fagin
Philadelphia, August 20, 1996

The writer is dean emeritus of the Pennsylvania University School of Nursing.

Claire Fagin's letter to the *New York Times* attracted a great deal of attention. Among other reactions, a prominent physician contacted Fagin to express his concerns about what was happening to nursing care. He conveyed his personal experience with hospitals that had cut nursing. He was so concerned that he introduced Fagin to the head of a private foundation, which then funded a research project on the erosion of nursing care and the resulting burdens on caregivers and patients.

Pointers on Submitting Letters to the Media

You don't have to be a specialist in the field to respond to coverage. If you have something to say, write a letter and say it.

- For newspapers and magazines, address your response to Letters to the Editor, and state that it is for publication. Include your name, address, telephone and fax numbers, and e-mail address. Publications do not run anonymous letters, and many call or send a letter to verify that you are the writer. Under some circumstances, the publication will withhold your name if you ask. But the point here is to get your name published along with "RN" if possible, and reference to your credentials, "As a nurse…"

- Make sure your letter conforms to the style of the paper, journal or magazine to which it is being submitted. "Brevity and clarity," Jurkowitz says, are the key ingredients to success. The standard length of most published letters is 200 words. If a newspaper prints letters that are only two or three paragraphs long, don't submit a four-page letter. Editors expect to trim a paragraph or two, but not much more than that. If a publication favors letters that are heavy on facts and statistics, follow suit. The best way to find out what kind of letter a news outlet will print is to read it.

- Respond in a timely fashion. If an article appears on December 2, don't wait until March to write. With e-mail and fax available, a newspaper may run letters pertaining to an article within two or three days.

- A letter that contains "news values" will be more publishable than one that doesn't.

- If you are responding to a particular article or articles, include the name of the article and date that it appeared.

- Make sure your facts are accurate. Some publications will actually fact check letters to the editor.

- A publication may ask you to condense your letter, or will do it for you. An editor may ask you for additional information. Some may edit your letter and publish it without informing you of the changes.

- Send copies of the letter to the reporter who wrote the story, to the editor of the section in which it appeared, and perhaps to the ombudsman if there is one. You can find out the names by calling the publication. If you're writing about a very serious issue, you might also want to send copies to the editor and the managing editor whose names are on the publication masthead.

The following letters are examples:

Vancouver Sun, January 13, 2000

LETTER OF THE DAY
Broken Legs or Broken Condoms, the ER Staff Cares

Crisis in the emergency department! This is news? It exists, but it is far from new.

As nurses working at St. Paul's emergency department, we have, for many years, had to battle overcrowding, struggling to care for patients expediently while attempting to assuage our guilt about making patients wait. However, there are many reasons to be proud of working at Vancouver's inner-city hospital. We would like to express a more positive view than has been recently portrayed in the media.

We have a highly educated nursing and medical team who are supportive, caring and collaborative in their approach to treating a diverse community of patients. Despite it being a challenging environment, staff who have left often choose to return to our unique department.

Patients can expect to be treated in a non-judgmental way whether they seek treatment for a broken leg, a broken heart, a broken condom or a broken needle in their arm. We provide a safe, albeit noisy, environment with humour and warmth.

Certainly from the trenches the solutions seem evident:

1. Build more extended care facilities for convalescent and geriatric patients.
2. Increase home-care services.
3. Open a temporary unit in each hospital for overflow emergency patients.
4. Increase the admission capacity of nursing schools.
5. Make nursing a more attractive career choice through public education, increased compensation for shift work and more opportunities for growth and development within the profession such as advanced nursing practice.

Lisa Moralejo and Michelle Gilbertson
Vancouver

The Boston Globe, February 22, 2000

Nurses Join Doctors in Calling for Reforms

In his February 8 column, "The doctors revolt," David Warsh seriously mischaracterizes the ad hoc ballot initiative. First, far from simply being doctors in revolt, the petition is signed and supported by health care professionals like nurses, social workers, and psychologists.

The 20,000 members of the Massachusetts Nurses Association support sweeping reforms of the current health care system. The association's longstanding "safe care campaign" and recent passage of whistle-blower protection for health care workers are just two examples of that commitment.

The petition calls for universal access to health care for citizens of Massachusetts, a moratorium on for-profit conversions, a patients' bill of rights, a cap on revenue expended on administrative costs, and a requirement that 90 percent of revenues be spent on patient care. Warsh suggests that this initiative would in itself create a crisis. It is our position that in the absence of needed and urgent reforms, our health care system will continue to deteriorate.

This initiative doesn't represent, as Jon Kingsdale of Tufts Health Plan suggested, "a law requiring water to run uphill," but rather places these questions before the citizens, many of whom join us in the call for a serious overhaul of a system that fails those in real need.

Karen Daley, RN, MPH
President, Massachusetts Nurses Association
Stoughton, Massachusetts

If you find you have enough material for a 750-word essay, by all means write an op-ed. Many a letter to the editor has evolved into an article.

The Birth of a New Forum

The op-ed page emerged as a contemporary journalistic form in the early 1970s when the news media were being pressured to grant greater access to "non-establishment" points of view. The political movements of the 1960s and '70s for expanded civil rights, an end to the war in Vietnam, and women's liberation challenged the status quo of many institutions including the news media. Some of this dissatisfaction with the news media came from journalists themselves. In a rash of new journalism reviews, reporters accused the mainstream media of representing mainly those who had power rather than functioning as a democratic forum for diverse, and even unpopular, views. Advocacy groups from the larger community and from journalism as well, demanded greater public access to news and editorial sections. The op-ed page was one of the most notable results.

Although the first op-ed page seems to have appeared in the *New York World* in the 1920s, it was limited to pieces by professional columnists.[5] The *New York Times* can thus claim credit for creating the open-access op-ed page. On September 21, 1970, readers who normally found the obituaries opposite the editorial page, instead found columns by W. W. Rostow, a political scientist, Han Suyin, a Chinese novelist, and Gerald W. Johnson, a Baltimore journalist. A *Times* editorial explained that the page would provide a place for contributors with "no institutional connection" with the *Times* to present political, social and personal views that would "very frequently be completely divergent from our own."

In 1990, in a commemoration of the 20th anniversary of the *Times* op-ed page, Robert B. Semple Jr., who had served a term as editor of the page, wrote that editors initially had no idea how many submissions the page would get. An early trickle quickly turned into a flood of manuscripts—some 60 a day. In 20 years, Semple wrote, more than 350,000 manuscripts had been submitted to the *New York Times* op-ed page. Some 21,000 were published.[6]

Semple described the process of selection: "Each incoming manuscript is read by several editors; even the articles solicited by the editors are not guaranteed publication. And those chosen for publication nearly always undergo editing.

"Long odds—but not, obviously, a significant deterrent to anyone with something to say. Nor has anyone been deterred by the fee, which, for a standard 750-word article, has remained at an inflation-proof $150 for at least a decade."

The popularity of the op-ed quickly spread to other newspapers and to magazines. They varied greatly then, and still do, as to the types of pieces they prefer and what they pay to contributors ($0 to roughly $300; with higher fees for longer Sunday "think" pieces). Today this essay form is found in weekly newspapers as well as dailies, and some newspapers even provide additional slots for op-eds in their business, health or other sections. *Newsweek's* long-lived "My Turn" column and *Maclean's* biweekly "Over to You" are notable magazine examples. The *New York Times Sunday Magazine* has its "Lives" column in which contributors reflect on a wide scope of personal experiences. Women's magazines sometimes contain columns written by non-staff members from various walks of life. Although the *Times*, like many big-city newspapers, regards its op-ed page as a magnet for policy analysis, from the beginning of the page, according to Semple, "there was a conscious effort to leaven the relentless discussion of geopolitics with offbeat and sometimes whimsical essays."

Even with stiff competition for access, the op-ed remains a forum of choice. For nurses, time dedicated to learning how to compose op-eds will be well invested. It may be necessary to submit an essay to more than one outlet, and to rewrite it several times. But there is a good chance that the article will be published in a newspaper or magazine.

The Nuts and Bolts of Op-ed Writing

An op-ed is only 750 words long, 2 1/2 to 3 double-spaced, typewritten pages. The standard form consists of four parts: lead, focus, elaboration, kicker.

1. The opening paragraph, or lead, sets the scene and tone for the reader. It may state the main point, or direct the reader toward the point. The lead could be in the form of:
    *   an anecdote or scene-setter;
    *   a summary of what has happened before;
    *   a direct statement calling for a specific action.

2. The second paragraph usually contains the focus of the piece (if it isn't already in the lead). The focal paragraph is known in journalistic jargon as the "nut graf" (meaning the core paragraph or "graf" for short), or "billboard," (meaning the paragraph that "advertises" to the reader what the article is about). Every op-ed, indeed every type of article, must have a nut graf. If you start submitting articles for publication, sooner or later an editor will ask you about your "nut graf" in just those words.

3. The rest of the article elaborates upon the focus and moves from point to point in an interesting manner using:
    *   factual statements,
    *   statistics,
    *   examples,
    *   quotations,
    *   anecdotes,
    *   explanations.

4. The kicker, or the last paragraph, wraps the article and ties it with a bow. The kicker could be:
    *   a different, dynamic or snappy restatement of the point;
    *   a direct call to action;
    *   a quotation;
    *   an anecdote;
    *   a warning.

The Op-ed Format

An op-ed must address a timely issue, one that has been in the news but has not yet been talked to death. It must, first of all, confidently express an opinion. Unlike a news article, an op-ed is not designed to present only the "facts," or take a wishy-washy "on-the-one-hand, on-the-other-hand" tone. An op-ed requires a forcefully articulated point of view.

The op-ed must also be concise. The form is strictly limited. Most op-eds run no longer than 750 or 800 words, but some, like those in *USA Today*, may be only 400 to 600 words. Submissions that vastly exceed the standard length run the risk of rejection on that basis alone.

The first and second paragraphs of an op-ed must engage the reader by offering, if not a novel approach, at least one that is non-predictable. An editor sifting through submissions may not read much beyond the first two paragraphs before consigning a manuscript to either the "further consideration" or "reject" pile.

Some editors may be so intrigued by a strong point of view that they will go beyond the normal editing and offer to help cut or reshape the piece. This is rare though. Longer commentaries—those between 1,000 and 1,500 words—should be directed to sections that accept that length.

An op-ed—even a humorous one—must address something that people care about or should care about. Health care certainly offers enough facets to keep op-ed writers busy for years. Precisely because of the broad nature of health care, however, the op-ed writer must resist the temptation to address several major points in one essay. While an op-ed can be about any number of things, the successful op-ed is only about one. The secret to op-ed writing is to organize the article around a particular point and only that point.

What Are Op-eds About?

- An op-ed can propose a solution to a pressing problem.
- An op-ed can present an unaddressed aspect of an issue or give a unusual twist to the discussion.
- An op-ed can expand on news coverage.
- An op-ed can present a personal experience that relates to a public issue.
- An op-ed can be a dramatic anecdote or narrative that describes what nurses do.

The column by Linda Aiken and Claire Fagin demonstrates how an op-ed can be employed to propose a solution to a pressing program and/or to critique an existing policy or proposal.

In early 1993, the shortage of primary-care physicians in the US became a major news story. The country's declining proportion of doctors in general

New York Times, March 11, 1993

More Nurses, Better Medicine
They need more authority for primary care

By Linda Aiken and Claire Fagin

Philadelphia—The US has a shortage of primary-care physicians. This limits the options for improving access to cost-effective health care. Nurses are a national resource with the potential to met this challenge.

Since the late 1960s, federal policy has promoted two strategies to increase primary care. The first included federal support for establishing a new physician specialty in family practice. It has not yet been successful. Between 1970 and 1990, the proportion of doctors in primary care declined, and the rate of decline is accelerating.

In contrast, the second strategy—employing advanced-practice nurses (nurse practitioners, clinical nurse specialists and nurse midwives)—has been enormously successful. Two decades of research, summarized last summer in the *Yale Journal on Regulation*, gives clear evidence that advanced-practice nurses provide care of comparable quality and at a lower cost than doctors do.

Advanced-practice nurses can safely substitute for physicians for up to 90 percent of primary care needed by children and 80 percent required by adults. The Yale report concluded that significant financial, legal and professional barriers prevent the effective use of nurses.

Yet nurse practitioners and nurse midwives prescribe fewer drugs, use fewer tests and select lower-cost treatments and settings.

Historically, nurses have been more likely than doctors to practice in areas where there is insufficient health care. Nurse anesthetists deliver 85 percent of anesthesia services in rural areas. Approximately one in five nurse practitioners and midwives practice in rural areas, and close to 50 percent of them work in inner cities.

International comparisons suggest that at least 75 percent of all prenatal care and delivery of babies could be safely provided by nurse midwives. But in the US, nurses deliver less than 4 percent of births.

The following ideas would lead to the more productive use of nurses:

- To increase primary care for Medicaid recipients, nurse practitioners and certified nurse midwives should qualify for direct reimbursement at the same rate as physicians. Bonus payments should be given to doctors and nurses in underserved rural and urban areas.
- Where fee-for-service arrangements exist, qualified nurses should be eligible for direct reimbursement by Medicare. This would save costs, not increase them.
- Hospitals must be required to offer admitting privileges to nurse midwives and nurse practitioners as a condition of participation in Medicaid and Medicare. Without admitting privileges, nurses cannot practice under state, Medicare and Medicaid legal guidelines.
- The high cost and uncertain availability of malpractice insurance for nurse midwives impede the growth of the midwifery practice. Malpractice insurance reform and possibly tort reform are required.

America needs a collaborative system where health care professionals are used appropriately and cost effectively. By better using nurses for primary care, the goals of national health care reform—improved access to appropriate services at affordable cost—can be achieved.

Linda Aiken and Claire Fagin are professors of nursing at the University of Pennsylvania. Professor Fagin is president of the National League for Nursing.

practice compared with those in specialized practice emerged as a leading concern. References to the lack of primary care in the US subsequently appeared in all sorts of stories on health care.

Few articles, however, mentioned nursing as playing a role in the solution. It was up to nursing to make the link.

In their *New York Times* op-ed, Aiken and Fagin covered a lot of ground in only 467 words.

In standard op-ed form, they led with a statement of the basic problem— the US has a shortage of primary care physicians.

The "nut graf" is the third sentence: "Nurses are a national resource with the potential to meet this challenge." Everything that follows flows from that focal point.

In their elaboration, the authors give background on the current policy and advance their argument that nurses should provide more primary care. They cite a study (that may have been the impetus for the piece) to buttress their case and to give a picture of the care that advanced-practice nurses already provide in under-served locations. In four bulleted paragraphs, they recommend specific policy changes that "would lead to the more productive use of nurses."

Their kicker is a restatement of their argument in the form of a declaration of what "America needs," and how its health care needs can be met by using nurses.

In op-ed writing, timing is everything. Aiken and Fagin took advantage of reports on the need for more primary care. Their arguments were not new in nursing. However, if they had written their op-ed when primary care was not in the news, it might not have been published. Its appearance in the most prestigious newspaper in the US indicates that the best time to get published is when the news media are paying attention—not before the issue has been raised, and not after it has crested.

New York Times, February 23, 1991

The Feminist Disdain for Nursing

By Ellen D. Baer

Philadelphia—At a recent party, a lawyer friend with whom I've shared feminist causes introduced me to her house guests as "almost a doctor."

"No," I protested. "I am a nurse"—to which she replied, "Oh, no, Ellen, you're more than a nurse."

I know her intent was to enhance my status in her friends' eyes by describing my expertise in non-nurse terms, to rescue me from the indifference or even denigration that being "only" a nurse often engenders.

This has happened so often over the years that it has come to exemplify for me the terrible paradox of feminism, which glorifies women who emulate masculine behavior while virtually ignoring women who choose traditionally female roles and careers.

I consider myself a dedicated feminist, but I refuse to accept a sort of feminism that abandons feminine caring roles in order to achieve progress. Such capitulation to masculine definitions is unacceptable and extraordinarily disappointing, when promoted by women.

I believe this has occurred with nursing because many feminists have found it too painful to look seriously at nurses' experience. It has been easier for them to hope that the fault lay within nursing, blaming the victim as it were.

The term "feminism" has come to mean "women doing what men do." If a woman merges and acquires, negotiates or forecloses and wields an ax or scalpel with the same effect as a man, she is judged to be liberated. I know it is important to struggle for a woman's right to choose to be a neurosurgeon, a lawyer or a banker. But why should that also mean that millions of us, who choose to be nurses, teachers, librarians, mothers and homemakers, are depicted as dumb, unliberated or prisoners of patriarchy?

It isn't surprising when men denigrate nurses. But when ostensibly liberated women do so, it is infuriating. I look at the shelves of libraries and bookstores, or at television, and get angry.

How dare Robin Norwood argue in *Women Who Love Too Much* that women from dysfunctional families are "over represented" in fields like nursing? Why did *Working Women* magazine list nursing, teaching and social work in its 1988 "Ten Worst Jobs" report? And why didn't Esther Shapiro of Spelling Productions correct the dumb and oversexed nurse image portrayed on the now defunct television series, "Nightingales"?

The answer is that, in general terms, nurses are women whom people can denigrate and still get away with it. No angry feminists write books protesting the poor treatment of nurses. I think that nurses and other "caregivers" are women about whom many feminists like to feel superior.

For 100 years, periodic nursing shortages have generated flurries of newspaper articles, salary increases and image-enhancement campaigns that yield some new recruits. But there will be no fundamental changes until people, including feminists, realize the critical importance of nurses in health care.

Professional nursing requires brains, education, judgment, fortitude, inventiveness, split-second decision-making, interpersonal competence, and day-after-day determination. When feminists or their families are sick, they want their own nurses to have all those traits, but they don't assign those attributes to the group as a whole.

Yet the fact that more than two million people—97 percent of them female—choose to be nurses in the face of hostility and contempt testifies to the tremendous appeal of nursing, an intellectual challenge with exquisite personal satisfaction.

Just imagine life without nurses. If some feminists have their way, and all the smart women end up in law firms, banks and boardrooms, what will become of the quality of our lives?

Lewis Thomas, the eminent physician and biologist, has described nurses as the "glue" that holds the health care system together. But that glue is losing its grip because the attitudes expressed by the women's movement cause many young people not to choose to be nurses, hospital boards not to include them in decision-making, doctors not to act like colleagues, and politicians not to support their education or reimburse them for their services.

To fully comprehend how much nurses know, how important their work is and how little they are credited is to understand the depth of the negative status of women in this society. It is imperative that real feminists address the needs of women doing "women's work."

Feminism will have succeeded not only when women have equal access to all fields but when traditionally female professions like nursing gain the high value and solid social respect they deserve.

Ellen D. Baer is associate professor at the University of Pennsylvania School of Nursing.

Like Ellen Baer's "Feminist Disdain" essay in the *New York Times,* an op-ed can elucidate an aspect that has been left out of a discussion and can give a familiar subject a new twist.

The behind-the-scenes story of her op-ed—which generated rave reviews from nurses, feminists and writers—is a story in itself about the value of persistence and networking.

Baer had written occasional letters to the editor "bemoaning," as she says, the feminist movement's lack of interest in nursing. After reading a cover story in the *New York Times Sunday Magazine* entitled, "Who Says We Haven't Made A Revolution? A Feminist Takes Stock," Baer was outraged.[7] She wrote the following to the letters section of the magazine:

> The sad irony of the feminism described by (writer Vivian) Gornick ... is that it glorifies women who emulate masculine ideals, goals, behaviors, and models. It does not admire, support, or promote societal regard for the importance of the work of women like me — wife, mother, professional nurse, teacher. In fact, the "feminists" of this revolution have tried to convince me and my peers to abandon our "women's work." As a result, the exhilaration and excitement I experienced in my 1970s consciousness-raising group turned to ashes. It's time for the women's revolution to celebrate women's work (as it has traditionally been defined). When female values command respect equal to men's, then we will have made a wonderful human revolution.

The letter was printed, but in an abbreviated form. Disturbed that the heart of her criticism had been eliminated, she wrote to the *Times* protesting the editing of her letter. A *Times* editor called, and after discussing her complaints, said that a letter to the editor could not accommodate the complexity of her argument. She should, he suggested, submit an article on the subject to the "Her's" column that then appeared in the *Times Sunday Magazine.*

Baer quickly submitted a column. She received no response. So she called the *Times.* She says she was told that the article was too polemical and was advised to rewrite and resubmit it. She did. Again the article was rejected.

Several months passed and Baer was discouraged. She expressed her feelings to Claire Fagin, then the dean of the University of Pennsylvania School of Nursing, who urged her not to give up. Fagin suggested that Baer contact us. When we saw the manuscript, it was obvious that it needed an anecdotal lead.

Baer recounted her experience of being introduced by a female, professional friend to other professionals. "Use that as your lead," we suggested.

It was important that Baer make a strong statement in the piece about her commitment to feminism if she did not want to be perceived as bashing feminism. The op-ed called for evocative, pointed language, which Baer employed.

Baer returned to the computer, redid her lead, added dramatic examples and submitted the article to "Her's." Again no success.

Several months later, Baer attended a wedding where she was seated next to a *Time* magazine columnist. She told him her frustrating story. The columnist offered to look at the piece. He said he loved it and passed it on to a friend— the editor of the *New York Times* op-ed page. The editor accepted the article.

"I fixed it up in a couple of places, and it was all set to go," Baer recalls. "Then the Gulf War started. So they called to tell me that since it was not a time-limited piece, it would go on the back burner. It was finally published on February 23, 1992. I didn't know that was going to happen until February 22 when someone from the *Times* called to suggest a few more cuts. I had to battle to keep certain things in.

"I'm very glad that other people insisted I had an important message to send to the wider world and helped me to send it."

Conveying Real-life Experiences and Describing What Nurses Do

Snapshots of physician practice are a staple of op-ed pages. Many physicians contribute stories about their moral dilemmas, relationships with patients, and successful, and unsuccessful, interventions. These narratives position physicians as the primary actors in weighing and resolving the ethical dilemmas that confront our advanced technological societies.

If nurses are to convince the public that they too are storehouses of human insight and health care expertise, they must dramatize this fact with compelling narratives. This is what nurse Jean Chaisson did in her op-ed-style article for *Technology Review*, a magazine published by the Massachusetts Institute of Technology (see reprint at the end of chapter two). It ran as a sidebar to a longer piece on contemporary nursing.[8]

In it Chaisson contrasts the nursing model with the medical model. Rather than elaborating this point theoretically or polemically, she uses an experience from her practice to describe the distinction. The approach tells the reader something he or she probably didn't know, that nurses, not just physicians, serve as expert witnesses in legal disputes.

Chaisson's depiction of the differences between medicine and nursing is never shrill. It is unlikely to be construed as "doctor bashing." She does, however, stand up for her profession. Through metaphors like "with physicians as the lens and disease as the definition of the field," she gets to her point that nurses look at the whole human being not just at their angry scars and aching joints.

Placing Your Op-ed

Compose your op-ed with certain publications in mind. For each one:

1. Find out the name of the op-ed editor and contact information. If it is not given in the publication, call the op-ed department.

2. When you have written the op-ed, mail, e-mail or fax it directly to that editor, preferably with a note briefly citing your credentials or experience with this issue.

3. Give the editor a few days to read it and follow up with a phone call. If you are successful in reaching the editor, be prepared to answer any questions, address any reservations and enthusiastically "sell" the idea and its importance.

4. If you can't get an editor on the phone, persist in calling. If your calls aren't returned, don't assume it's because the editor isn't interested. Encourage the editor to use it, but then get an answer as to whether it will or won't be used. If your article is rejected try to find out why so that you can alter your approach if necessary to increase your chances of success at another publication. Large papers get so many submissions that they usually send a form rejection. It's unlikely they will take the time to discuss your piece with you. Smaller papers might give you useful feed-back.

5. If you are trying to get a response to an idea for an op-ed, explain who you are, why the issue is important, and why your point of view will add to the debate. In many cases, an e-mail query will work better than a phone call. Sometimes editors won't respond to either. In that event, send in your written essay.

6. If you have any personal contacts that can be useful at a publication—a reporter in another section, a neighbor who knows an editor at the paper, or a fellow wedding guest—don't be shy about using them.

7. Since all op-eds are "on spec," which means that editors do not guarantee publication, if an editor is interested he or she will suggest that you submit it for consideration. Don't be discouraged by the lack of a firm commitment.

8. Unless you have a commitment from an editor, you can certainly submit your op-ed to any number of publications.

9. Acceptance is not the end of the process. Editing comes next. Editors may make suggestions for revisions. Be prepared to accept good suggestions and argue against those that seriously alter your meaning or tone.

Chaisson shows that doctors aren't the only ones who diagnose patients' problems. Without condemning physicians, she allows salient facts to emerge from the narrative: doctors not only abandoned this patient to her pain, they were unable to help her secure even the meager disability payments she needed to survive. Chaisson introduces another person, the patient's son, to pay tribute to nursing. "Nobody has ever asked her about these things before," he says. "Nobody has cared what it is like for her."

In her kicker, Chaisson speaks from her own agency to assert that a health care system that ignores the human experience of illness can produce neither health nor care. Without being boastful, she underlines her contribution to this woman's care and, by extension, teaches the reader what nurses have to offer: "Other health care professionals had talked about her disease: I asked about her life."

Revising a Nursing Journal Article

An op-ed can be a piece from a nursing journal that is revised or shortened for a general audience.

Critical-care nurse Marjorie Funk wrote a poignant account of her father's death in a critical-care unit for *IMAGE: Journal of Nursing Scholarship*. The article, "Caring," appeared in an op-ed type forum in the nursing journal. It was an ideal candidate for an op-ed for a general audience as well. Even though Funk is a critical-care nurse who worked on the unit where her father was hospitalized, her anguish while trying to decide what would be in his best interests linked her experience to those of other sons and daughters concerned about the quality of their parents lives and deaths. It was the kind of human interest piece that newspapers are eager to have.

Funk's article is very well executed. Her repeated use of the phrase "...and said no," draws the reader's empathy to her deliberation, decision making, and sadness. Two sorts of revisions made it more marketable for a general audience

The first was the conversion into everyday language of initials (MI, GI...), nurse-speak ("relative contraindications"), and the names of drugs (nitroglycerin, heparin) so that a lay audience could understand what these things meant.

The second was the addition of a clear explanation of why she deemed the available technology inappropriate for her father. She further connected her experience to that of others by showing empathy for lay people who must go through this trial, and by pointing out the obstacles posed by managed care.

When she submitted the revised piece to the *Boston Globe*, it was accepted.

IMAGE: Journal of Nursing Scholarship, Summer 1992

Caring

By Marjorie Funk

On Saturday, April 27, 1991 my father had chest pain. He was evaluated in the Emergency Room of Bristol Hospital, where they determined that he was having an acute MI. They discussed giving him thrombolytic therapy to dissolve whatever clots might be occluding his coronary arteries. His history of GI bleeding and TIAs were relative contraindications to this type of therapy—but the decision was mine. I thought about it carefully ... and said no.

Because there were no ICU beds available in Bristol Hospital, he was taken by ambulance to Yale-New Haven and admitted to the Coronary Care Unit. He arrived about 10 p.m. The issue of thrombolytic therapy was again raised. Again, I deliberated ... and said no.

He was attached to a monitor, had his vital signs taken frequently and received continuous infusions of IV nitroglycerin and heparin—all usual care for patients with acute MIs. He continued to have intermittent chest pain. They gave him a little morphine. He seemed to be having a little trouble breathing and his oxygen saturation dropped. Maybe he was going into congestive heart failure. A pulmonary artery catheter would provide the necessary data to guide further therapy. They suggested taking him into the Procedure Room and inserting this device. I considered it ... and said no.

A little later we discussed whether he should be resuscitated if he arrested. I carefully considered this ... and said no.

I stayed at his bedside all night. He slept some. Although his breathing seemed a bit labored at times, he did not appear uncomfortable. About 7 a.m., his blood pressure dropped and he suddenly became unresponsive. For a brief moment, I shifted gears—I had worked as a nurse in that unit for years. I knew exactly what to do. Lower the head of the bed, call for the code cart, get the arrest board under his back, begin CPR, prepare to administer ... They asked me if I wanted them to do anything. I took a deep breath ... and said no.

I continued to hold his hand. A number of people gathered quietly in the room—nurses, physicians and even some of my students—my friends. He died about five minutes later.

I was alone. My favorite person in the whole world had just died. Where was the rest of my family? Mom was back in the convalescent home where she shared a room with Pop—they both had Alzheimer's disease. She would never know that he died. My brother was home sleeping—he was planning to come in a little later to be with Pop so I could go home to sleep.

No, I wasn't alone—my friends were there. They hugged me, some cried. I felt caring and support.

They seemed to support my decisions to forgo all the technology. How ironic—my professional life had been centered on the highly technical critical care environment. In my practice, I had worked to master the technology. I had tried to teach my students the technical skills necessary for the delivery of proficient care—maintaining that being technically competent was one of the most visible ways a nurse can exhibit caring. My own research concerns the safe and appropriate use of technology.

Over the last 12 hours, I had deemed just about all the available technology inappropriate for my father. Will I ever be totally at peace with these decisions, made alone, but deliberately and contemplatively ... ?

Marjorie Funk, RN, MSN, CCRN, Delta Mu, is Assistant Professor, Yale University School of Nursing, doctoral candidate, Yale School of Medicine, Department of Epidemiology and Public Health and staff nurse in the coronary care unit, Yale-New Haven Hospital.

Boston Globe, May 30, 1994

Doctors, Nurses, Don't Forget the Human Touch

By Marjorie Funk

Late on a Saturday afternoon my 88-year-old father, who had Alzheimer's disease and had been in a nursing home for three months, developed chest pains. He was rushed to the emergency room of our local hospital, where physicians determined that he was having a heart attack. They discussed giving him medicine to dissolve the blood clots that were presumably blocking his coronary arteries and causing the heart attack. His history of small strokes increased the danger of this type of therapy—but as his daughter, with power of attorney, the decision was mine. I thought about it carefully and said no.

Because there were no intensive care beds available in the local hospital, he was taken to a nearby urban teaching hospital and admitted to the coronary care unit, where I worked part-time as a staff nurse and taught students as a professor of nursing. The issue of administering the clot-dissolving medication was again raised. Again, I deliberated and said no.

He was attached to a monitor, had his vital signs taken frequently and received intravenous nitroglycerin and heparin—usual care for patients with heart attacks. He continued to have intermittent chest pain. His nurse gave him a little morphine. He seemed to be having a little trouble breathing, and the oxygen level in his blood dropped. The doctors and nurses worried that he might be going into congestive heart failure. A pulmonary artery catheter would provide the necessary data to guide further therapy. They suggested inserting this device. I considered it, and said no.

A little later we discussed whether he should be resuscitated if he had a cardiac arrest. I carefully considered this, and said no.

I stayed at his bedside all night. He slept some. Although his breathing seemed a bit labored at times, he did not appear uncomfortable. About 7 a.m., his blood pressure dropped and he lost consciousness. For a moment, I shifted gears. I had worked as a nurse in that unit for many years. I knew exactly what to do. Lower the head of the bed, call for the resuscitation cart, get the arrest boards under his back, begin CPR. The staff asked me if I wanted them to do anything. I took a deep breath, and said no.

I continued to hold his hand. A number of people gathered quietly in the room—nurses, physicians, some of my students—my friends. My father died about five minutes later.

For years, my professional life has focused on the highly technical critical-care environment. In my nursing practice I have worked hard to master the technology. I have tried to teach these technical skills to my students. I have long maintained that being technically competent was one of the most visible ways a nurse could exhibit caring. Even the research I have been conducting concerns the safe and appropriate use of technology.

Yet over 12 hours, I had deemed just about all the available technology inappropriate for my beloved father. As an experienced health care professional, I had a realistic sense of the odds. I knew that after a massive heart attack there would be little chance of full recovery. I knew that dependence on medical technology, such as a ventilator to assist his breathing, would have increased the confusion of his Alzheimer's. I was aware of myriad possible complications. Even knowing all this, I agonized. I needed all the support I received from the nurses and physicians, who also happened to be my professional colleagues and friends.

As I reflect on my own experience, I am struck by how difficult it must be for the average person, with no medical background, to make these decisions. We health care providers hide behind our legalistic strategies of living wills, advance directives and health care proxies and assail patients' families with statistical data on the probability of recovery. We assume that people who are facing the most frightening decisions a human being can confront and who have entered an alien medical culture can somehow engage in a complex series of rational deliberations. My decisions were made a bit easier not just by my familiarity with the highly technical hospital environment but also by the support I felt from the hospital staff. Somehow, we as health care professionals have to extend that level of understanding and attention to all patients and their loved ones. We need to encourage dialogue about options, and we need to create systems that enable this to happen.

It is alarming to realize that the managed care that has become so pervasive may be doing just the opposite. We seem to be racing patients through the system and denying providers time to work with and support them, as my colleagues worked with and supported me. As we design and debate health care reform, human exchanges aimed at understanding must be valued as much as heroic interventions aimed at cure.

Marjorie Funk is an associate professor at Yale University School of Nursing and a part-time staff nurse in the coronary care unit at Yale-New Haven Hospital.

A Deeper Perspective

Suzanne Gordon's article for the *Gazette* in Montreal is an example of a critique of a policy proposal that adds depth to the discussion. In this case, Gordon adds an international and feminist perspective to what appears to be a local issue. The op-ed editor decided not to trim this 1,100-word-plus article, which might have also found a home in a Sunday section.

The lead sets up the dilemmas that nurses—and by extension—patients face because nursing education is not taken as seriously as medical education.

Paragraph two sets up the focus by providing a historical context to the issue at hand—Quebec's move to cut off access to nursing through university schools. It conveys the idea that what is going on in Quebec is illustrative of a larger dynamic.

A great deal of the piece concentrates on the historical underpinnings of the current debate. In paragraph 9, Gordon gives Canada credit for being a progressive global force in nursing education. She then links that forward thinking to what nurses actually do in hospitals. Later the author introduces readers to nurses' work in the home and community.

Paragraphs 14 and 15 bring us into the ever-changing world of health care, further explaining why university education for nurses is critical.

In the kicker, Gordon uses the government ministers' own words to advise them to reconsider their recent decision.

The Gazette, Montreal, March 30, 1998

COMMENT

Grim prognosis discouraging university-trained nurses threatens health care

By Suzanne Gordon

One of the great paradoxes of Western health care lies in the fact that our industrialized societies have given a large group of women—and some men—responsibility for the care of the sickest of our citizens without simultaneously giving them the education, authority, respect, and resources needed to fulfill this mission. In Canada and the United States, and most other Western nations, nurses are the largest profession in health care, outnumbering doctors almost four to one. Yet, for over a century, nurses have been struggling to obtain the kind of high-quality education doctors take for granted.

Indeed, the history of nursing education is one of the longest running feminist struggles in any profession in either Canada or the United States. When nurses try to win public support for this struggle, they have often been confronted with hostility, indifference and lack of understanding when they appeal for help from public officials. The recent move by the Quebec's minister of education to close off direct access to nursing through university schools of nursing is a sad case in point.

The decision to close the university as one of the two routes to nursing, and by forcing nurses to enter the profession through the college route, as well as by assigning nursing assistants responsibility for the elderly and chronically ill in nursing homes and long-term care facilities, demonstrates yet again politicians' lack of understanding of the non-negotiable elements of high-quality care for the sick.

Mistakes of the Past

One would have thought politicians and health policy experts would have learned from the mistakes of the past.

At the turn of the century, the status of nurses relative to doctors was far less inferior than it is today. In the ensuing decades, physicians were able to create a coherent system of academic medical training and gain control of medical practice. Nurses were unable to do the same.

In the early 1900s, nurses were trained in schools which were wholly owned and operated by hospitals and which were adamantly not educational institutions. Offering young women room and board and a rudimentary introduction to physiology, pharmacology and other scientific principles, they viewed student nurses as a cheap labor force, not as learners. Members of this cheap labor force would be expected to log 12-to-14-hour days and then remain awake for a few classes at night. Hospitals limited nurses' occupational mobility by tying their educational credentials to a particular institution, that is, a hospital school or training program and its needs.

Hospitals also successfully gained and maintained control over the money used for nursing education. Thus, nursing was effectively tethered to the institutions that purchased nursing services.

In Quebec, the hospital schools stopped admitting students only in 1969 and were replaced by the CEGEP system of three-year nursing programs. Nursing leaders have, however, fought to make entry into the profession at the university level with a minimum baccalaureate degree.

Canada has been one of the world's leaders in the effort to give nurses the education necessary to provide high-quality care of the sick and, with the exception of Ontario and Quebec, most other provinces have taken steps to make a university degree a minimum requirement for the practice of nursing.

They do this because they know that caring for sick patients today is an enormously arduous endeavor that demands a great deal of education. In hospitals today, nurses are caring for patients who often have multiple diseases: a patient in congestive heart failure who also has a history of chronic kidney disease, a diabetic man with an amputation who is now admitted with a gall bladder attack, or a woman with heart disease whose breast cancer has just recurred. These patients are taking a variety of medications, increasing the chance of untoward drug interactions, and they may be monitored using high tech machinery that requires sophisticated training to comprehend and manipulate.

Aggressive Therapies

To treat their diseases and disorders, medicine mobilizes toxic, invasive and aggressive therapies that can not only cure but kill. Nurses help insure that patients survive these therapies, while at the same time educating patients about their illnesses and treatments, dealing with their emotional concerns and helping their families cope.

In hospitals, nurses are the ones who make sure the 72-year-old man who has just had a stroke does not have an impaired gag reflex and can be safely fed, thus preventing the kind of aspiration pneumonia that will put him in the intensive care unit and add thousands more dollars to the cost of his care. They are the ones who make sure the woman recovering from a compound fracture in her leg after a skiing accident doesn't develop a blood clot in the leg that can lead to pulmonary embolus which can be rapidly fatal. It is nursing care, not doctors' care, that prevents the kind of horrendous bedsores that can cost up to $50,000 to heal.

Provide Primary Care

In the home and community, nurses are the ones who assure the safety and provide the primary care for the 85-year-old patient who has a slow-growing prostate cancer as well as coronary artery disease, and they are the ones who help the 80-year-old woman crippled by rheumatoid arthritis as well as a heart condition take care of her 82-year-old husband who has just had a stroke, has diabetes, can't walk or speak, and is incontinent.

As medical science has advanced over the past decades, nurses must understand patho-physiology, high tech interventions, the kind of complex surgery and invasive procedures that patients will undergo. Today, patients on a regular hospital floor are on ventilators, receiving dialysis and getting other treatments that would have only been given on intensive-care units 20 years ago, while patients in clinics and at home are treated with the kind of therapies that would only have been administered in the hospital on an in-patient basis.

Today, nursing has been transformed not only by medical and nursing science and research but by changes in health policy that move sicker patients in and out of the hospital more quickly and push care into the home and community.

When health minister Jean Rochon and education minister Pauline Marois say that the situation has changed in health care and the social services, they are absolutely right. That is why nurses today need more education, not less—and why the ministers immediately should reconsider their decision to close university education and help advance the cause of patient care.

Suzanne Gordon is a Boston-based journalist who writes about nursing and health care. She is adjunct professor in McGill University's school of nursing.

Try and Try Again

In writing letters, op-eds and longer articles, the main thing to remember is that you can't succeed without trying. There are many publications—major newspapers, regional newspapers, small town dailies or weeklies, news magazines, women's magazines—that are looking for intelligent, new points of view.

Nevertheless, nurses who are frequently published in letters pages or op-ed sections, rarely have all or even most of their work accepted.

"I've had many letters to the editor published in major newspapers like the *New York Times* or *Philadelphia Inquirer*," says Claire Fagin. "I've succeeded because I've written so many. When I see something I like, I write to compliment the reporter. When I see something that concerns me, I go to the computer and express my views. Because people see me in print, they think that my scorecard is better than it is. For all the pieces I've had published, I've had many more rejected. In fact, I could publish a volume called The Unpublished Letters and Articles of Claire Fagin. My advice is just keep writing."

Endnotes

1. M. Jurkowitz, "A Drawbridge of Letters," *Boston Globe*, 29 May 1995, p. 13.

2. M. Jurkowitz, "Getting Through to the Globe," *Boston Globe*, 30 October 1995.

3. Jurkowitz, "Drawbridge of Letters," p. 13.

4. A. Goldstein, "Telling the Doctor Where It Hurts," *Washington Post*, 26 March 1991.

5. C.M. Antin, "Letter: Where First an Op-ed Page Was Seen," *New York Times*, 15 October 1990.

6. R.B. Semple Jr., "Op-ed at 20," *New York Times*, 30 September 1990, p. 4A.

7. V. Gornick, "Who Says We Haven't Made A Revolution? A Feminist Takes Stock," *New York Times Sunday Magazine*, 15 April 1990, pp. 24–27, 52–53.

8. S. Gordon, "The Importance of Being Nurses," *Technology Review*, October 1992.

Chapter 10
APPEARING ON
TELEVISION
AND RADIO

Radio and television offer limitless opportunities for nursing to become better known. This chapter covers the essentials of appearing on interview programs and talk shows.

One fall morning, Cindy Dalton, a nurse who works in a Montreal community health center, the CLSC Metro, was about to make her television debut. As she waited in the "green room" near the set of the program "Montreal Today," she reflected upon the fact that the sum total of her media experience consisted of being interviewed for five minutes on the radio. Now she was about to appear on a major television show to talk about the nursing crisis in Quebec. Her fellow guest was Suzanne Gordon. Dalton told Gordon that she was nervous. Gordon suggested that she rehearse. Gordon pointed out that the segment on nursing would be only six minutes. "Deducting the time spent on questions from the host, we'll each have about two and a half minutes," she said. She suggested that Dalton prepare an anecdote so that she could use that time to convey the importance of what nurses do.

Dalton thought for a moment. "I work as a community health nurse in the area of family health," she began. "I begin working with families during pregnancy and continue until the kids are six years of age. The other day a pregnant Chinese woman had trouble getting her needs across when she visited the obstetrician. Doctors don't have much time these days, so it's important to ask them the right questions. I worked with her to prioritize her questions and make a list."

Since it was close to airtime, Gordon interrupted. "The problem with this anecdote is that it doesn't focus on you, the nurse," she said. "It focuses on the physician, on the busy man or woman who has no time. You want to highlight the importance of nursing. Is there another anecdote you could use?"

Dalton considered the question. Then she described her home care work with a multiple sclerosis patient who could no longer walk on his own. The man spent his days sitting on the sofa while his wife cared for their two children, a two-and-a-half-year old and an infant. Although he was unsteady using a walker, the patient refused to use a wheelchair or modify his home to accommodate his condition. He was depressed because the only thing he could manage was to go to the bathroom. He was so afraid he would drop his infant that he wouldn't even hold the baby. As she began explaining how she helped this patient, Dalton suddenly stopped.

Gordon asked her why.

Dalton looked frozen. "I can't use that anecdote. It's private," she said. "The patient might listen to the show. Telling his story would be a breach of patient confidentiality."

"Just change the details," "Gordon said. Make him a woman, change the ages of the children."

"But if I do that, I'm lying," Dalton protested. "Then I'm going to have trouble being truthful while I'm on the air." Dalton said she was also concerned that if she pared her story to a few sentences, people would not "hear the nursing."

Gordon assured her that she would feel more comfortable with a little practice and that if she talked about her nursing work, listeners would not miss the point.

As the two approached the set, Gordon coached Dalton to "take advantage of whatever opening the host gives you to bring up your anecdote."

When the cameras rolled, host Leslie Roberts immediately said to Dalton: "Tell me a bit about your work if you can. You've been a nurse for 12 years. Is it getting worse? Do you see the crisis or is it being blown up by the media?"

"Definitely, nurses are more challenged in the present health care system," Dalton said. "Every time there's a challenge you have to adjust to it and today the challenges are coming more quickly and the period of adjustment is shortened."

The host had been asking for a general description of nurses' problems. But Dalton astutely took advantage of the opening he gave her to bring the audience into the world of daily nursing practice.

"I can give you an example of the kind of work I do," she continued. "At the moment I'm working at a CLSC with families with young children. But I also work with people who have chronic illnesses. When I went to visit one family in their home recently, I found they had a newborn baby and the wife had multiple sclerosis. It was a challenge for me to work with her because she was very depressed. The husband was taking on more and more work with the newborn baby. For the first time in her life, the wife couldn't walk but was reluctant to use a wheelchair. I knew she could fall and if she fell, it would cost more health care dollars because she would need more services. I was also concerned about the baby. I had to take on a very important role in taking care of her."

After this anecdote, Roberts asked Gordon to talk about the problems nurses face in the United States. Another guest, Pierre Salinger, who had been press secretary to President John F. Kennedy (and who had addressed the Clinton/Lewinsky scandal in his segment moments earlier) broke in citing statistics about the scandalously high number of uninsured citizens in the US. Turning to Dalton, Roberts asked if Canadians should solve their health care crisis by becoming more like the United States.

Although Dalton is not a health policy expert, she did not hesitate to voice her opinion. "No," Dalton answered. "The solution is to strengthen the present health care system. My own personal opinion is that under privatization there would be people who need services and couldn't afford them or would not get good services."

Roberts argued that Canada already has a two-tiered health care system with some people getting better care than others. Dalton agreed that while "there are some services you can pay for and get quicker, we still have universal health care and we should maintain it. It's very important."

Then she bridged to more discussion of nursing.

"Nursing is also very important," she explained. "When you go to the emergency room, the first person you see is a nurse. When you're going to have an operation, the person who prepares you before surgery is a nurse. What's the first thing that happens when you open your eyes? Who are you going to see at your bedside? A nurse. When you're going to ring your call bell at night for help because you're in pain, or you're worried about being sent home the next day, who's going to come to your room? A nurse." Roberts and Salinger were riveted.

After the show Dalton was exhilarated. "As I started to talk about nursing, I became more and more energized," she said. "At first I was preoccupied by the set, the lights, the people walking around making strange signals to one another. Because the host kept nodding his head, I was worried that I was taking too much time and that he wasn't interested in what I had to say. I was too focused on his agenda. I was letting the setting paralyze me.

"Then I remembered why I was here. I was here for a purpose—for nursing. I realized I had to focus on my agenda. Once I got comfortable, the ideas started coming to me. At the end, I felt I could do this again. If I did, I would be much better."

With preparation, a sense of purpose, and the conviction that nurses have a right to speak for themselves and their profession, most nurses will find that it isn't all that hard to speak on television or radio or in front of a live audience.

The basic rules are:

- Prepare, prepare, prepare.
- Create three "bumper stickers."
- Be credible.
- Be accessible.
- Be enthusiastic.
- Speak with conviction.

How to Feel in Control

As with patient care, the best way to feel you're in charge is to get as much information as possible in advance.

If a reporter or producer calls you to arrange an appearance on a radio or TV program, ask the name of the show and of the host who will be interviewing you. Producers rather than the on-air reporters or talk-show hosts usually make the initial contact.

Find out if the show is on health care or public policy. Is it an entertainment show? Is it a Rafe Mair or a Chris Matthews style show that encourages conversational dueling? This will tell you what kind of audience it attracts and how to prepare.

There are many different kinds of television and radio programs. Some are fast-paced entertainment shows that rely on glib retorts. Some try to generate controversy for controversy's sake. Others are more interested in drawing out solid information on a particular problem. You can find out about these shows by asking the host, a friend, an organizational PR person, or by tuning in yourself. It's a good idea to observe the format of the show, particularly if you don't have a great deal of on-air experience.

You'll need to know if a show is live or taped. Some shows are taped in advance and aired later. You will want to know if the show has call-ins. This means that members of the listening or viewing audience will be calling to ask you questions or to offer their opinions (many of which will be uninformed). Callers' comments limit your time on-air. In addition, you'll have to respond to differing perspectives and to a wide and unpredictable variety of questions.

Ask the producer or interviewer if there is a particular slant to his or her thinking on the subject that will be addressed. Ask if you will be appearing or speaking alone, or if you will be joined by other guests. Ask how many and who they are. Get a sense of their area of expertise or point of view. If you know you will be debating someone with an opposing point of view, you can try to find out from other sources what they are likely to say. Find out how long will you be on the air. You need to know whether you will have two minutes or an hour in which to make your points.

Many shows do a pre-interview to screen potential guests. This is useful to both you and the show's producers and reporters. How you respond to questions and your "stage manner" will help them decide if they want to have you on the program. In this pre-interview, you will get an idea of the slant and you will be able to rehearse your comments.

Your attractiveness as a guest will depend upon your ability to get your points across vividly and succinctly. Syndicated newspaper columnist Ellen Goodman once told us that when she is unenthusiastic about being on a show, she tells the pre-interviewer that the subject has many facets and then she starts to elaborate on all of them. Interviewers quickly terminate the call.

It's important to know how a show plans to use nurses—for their clinical or health care expertise or for entertainment value.

Several years ago, for example, Sally Jessy Raphael planned a show on the care of her son who had been in an automobile accident and hospitalized for a month. A group of nurses was invited to the program. To thank the doctors and nurses who had cared for her son, Raphael presented video clips of his hospital stay and asked the experts to talk about his treatment.

The "experts" were all MDs. Dressed in suits and ties, they sat on the show's main set and conversed with Raphael. The young man's nurses, on the other hand, had been invited en masse. Dressed uniformly in scrubs, they sat in the audience where they dutifully applauded or laughed on cue. None was asked to speak about the nursing issues that were involved in the complex case.

David Letterman's treatment of six physicians and two nurses who appeared on his show after his heart surgery was quite different. He joked with each individual but also thanked all of them and said they were the people who "saved my life." He got a laugh when he said that one of the nurses had given him a bath, but there was no lewd implication. He simply stated that the nurse took care of him when he was much too sick to care for himself.

In response to Sally Jessy Raphael's request, the hospital public relations and nursing department should have insisted that at least one nurse be on the panel to talk about nursing care. That should have been the condition for nursing's participation. If Raphael refused, the nurses should not have appeared. Nurses had the power to embarrass a daytime woman's show host whose son was saved by nursing yet wouldn't allow his nurses to appear on a panel of experts. This would have been a good story to leak to the news media.

Using nursing's leverage in this way may sound risky. Nurses may be concerned that they will alienate the media—or their institutions—if they do so.

Hospitals that want free publicity may pressure nurses to cooperate with media requests that demean nurses. But why should nurses agree to reinforce traditional stereotypes? Nurses have a right to negotiate the conditions of their participation in media discussions. And, they have a right to refuse to participate. Exercising this right when necessary will teach reporters and institutional PR staff to show more respect toward individual nurses and their profession.

Being Interviewed at Home or at Work

Some shows will ask you to come to their studio. Others will interview you at your home or workplace. Communication satellites make it possible for radio programs originating across the country or the globe to set up a telephone conversation that sounds as though everyone is in the same room. It is not unusual for television programs to bring their cameras to you.

In the case of radio, if an interviewer calls for a comment and you are in the middle of something or just feel unprepared, ask them to call back in a few moments to give you an opportunity to get your thoughts together. Sometimes interviewers will be on deadline and will want you immediately. Buy a little time to think by asking a few questions about the show.

If you don't feel ready, you don't have to agree to the interview. But remember, you're the health care expert. The program is seeking your expertise. Try to compose yourself and speak from your heart about what you know. Most of the time people sound and look much better on radio and television than they think they do.

If you have advance notice of an interview that will take place at your home or workplace, give yourself a little breathing space. If you've just seen ten patients and are stressed and harried, don't go directly from those patients to the phone. Try to take a fifteen-minute or even a five-minute breather. Take some deep, relaxing yoga breaths and collect your thoughts.

Do the same if you will be receiving a call at home. If the kids have just been fighting, take a moment to catch your breath and organize your thoughts. If it's an early morning show (you'd be surprised by how many are) set your alarm to wake you at least a half-hour before you're supposed to be called. Have a cup of coffee or tea. Put on your clothes. It's amazing how talking on the radio in your bathrobe at six in the morning can undermine your professionalism even though no one can see you. Some people like to stand up to give radio interviews because it makes them feel more dynamic and authoritative.

If you are going to a radio or television station for an appearance, give yourself plenty of time to get there. It's better to arrive 15 minutes early than exactly on time but frazzled. Air times are locked in stone. If you're five or ten minutes late, you may miss the opportunity to be on at all.

Appearance

How you appear and behave on radio and television will influence how the audience receives your message. Whether you're a staff nurse or a prominent researcher, you want to appear knowledgeable and credible. Your dress and the body language you use will help or hinder this effort.

Look professional. Wear neat, tailored clothes. Don't be bland, but don't be jarring. You should have some color in your attire, but bright reds and oranges go neon on the screen. Whites tend to fade out. Keep away from checks, herring bone tweeds, small stripes, and other small patterns that tend to wiggle on TV. Avoid flowered, sweet or cute clothing. Men should wear suits, or sports jackets, and ties.

Since television's bright lights tend to wash out even the rosiest complexion, it helps to wear some makeup. Foundation, rouge and powder will do. Men may also want to apply at least some powder and perhaps foundation too. Some national shows have professional make-up people on staff who will make you up. Assume, however, that you won't be made up and apply your own cosmetics before you go to the studio. If you are going to appear on television a lot, you might want to invest in a lesson from a make-up artist. (When digital television, which produces a more natural picture, becomes widespread, television makeup will be a thing of the past.)

Avoid excessive jewelry, particularly the clanking variety. You don't want necklaces or bracelets to jangle against sensitive microphones or strike desks or chairs. Dangling earrings are a distraction. So are long, Barbara Streisand-type nails. The grunge look or an elaborately teased hairdo also compromises a credible presentation.

When you are seated on the set, try to look alert but relaxed and comfortable. Don't slump over. Sit up straight and lean forward slightly. This is an attentive posture. Make eye contact with the host. Don't worry about the camera. It will follow you, you don't have to follow it. Try not to be distracted by camera people and producers who are signaling one another or the show's host. These people are not signaling because you've just made a terrible mistake. They are communicating with the host or each other about timing and production details. If the host looks at people in the studio while you are talking, or reviews his notes, or seems to be listening to what someone is saying in his ear piece, he knows the camera is on you and he is counting on you to continue talking.

With today's automated sets, you might find yourself in a booth with a remotely operated camera situated in a corner of the main set or in a separate room. This will also be the arrangement if you go to a studio to be interviewed for a program based in another city. Your "face-to-face" with the host will be via his image on a monitor or his voice in your earphones, and you might not get even that much human contact. This can be unnerving. Keep in mind that on television it will look like you are actually having a conversation with the interviewer. Your job is to regard the robotic camera (which may advance eerily and back away all by itself) as though it were a human being and talk directly to it. You will get an indication of when the show has gone to a commercial and you can relax for a moment. But, when the discussion is going on, don't assume that you are not on camera just because someone else is talking. Your camera may be taking reaction shots of you. This is such an artificial environment, you may feel as though they have put you in isolation and forgotten about you. But you are very much part of the program. If you have something to say, and no one has given you a chance, politely, but assertively, interject.

When you are asked a question, don't roll your eyes toward the ceiling as if waiting for the angels to send you an answer. Keep your eyes on the host (or robot camera). Some people blink rapidly when they are working their way through an answer. If you have this tendency, consciously override it so that you have a steady look. If you're responding to another guest on the show, look at him or her (or at the robot camera as though it were he or she). Make hand gestures, but don't let them get out of control. You want viewers to listen to what you say, not get caught up with your mannerisms.

When someone else is talking, look interested, even if you are not. Don't scratch your head, scowl, roll your eyes, or snicker if you think what the person said is absurd. The camera might pan toward you at any time and catch your reaction. When someone is asking you a question or making a statement, resist grunting or uttering affirmative "uh-huh" sounds. Similarly, don't automatically nod your head. Women seem to do these things more often than men. They are intended to show the other person that you are taking in what he or she is saying. However, on radio or television, the sounds are a distraction. In addition, affirmative sounds and nods give the impression that you agree with what the person is saying even if it is outrageous or contradicts your argument. Just looking attentive is sufficient. This is also the correct demeanor for participating in a panel discussion or engaging in questions and answers from a lecture podium.

State Your Qualifications and Set Ground Rules

Before you go on air, establish how you will be identified and how the host and other guests will address you. This is essential for nurses to do. Tell the producer of the show exactly how you want to be identified.

Give the correct spelling of your name and title for the identifier that will flash on the screen when you are talking. Make sure "RN" or "nurse" is included in the identification. If you have another title, like professor, your nursing identification may disappear unless you insist upon it being present. Identifications in radio and TV land (and even in most mainstream publications) are short, so get in the essentials, and accept that no one is interested in the fact that you are the Florence Nightingale/Lavinia Dock/Lillian Wald professor of physiological and anatomical nursing at the university of such and such school of nursing. What they need to know is that you are an expert on a certain subject and a professor at the University of such and such school of nursing.

Make sure you establish ground rules for oral introductions. Ask to be introduced with your specialty and perhaps the number of years you have been a nurse, as in: "Joanne Clarke is with us today. She's been a psychiatric nurse for 20 years and works with adolescents." If you are a staff nurse, provide additional details too. For example, you might want to be introduced as "Tom Smith, who has been a medical-surgical nurse at General Hospital for ten years. Nurse Smith works extensively with elderly patients."

If you're a PhD nurse, beware of being called "doctor" over and over again. The audience will probably think you are a physician. If you use your "Dr." title, be sure to preface statements with, "As a nurse … "

If you are not a PhD and you are going to be on air with MDs or PhDs, insist upon being addressed as Mrs., Miss, Ms., or Mr. (last name) or Nurse (last name). Unless you intervene, hosts will call doctors "Dr.," professors "Professor," and you Joan or Jim. Even if you have to intervene while on the air, do not allow yourself to be called by your first name while others are being addressed with titles that convey expertise.

Tone of Voice and Interview Etiquette

Tone of voice is important, especially so on radio. Maintain an even, measured tone of voice even if you are provoked. Don't get riled by what a caller, another guest, or the host has said. Maintain your composure just as you would with a difficult patient. Combat their comments with a powerful argument, not by raising your voice, making personal attacks, mocking, or being sarcastic.

It may require an act of will to pretend that a stupid question is not stupid. Carl Golden, press secretary to New Jersey governor Christine Todd Whitman, advised her to resist remarking on the vapidity of some questions she is asked. Some questions, Golden said, "are just remarkably stupid. I mean, there are reporters, the Nobel Prize for physics isn't in their future." Golden told Whitman, "If you want to smile, that's fine, but the worst thing you can do is show up a reporter in front of his colleagues … They don't need you to say, 'What a dumb question.' They know it's dumb. You just answer it."[1]

To be polite and still make your point, you can say, "That was interesting, but let's think about this aspect of the issue," and move on to your message.

The effective way to deal with negative and insulting comments is to regard them as opportunities to make your own points. For example, if a host says, "It's surprising to me that you nurses know so much about diseases and medications," pick up on the host's language and respond, "You know, what's surprising is that you're surprised." Then describe what nurses know.

If you're talking about the consequences of a shortage of nurses or understaffing on hospital floors, a host might concur in a way that subtly demeans nurses. "So what we're missing in health care," he might offer, " is the TLC nurses bring."

To this, you can reply: "Nurses definitely bring a great deal of caring and compassion to their patients and to their patients' families. But the real problem with a shortage of nurses is that there won't be anyone in hospitals to rescue patients from complications that could lead to death. That's what nursing is, a matter of life and death."

If you're on a show where the host or his guests are constantly interrupting and shrieking at one another, your challenge will be to resist retreating into frustrated silence or joining in the shouting match. Try an amused tone to interject: "Well, if I could just get a word in edgewise," or "If one of you would just let someone finish a sentence." When someone interrupts, you can say firmly, "Excuse me, it'll take less than a sound-bite for me to finish my sentence."

The most important thing is to be interested, enthusiastic and cooperative rather than withholding and monosyllabic. When Dick Cavett had a conversation show years ago, we watched him interview a famous Russian ballet dancer (we're pretty sure it was Rudolph Nureyev). Cavett asked the dancer an intelligent question, to which he responded "yes." Then Cavett asked another excellent question, to which the dancer responded, "no." Another perceptive comment received a terse, "yes," followed by "yes," "yes," and "no." After the first few minutes, it must have been agonizingly clear to Cavett that he was living the interviewer's worst nightmare: he had to fill up air-time with a talk-show guest who refused to talk.

If you're nervous, or suspicious, don't pull a Nureyev. The way to deal with this is to be prepared, and then talk your way out of your anxiety.

Be Prepared

You must know in advance which points you want to make. Years ago Christopher Lydon (now the host of "The Connection" on American public radio) told Bernice Buresh before interviewing her on television that she should think of her points as "bumper stickers." This is a very useful image that we have repeatedly passed on to others. "Bumper stickers" represent the essence of your message and are easy to remember. You can embed your bumper sticker into an anecdote, example or rejoinder. But the main point must be short and clear. Realistically, you may not have time to make more than three points, and, in fact, you may only get a chance to make one, but you can make it count.

In chapter four we talked about preparing three anecdotes on nursing. For television and radio, these anecdotes must be boiled to a few sentences that can be delivered quickly in a conversational style and still make the bumper sticker point. Write down your points, and the statistics or facts that will bolster them, on small cards and take them with you to the studio. Review the points before you go on air.

Translate jargon into ordinary language: critical care unit, not CCU; cancer, not CA; heart attack, not MI or myocardial infarction.

Bridging

Bridging is a technique for getting to your bumper stickers. It means using a question or comment as a bridge to make your point.

That's what Cindy Dalton did on "Montreal Today." She briefly answered the host's question then seized the opportunity to describe the challenges nurses face in their daily practice. Later, when the discussion turned to health care policy, she directed the conversation back to the nursing component.

A bridge is merely a transitional statement such as:

"You know that's an interesting issue, but so is this … "

"Let me tell you about …"

"While we're talking about what's important to patients, consider this …"

"The real issue is …"

"Here's another factor that hasn't been mentioned …"

Questions come in various forms. Some of the following may be surprising.

1. The flattering or gift question

An interviewer might say: "Oh, nurses are wonderful people. They do such important work." Or, "It's just terrible what's happening to nursing."

These "non-questions" can derail you because it's hard to know how to respond. Consider them a gift. "Thank you," or "Yes, that's true," are reasonable prefaces to a follow up like, "I'm glad you feel that way. Nurses hope the public will transform private gratitude into public support for nursing. Those listeners who share your views about nursing may want to call their political representative to support increased funding for … " Here you can fill in the blank: nursing research, nursing staff in hospitals, nurse-run community clinics. This type of question can be regarded as an invitation to take the conversation in the direction you'd like to go.

2.   The open-ended question

"What's it like to be a nurse?" Taken too literally, this type of question can have you chasing all over the landscape. Regard it also as an invitation to tell an anecdote that contains one of your bumper stickers.

3.   The double-bind question

By confronting you with two untenable options, these questions are a classic Catch-22.

An example: "Did you become a nurse because you didn't have what it takes to get into medical school, or because you're just too nice to be a doctor?"

Without repeating the question, one answer would be: "I became a nurse because I wanted to apply my intelligence to caring for the sick and vulnerable. Here's how I do it… " Then bridge into your messsage.

4.   The erroneous assumption question

Like the double-bind question, this query throws negative material at you. The challenge is to quickly dispense with the negative and turn to the positive.

A Canadian radio interviewer once interrupted a guest who was describing the burdens being placed on nurses with: "So if nurses don't get enough respect, why don't they just all move up the food chain and become doctors?"

To which the guest responded: "In my view, nurses are already at the top of the food chain. Think about it, if all the nurses become doctors, who would provide 24-hour care of the sick?"

Never be afraid to challenge erroneous assumptions or misinterpretations of nursing. You are being interviewed because you are the expert, and therefore, it is your role to correct mistaken ideas about nursing. Be prepared to do so.

Several years ago, nurses being interviewed by journalist Bill Moyers for a documentary series, "Healing and the Mind," seemed taken aback when Moyers misidentified their work.

In the documentary, Moyers observed nurses working with fragile premature infants and their teenage parents at Parkland Memorial Hospital in Dallas and talked with the nurses about what they were doing. Clearly impressed, Moyers nonetheless demonstrated at the end of the segment how even the most intelligent and sensitive people can become confused about nursing. "You're *more* than nurses, you're *more* than technicians," he exclaimed.

Then placing their work in the context of innovations in medicine, Moyers declared: "That's what *medicine's* about today."

Moyers's response was startling. But imagine the effect the nurses would have had on millions of viewers if they had been ready for such a predictable misinterpretation. They could have politely, but firmly, responded: "No, Bill, what you have just seen is the very essence of nursing."

5.   The absent-party question

The interviewer may use a comment made by a general or specific absent party to inject controversy or discredit your arguments.

"Many people are now saying that nurses have become too vociferous in their demands," is the way one of these questions might go. To which you might respond, "Most people tell us quite the contrary. They are glad that nurses are standing up for patient care."

A variation of the form might be: "I have a friend who teaches chemistry at a prestigious university and he says that nursing students are the dumbest ones in his class."

This technique is insidious because you know neither the person nor what he really said. Yet, the absent party is set up as an authoritative commentator. To this particular statement, you might reply by describing the rigors of nursing education.

6.   The question with a loaded preface

An interviewer might say, "I know your organization doesn't represent many people and has not established a track record in this area. What is its mission in this campaign?" Take a mental breath and use the question to describe the importance of your organization and its key role in the current issue.

7.   The irrelevant or non-sequitur question

"My mother-in-law just loves the nurses on ER," an interviewer might begin, and, with no warning, move on to a completely different subject. In this case, you might say, "Yes, the nurses on ER are great," and move to the real point.

8.   The direct accusation question

How about getting hit with this? "You're complaining about violence against nurses. What about all those nurses who kill their patients?"

You might reply by saying: "There aren't many nurses in the second category, but the statistics indicate that more must be done to protect nurses from violence," and then marshall the facts to make your point. Whatever else, do not repeat the phrase "nurses who kill their patients."

Similarly, a nurse practitioner might be told, "What you are really saying is that nurses want to practice medicine."

To this ubiquitous accusation, you might respond that "nurse practitioners practice nursing." Then present a brief example of the difference between the services of an NP and those of a physician.

Nurses and other caregivers are often attacked when they "break frame" by asking for something for themselves or by going on strike. Journalists may pepper them with questions that imply that nurses are being selfish.

Nurses might be accused of hiding behind the patient care issue to get something for themselves, as in the question: "Are you really trying to protect your patients, or are you just trying to protect your job?"

A discussion of the need for lunch breaks and the end of mandatory overtime might be answered with a retort such as, "But it isn't a hospital's job to protect nurses. It's the job of nurses to protect patients."

A picket line interview during a strike might produce: "Why are you abandoning your patients? Isn't your job to be at the bedside no matter what?"

Because nurses don't want to be perceived as selfish and uncaring, their tendency is to spend time trying to prove how unselfish and caring they are. A better tack might be to answer forthrightly:

"We certainly do want to protect our jobs. That's because our job is to save your life."

"A hospital's job is to care for patients and to support and sustain the people—professional nurses and other staff—who provide that care 24 hours a day. Because hospitals have cut too many nursing jobs, staff nurses are frequently asked to work two back-to-back ten-hour shifts. The nurse may be exhausted, have no time to go the bathroom or take a lunch break. How can she provide safe care under these conditions?"

"When nurses adapt to unsafe conditions they're putting patients at risk, not helping them. We are working to assure that there will be enough nurses at the bedside to take care of patients."

---

9.   The inconsistency question

This type of question suggests that you are unable to make up your mind and thus can't be trusted.

An interviewer might say, "Five years ago nurses were all for managed care. Now some of you are its worst critics."

To which the response might be, "Times and circumstances change. Today, unfortunately, insurers and governments aren't really managing care, they're managing costs. This is giving the genuine management of care a bad name."

Or, an interviewer might argue, "First you wanted to care for people in the hospital. Now you want most nurses to work in the community. Can't you make up your mind?"

Calmly, and firmly explain that "visiting, home care, and public health nurses have given care in the community for over a century. We want a system that funds both community and hospital care."

10. The question you don't know the answer to

Sometimes interviewers will ask you questions you simply can't answer. If you're an oncology nurse an interviewer could come from left field and ask you a question about the treatment of diabetics or the latest proposal for health care reform. If you, in fact, know about diabetes or have an opinion about the latest health care reform proposal, by all means voice it. If you don't, don't take a stab at it. Simply say, "That's an interesting question, but it's not my field. You might want to talk to a nurse who specializes in diabetes," or "You can get a lot of good information on health care reform by talking to people at the American or Canadian Nurses Association. Then, use the question to bridge into what you do know about.

Interview Tips

- Find out in advance what the interview will be about.
- Prepare three "bumper stickers." Look for opportunities to use them.
- Don't be a captive of the question. Use a transition to bridge from the interviewer's question to the points you want to make.
- Use anecdotes, personal stories, statistics, sparkling language.
- Avoid jargon, technical terms and alphabet soup.
- Tell the truth; don't exaggerate to win an argument.
- Don't repeat a negative question or offensive words.
- Know in advance what you will not divulge. Whether it is personal or has to do with your institution or profession, make sure you know how far you are willing to go and go no further.
- Assume everything is on the record. Don't comment if you don't want your comment to be aired.
- If you don't know something, say so. Then talk about what you do know.
- Be cooperative and communicative. Enjoy your experience on air.

Beware of repeating negative statements. While it's a normal response for people to repeat the negative to refute it, you may inadvertently give it more weight than it deserves. If an interviewer asks you about "nurses who kill their patients," and you say, "nurses don't kill their patients," the listener has just heard the words "nurses ... kill ... patients" twice.

When people are under stress they might even introduce a negative suggestion themselves as Richard Nixon did in 1973 in the statement that became emblematic of his unraveling presidency: "People have got to know whether or not their President is a crook. Well, I'm not a crook."

If other people make allegations, simply refute them without repeating them.

Call-in Shows and Nurse-run Shows

Thanks to the myriad call-in shows that are on television and radio, you can use the electronic media to make your point even if you are never invited to appear on a show. If you are at home, at work, or driving in the car and you hear people discussing health care, listen carefully. If you're thinking "I have something to say about that topic," dial the number and express your point of view. People who call in to shows are generally not asked to give their last names. So if you're worried about retaliation, this is a perfect forum.

We've been on a number of shows where nurses have called in spontaneously. Some have recounted heart-wrenching experiences. Some have talked about the work they do with patients. Others have discussed their research. All have significantly advanced the discussion.

The show doesn't have to be on nursing to allow you, as a nurse, to contribute. It can be about health care reform, about legislation, about a political candidate's stand on issues, about women and gender, or education. If you are listening and feel that something should be added, you're just the one to do it.

Nurses, as well as doctors, can become health care experts and hosts on TV or radio. Local cable television shows offer an excellent way to enter the television market.

In Rhode Island, Nurse Katherine Lukas has been the host of a cable television show on children, "Kids 1st," since 1998. Lukas, who works on the coronary care unit of Rhode Island Hospital, began her TV career when she was doing a clinical rotation for her masters' degree. A community liaison pediatric nurse at Newport Hospital asked her to help assemble focus groups on children's issues for a number of social service agencies. Lukas, who has an undergraduate degree in public relations, volunteered to contact a local cable television station to find out if it had a public affairs program on children's issues. Members of the coalition, she suggested, could go on such a show and solicit participants for the focus groups. She contacted the person in charge of community programming for the Cox Communication station, who responded that he was just putting together a show on children but had no one to host it. "I can do that for you," Lukas offered.

After Lukas finished taping interviews for the show, she was asked if she would host another. That led to a monthly program. Although the program doesn't concentrate exclusively on health, "RNs make excellent guests," Lukas says. "In our jobs, we communicate with all kinds of people. So we're careful to use language that lay people can understand." Lukas encourages other nurses to look for cable TV opportunities.

Diana Mason, the editor-in-chief of the *American Journal of Nursing*, has co-hosted the radio program "Healthstyles" on WBAI in New York City since 1985. Mason began her talk show work as a guest on the program's predecessor, "Everywomanspace," when it was produced and hosted by two other nurses, Diane Mancino and Paula Tedesco. Mason and Barbara Glickstein, director of clinical services for the Center for Health and Healing at Beth Israel Medical Center in New York, appeared on the show. When Mancino and Tedesco left the show, Mason and Glickstein took over the monthly hour-long talk show and expanded it to a biweekly production.

"When Diane and Paula started in 1979, one of their goals was to provide a place for nurses to gain experience with the media," Mason explains. Barbara and I continued doing that. Over the years, we've had a number of nurses act as co-moderators and producers. They've put together segments with interviews, music and sound-bites, that we, as volunteer, unpaid producers, did not have the time to produce."

As the nurses became more media savvy, their goal was "first and foremost, to produce good radio. If nurses aren't well-focused, expert and articulate," Mason says, "we can't produce good radio and we also can't make nursing look good."

The program, which has received several awards, was one of the first in New York to talk about the politics of AIDS and the resurgence of TB. "This is because we talked with public health nurses in the field who described their experiences," Mason explains.

"Nurses," Mason advises, "shouldn't underestimate the skills they have communicating with the public. Nurses know how to interview people. They know how to analyze a situation. And they have an understanding of issues grounded in clinical practice."

Mason is also impressed with the qualities that nurses bring to the program as expert guests compared with those of some physicians. "We did a program on urinary incontinence," she recalls. "We got a glitzy press release from a urologist in the city and had him on with a nurse who is a national expert on incontinence. The nurse showed up on time. The doctor was 30 minutes late, but nonetheless tried to assume the mantel of authority.

"When a man called to discuss the embarrassing problem of his mother-in-law's incontinence, the doctor—in an intimidating manner—asked him if he had taken his mother-in-law for medical work-ups. He made the man feel incompetent," Mason explains.

"The nurse, on the other hand, gently asked the caller a number of questions to find out if he and his wife had discussed this sensitive issue with his mother-in-law. He said he had not because his wife also had problems with incontinence. The nurse helped the caller rehearse a conversation he might have with his wife.

"This is a great example of the kind of skills RNs can bring to media," Mason concludes.

Endnotes

1. A. Weissman, *Christine Todd Whitman: The Making of a National Political Player* (Carol Publishing Group, 1997).

Chapter 11

PROMOTING
NURSING RESEARCH

The public will more readily understand the relevance of nursing to health and illness when nursing research becomes more visible. This chapter describes efforts to promote research done by nurses and suggests an overall publicity strategy.

Early in the year 2000, news organizations throughout the United States received the following news release:

NEW STUDY SUPPORTS "FAMILY PRESENCE" IN EMERGENCY DEPARTMENTS

Research Demonstrates Numerous Benefits during Life-Saving Procedures

New York, NY, February 17, 2000—In 1994, Theresa A. Meyers, RN, trauma case manager at Parkland Memorial Hospital in Dallas, Texas, made a split-second decision that went against her hospital's usual practice, and ignited a firestorm of controversy. Her actions—letting the parents of a dying boy into a critical care area while medical personnel tried to save him—focused attention on this controversial practice and have been debated ever since.

Now a study released in the February issue of the *American Journal of Nursing,* on "family presence" in the emergency department (ED) during invasive procedures (IP) and cardiopulmonary resuscitation (CPR), confirms that family members, nurses and physicians support the practice as positive and beneficial. Largely as a result of the study, Parkland Memorial Hospital implemented a policy and now offers the option for family presence during IP and CPR throughout the hospital.

With this dramatic lead, the *American Journal of Nursing (AJN)* initiated a bold approach to publicizing nursing research. It hired a public relations firm to distribute news releases on the "family presence" study reported in its February issue to hundreds of local and national print and radio outlets.

Additionally, a two-minute video news release (VNR) filmed at Parkland hospital and supplementary B-roll video material went out to television stations. Public relations staff followed up with phone calls to journalists and producers pointing out the story elements inherent in this research and its potential to transform hospital practices. They also offered to arrange interviews with researchers.

The *AJN* got another shot at coverage by notifying journalists of a Web cast on the study scheduled for February 29 during which the authors would answer questions submitted on-line or phoned in on a toll-free number.

Newspapers throughout the US picked up the story. *USA Today* did a cover story. Cable News Network, which is seen throughout the world, shot a feature. Shortly after its release, the VNR aired 75 times in 45 markets reaching an estimated 5.7 million people.

As a result of this promotion, the family presence study attained a high level of visibility. In the process, it may have raised the profile of nursing research itself, making a significant contribution to new efforts to publicize research conducted by nurses.

That was certainly the intention of *AJN's* editor-in-chief. In her editorial in the February issue, Diana J. Mason announced that the *AJN*, the official publication of the American Nurses Association, would be publishing (and publicizing) "compelling, original research that can transform practice." Mason accepted the position of editor-in-chief in 1998 only after *AJN* publishers Lippincott Williams & Wilkins pledged to support her intention to editorially strengthen the journal, make it more relevant and credible, and promote it not just within nursing but in the broader health care and public communities.

Although she says she had to fight hard to get what she regarded as a modest budget, she was determined to follow promotional models established by medical journals. Her publisher was pleased with the attention the family presence study received. The feedback indicated that the general public was now more aware of changing emergency department protocols and so were a greater number of nurses, physicians and other care givers. They hadn't learned about the issue through the journal's publication but through the mainstream news media. Mason had succeeded in finding the right study to promote.

Few research studies in nursing or medicine have as many strong news values as this one did. It featured a heroic working nurse, Theresa Meyers, who bucked the system to allow a mother and father to be with their dying 14-year-old child. It had controversy and conflict—some of the physicians, nurses and administrators at Meyers's institution at the time, and a large percentage of medical residents in general, opposed the presence of family members during invasive procedures and especially during CPR. The study was attractive because it refuted conventional wisdom: those family members who were permitted to stay were not disruptive and tended to appreciate, rather than judge, the work and life-saving attempts of the clinicians.

The study had impact for members of a broad general audience who might imagine themselves in this tragic situation. They learned that 97 percent of the family members who were permitted to stay felt they had a right to be present and said the experience was important and helpful. The research seemed to convince nurses, physicians and others on the interdisciplinary team that relegating families to waiting rooms during a code or invasive procedures might be too severe. Furthermore, the media appeal of the research had already been established. National radio and television news outlets did stories on the issue while researchers were testing the protocol.

The *AJN's* foray into high-test media relations is an excellent example of what can happen when nurses who conduct research tell the world about their studies and discuss the applications of their work.

Patients, families, and the health care system in general can only reap the benefits of research done by nurses if that research is disseminated and publicized beyond the nursing community. Public demand and pressure drives the funding and implementation of medical and health care research.

Funding for nursing research is a story of both achievement and unfulfilled potential. After a great deal of lobbying from the nursing community, the US National Institutes of Health (NIH) set up a National Center for Nursing Research in 1986 with an initial budget of $16 million. The Center was upgraded to a full-fledged institute, the National Institute for Nursing Research (NINR), on June 10, 1993. In fiscal year 1999, thirteen years after its founding, the institute reached a budget of $70 million. It was, however, the institute with the lowest level of funding in the NIH. Its allotment was less than one-half of one percent of the NIH budget.

The most visible and highly funded institute, the National Cancer Institute, had a budget of $2.9 billion in fiscal year 1999. The second lowest funded institute, the National Institute on Deafness and Other Communication Disorders received an allocation of $231 million. Most of the NIH Centers, which have less prestige than the institutes, had higher allocations than the nursing institute. While it received less money than the NINR, the National Center for Complementary and Alternative Medicine registered a more accelerated rate of funding since its founding in 1993. In six years it went from a budget of $2 million to $50 million.[1]

The NIH receives its funding from the federal government. The amount it and its member institutes will get is worked out in interplay between the US Congress and the President. These decisions are influenced by lobbying and by the personal interests of the decision-makers. As one observer pointed out, "Didn't you know that members of Congress are worried about getting cancer?" A presidential appointee who reviews the NIH budget told us there is no question that money flows more readily to those who make the case for the relevance of their research. Alternative and complementary practitioners have followed in the public relations footsteps of medical researchers. They have successfully mobilized patients and the public to pressure politicians for more money for research on alternative remedies. More vigorous PR for nursing research can only enhance the funding process.

Whether it is to maintain and enhance nursing research, to advance nursing practice, or to improve the organization of nursing services, public communication is key. Hospitals, nursing homes and other institutions must be convinced, or required, to hire sufficient numbers of nurses; to give them the time needed to master and apply practice innovations; to create an organizational environment in which nurses can work effectively; and, to encourage real collaboration among all the members of the health care team.

Research alone won't convince them to do this. "Whether it's to change policy or enhance practice, our research is meant to be used," says University of California nursing home expert Charlene Harrington. "It has to go beyond nursing publications. If we're trying to influence policy, we have to publish in policy journals like *Health Affairs* or *Medical Care.* And we have to reach out to the mainstream media, no matter where our work is published. If we keep this work a secret within nursing, neither practice nor policy will change."

Visibility around other aspects of nursing is critical. But because so much of health coverage is generated by research, if nursing is not present in this significant area, other efforts to improve nursing practice and nursing's image will be compromised. For every Darva Conger (the emergency nurse who married a multimillionaire stranger on prime-time American television), there must be scores of Theresa Meyers and other nurses visibly demonstrating the significance of the profession and the breadth of its accomplishments. (Indeed more than one letter to the editor raised the question of whether Conger's clinical judgment in the ER was as bad as her judgment about how to conduct her life.)

Medical Journals Have Paved the Way

Although medical research is now a large part of health coverage, only a few decades ago doctors had little incentive to communicate with reporters and the lay public. Until health care costs soared and research funds began to shrink, the idea that physicians had to be accountable to the general public was foreign to most MDs. Patients were far more passive in their relationships with their doctors. Medical organizations discouraged doctors from talking with reporters, equating this with advertising, an activity that used to be associated with quacks and patent medicine salesmen.

Over the past 20 years, several factors made it essential for physicians to communicate with the public. Insurers and government were no longer willing to write blank checks for health care services, and demands for reform of the system were increasing. If doctors were going to influence the funding and delivery of health care, they had to be willing to take their case to the public. At the same time, competition was growing for research funds and patients were becoming more knowledgeable and wanted more information and communication with their doctors. Medical organizations did a turnabout. They dropped their bans against advertising, encouraged physicians to raise their public profile, and taught them how to use the media effectively.[2]

Not all doctors are happy about the pressure to communicate, nor do all appreciate the coverage that results. Nonetheless, a critical mass engages in the process. Sixty percent of medical reporters surveyed for a special report on the relationship between journalists and physicians described doctors and medical researchers as highly accessible, and 38 percent said doctors were somewhat accessible.[3] A survey of medical researchers found that 86 percent of them felt that news reports based on their research were accurate.[4]

For many years, bioethicist Arthur L. Caplan (one of today's masters of the intelligent quotable quote) has urged doctors to learn how to express themselves so that they can gain public support. He has recently urged nurses to do the same. Caplan told nurse executives attending a University of Pennsylvania conference that it was essential to talk to the media to inform the public about current health care issues and to influence the democratic process of decision making. Caplan, who directs the Center for Bioethics at the University of Pennsylvania, advised nurses to "take tough positions, advocate your views and don't be wishy-washy."[5]

Medical journal editors have paved the way for those nurse researchers willing to follow this good advice. They have convinced journalists that dry, seemingly incomprehensible articles can be fascinating and worthy of media and public attention. They have made research findings reader-friendly for reporters who, in turn, have learned how to translate that research into understandable, everyday language.

Although George Lundberg, a former recent editor of the *Journal of the American Medical Association* (*JAMA*), is generally credited with making medical research a media staple, the editors of *JAMA*, in fact, have been recommending studies for coverage since the 1930s. In the 1940s, *JAMA* editor Morris Fishbein provided the Associated Press in Chicago with page proofs of the journal as long as no information was released until the journal's publication date.[6]

These days, news about health and medical developments swell mid week because of the orchestrated embargo system established by *JAMA* and adopted by the *New England Journal of Medicine*—the only two weekly medical journals in North America. To have time to prepare their stories, reporters get advance copies of the journals. But they must agree to hold their stories until the nominal publication date, thus giving doctor subscribers a chance to at least skim their journals before newly published findings hit the airwaves.

JAMA, which has a Wednesday publication date, releases its embargo Tuesday night to permit radio and television to break research stories then and newspapers to run their stories on Wednesday morning. The *New England Journal*, which publishes on Thursdays, does the same a day later. This system guarantees that "nobody can have a scoop. Nobody can jump the gun. Everybody has time to do it right," Lundberg has explained.[7]

The American Medical Association (AMA) sends news release packets, in print or electronically, to thousands of reporters and media outlets throughout the world. The typical print packet consists of six to ten pages highlighting the most newsworthy articles about to appear in *JAMA* or the other medical journals published or co-published by the AMA. Journalists receive these packets about a week in advance of publication. The editors keep an eye out for those rarer studies that are particularly rich in human interest or visual potential. These can be the subjects of video news releases. A VNR offers television everything it needs to do a report: a complete narrated feature, including interviews and dramatic visuals, that can run as is; a script if a station wants to use all or part of the feature but have its own reporter narrate; and B-roll sound bites and visuals for those who want to do their own report but need illustrations.

The process of selecting articles for media promotion begins some two months in advance of publication, according to members of the AMA's science news department. As advance make-up sheets for each issue get assembled and altered, PR staff members confer and receive editorial recommendations about which studies to highlight and which (a smaller group) would be the best candidates for video play. Lead time is needed not only to prepare the written releases but to line up interviews, shoot illustrative scenes, and write scripts for the VNRs that are fed by satellite to television stations in North America and elsewhere. A signal embedded in the VNR tape allows a monitoring organization to see how widely the tape has been used. According to the AMA, some hundreds of stations each week take excerpts out of the VNR to illustrate their own reports, or use it in its entirety.

The *New England Journal of Medicine*, published for nearly two centuries by the Massachusetts Medical Society, has striven to be *the* premier medical journal and has an eager audience awaiting each new issue. It does not engage in the same level of promotion that *JAMA* does, but will send advance copies of the publication to journalist subscribers as long as they observe the embargo.

Using sophisticated public relations techniques is standard operating procedure in medical research. This is why most journalists see medicine as cutting-edge, and dynamic, and the source of stories that must be covered. Journal editors may not always say so, but they actively court the news media. In 1990, *JAMA* even changed its publication date from Friday to Wednesday, a day earlier than the *New England Journal*. *JAMA* editor Lundberg candidly admitted news coverage was one consideration for the change after reporters complained that Friday was a busy news day and that it was hard to do follow-up stories. *JAMA* chose Wednesday after surveying reporters to find out what day would be good for them.[8]

Newspaper and television coverage varies widely in form and from week to week. Some studies get boiled down into a paragraph for inclusion in health news columns. Others may get full-blown treatment on the front page or the top of the newscast. Some never see the light of day. Some independent-minded reporters resent the AMA's newsworthiness evaluation. They claim that they toss the news releases and read the journal themselves to decide what to report on. The reports that annoy the AMA are those that are so truncated, they neglect to cite *JAMA* or another AMA publication as the source.

To get the best coverage, the AMA goes out of its way to accommodate the media. Although the news releases do not contain the text of the study in question, any reporter, or virtually anyone for that matter, can get the full article faxed to him or her by calling the AMA in Chicago. The AMA's media operation is expensive. Its rationale for its huge investment in media and public communication is that a large part of the organization's mission is public health education.

The *Canadian Medical Association Journal (CMAJ)* also expends considerable effort publicizing medical research. The *CMAJ*, which publishes every other Tuesday (except in December when there is only one issue), puts out a press release on every issue. The release is accompanied by a table of contents highlighting what the editors consider important studies. The releases, which are faxed to journalists, include contact information for the authors of the studies.

It is now established practice for medical researchers to engage in personal communication with journalists. Public relations specialists at research institutes, foundations that fund research, university medical schools, and hospital PR departments all try to get their researchers to talk about their work.

Doctors and other medical researchers can be very assertive themselves in reaching out to help promote, and fund, specific research. After actor Christopher Reeve suffered his severe spinal cord injury, researchers asked

Reeve to help raise public awareness and money for spinal cord injury research. Reeve's physicians helped him to reconstruct the medical treatment he received so that he could write his book, *Still Me*. As a result, Reeve has become an effective lobbyist for funds and the most visible bridge between the research community in this area and the public.

A similar process occurred after writer and publishing mogul Michael Korda contracted prostate cancer. Korda quickly became an advocate for the type of surgery his doctor performed and for routine prostate cancer testing for older men.

Journalists and Nursing Research

Journalists play a critical role in the dissemination of medical research. But many have been spared the knowledge that nursing research even exists, and others who may have heard of it harbor misconceptions.

Many say that they hear next to nothing from nurse researchers or their organizations. Judy Foreman, who writes the syndicated "Health Sense" column for the *Boston Globe*, says she is very open to nursing and would "love to hear from nurse researchers" and do stories on their work. But she doesn't get much usable material from nurses. "They seem to be new to the idea of peddling their work to the media," she says. "When they contact us, they tend to send PR material as opposed to news." Reporters will be wary of anything that looks like puffery rather than real news.

Some reporters have a limited view of nursing research. One told us he thought nursing research was probably "touchy feely stuff." Another imagined it was about "bedside things that only nurses care about and aren't important to readers."

There was a time when reporters didn't see the story value in medical research either. Then and now "a good story" is what is paramount. They claim they don't care what initials follow a researcher's name, as long as it's "good copy" from a credible source. Nurses have to sell reporters studies based on their value to patients or to the health care system, not because the studies are conducted by nurses.

Julie Marquis, who writes about health care delivery and public health for the *Los Angeles Times*, said that she rarely received material from nurse researchers until she was asked to speak on one of Sigma Theta Tau's media panels. After telling participants that she would like more information about nursing, she began to receive more. She finds material on the nursing shortage, nurse staffing and health care delivery particularly useful.

As journalists usually do, she became aware of nursing research through personal contacts. "I would be very receptive to stories about important research done by nurses," said Richard A. Knox, of the *Boston Globe*. "But since we have our hands full reading the major medical and scientific journals, someone has to call our attention to important studies if they want us to report on them."

When we asked Knox if he gets material or calls from nurse researchers or their organizations, he replied, "Very little."

We asked if he receives material from the National Institute for Nursing Research. "No," he said. "Does it exist?"

If nursing research is to receive the support it deserves, researchers will have to give journalists and the public a context for understanding what nurses do in health care research. The public will have to know that there are nurse scientists, just as there are medical scientists. People will have to understand that nurse scientists investigate a broad range of health and health care questions either within their own discipline or as participants in interdisciplinary studies. Their studies could be concerned with patient care, health promotion, or disease prevention, or with health care policy and systems of health care delivery. Nurses who work with patients also participate in research by collecting and recording clinical data for studies of experimental treatments and various other interventions. It's essential for the public to know nursing practice is based on what has been learned from research studies.

Nursing scholars tell us that while opposition still exists to faculty visibility in the media, attitudes are changing. In *How to Work with the Media*, Northeastern University criminologists James Alan Fox and Jack Levin strongly advocate that "academics broaden their audience—to bridge the cultures of academia and everyday society." They point out that writing for the popular media or appearing as an expert source or commentator is not "a substitute for solid academic research as the foundation for generating and testing ideas." However, Fox and Levin, who appear frequently on television, urge that "academics be not only responsive to the media, but proactive as well. In certain topics of vital concern, it may be our duty."[9]

Working with Institutional PR People

Some nursing schools and nurse researchers have built communications into their school or research project's budget. When Claire Fagin became the dean of the University of Pennsylvania School of Nursing in 1977 one of her top priorities was addressing the invisibility of the school. "I made a deal with the Hospital of the University of Pennsylvania to use their PR staff to work with the School of Nursing," Fagin recalls. "This reflected the hospital's high level commitment to promoting nursing. For a while it went very well. The hospital hired a very good PR specialist who had a mandate to work with the School. "

How to Encourage a Reporter to Cover Nursing Research

Approach #1:

Researcher: Hello. I am (full name,) a nurse researcher at the University of… I've been following coverage of health care research that you've run over the past several months in the *Daily Bugle*. My colleagues and I are concerned because coverage tends to focus exclusively on medical studies and excludes important work done by nurse researchers.

Reporter: Sorry you don't like our coverage. But it isn't our job to cover professions. We cover good stories. By all means call when you have one.

Approach #2:

Researcher: Hello. I am (full name). I'm a researcher on cardiac care at the University of… School of Nursing. We have a very important study that we think will help save people's lives after they have had heart attacks. I hope this will interest you and provide material for a good story.

Reporter: What kind of researcher are you? Are you a nurse?

Researcher: Yes, I'm a nurse and a PhD on the faculty of… I study…

Reporter: We've already done stories on treatments for heart attacks.

Researcher: And I've seen them. But what they're missing is how people deal with heart attacks when they have them. Our studies show they're never going to get the treatment you described unless they recognize that they need quick medical attention. Many people don't respond to their symptoms and don't go to the emergency room and may die or suffer serious heart damage as a result. That's what our scientific research is about. We've studied why people delay getting treatment when they've had a heart attack and what will get them to go to the hospital quickly.

Reporter: I've never heard of nursing research. Is this what you do?

Researcher: Precisely. What's important to people isn't just what happens in the operating room or in the doctor's office. It's the care they receive when they get sick, how they respond to being sick, and how they live during or after an illness. That's the missing story in health care.

After about five years, the hospital's priorities changed. They reduced their staff. "I decided the School of Nursing had to hire its own PR person, which we did on a part-time basis," Fagin says.

Since the mid 1980s the school has had several excellent public relations professionals, most notably Susan Greenbaum who, in her role as media relations officer from 1992 to 1999, helped to put the school's research activities on the map.

"In a city like Philadelphia there's enormous competition for journalists' attention," says Greenbaum. "People in the medical school are out there pitching to journalists who are inundated with health care material. My job was to be on the lookout for trends that would interest them."

In a 1998 conference on how to increase coverage of nursing research, Greenbaum described strategies that she said worked successfully at Penn.[10] Greenbaum called one strategy "educate, educate, educate," because "most reporters I have worked with are unaware that nursing practice is research based." Greenbaum said that she peppered her news releases with "buzz words" like "nurse researcher," "PhD," "federally funded research" because "these are words reporters associate with medical research. Their use in relation to nursing helps to put nursing research on an equal playing field in the heads of reporters."

Greenbaum also said that she tried to get all interviews to take place at the school or at one of its community-based practice sites. "I greet and accompany each reporter and before the interview I walk them around our building, introduce them to the dean, and describe the research of each faculty member we meet along the way. You never know what might pique a reporter's interest."

Norma M. Lang, who succeeded Fagin as dean of the school, made it clear to her colleagues at the conference that media relations is a high priority. "Susan has access to me, and to every faculty member, whenever she needs it," Lang said. "I understand the deadline-intensive nature of her work and make myself available whenever possible by phone, by e-mail, or by running down the hallway."

Charlene Harrington works with the public relations office at the University of California at San Francisco to arrange press briefings and to construct news releases when research studies appear. "You may have to help PR staff write the press release, but they're looking for things to promote," she says.

At McMaster University in Ontario, Gina Bohn Browne and her colleagues have integrated media work into their program. The McMaster System-Linked Research Unit on Health and Social Services Utilization compares the effects and costs of comprehensive care delivered by those in various disciplines. To inform those who can make use of this research, Browne and her colleagues created a plan to disseminate research findings to the media, patients, health care practitioners, policy makers, other researchers, and the public. Browne's group even hired a public relations firm to put two of the unit's project reports into "digestible form," and get them out to the media.

Nurse researchers who want to promote their work may encounter resistance in their institution. An argument that some faculty members put forth is that popularizing research can over-simplify, mislead or overstate what is actually known. Kathleen Dracup, dean of the School of Nursing at the University of California at San Francisco, elaborates on this problem: "Scientists are very reluctant to talk about the little nuggets that come from research that make a difference to people's lives. This is because, as scientists, they always want to replicate their findings before urging a change in practice. But then the problem becomes: When is there ever enough data? When can you ever feel comfortable taking the message to the public? We have to get over the tendency to wait too long."

Nursing research will only be seen as a dynamic enterprise in the same league as medical research if researchers are willing to comment, critically at times, on work by other researchers and stand up for their own findings when debate occurs. When science and medical journalist Ellen Ruppel-Shell was writing a magazine article on how *JAMA* and the *New England Journal* operate, she looked for a nurse knowledgeable about therapeutic touch to discuss the controversial "study" by a 9-year-old girl that *JAMA* published discrediting the therapy.[11] Ruppel-Shell, who is also co-director of Boston University's graduate program in science journalism, says that she wanted an expert to discuss the implications of such an article being published in the journal. "I wanted to get into the issues, but I couldn't because I couldn't get a nurse to talk to me about it on the record."

"Nurse researchers must assume the responsibility and authority that go along with being professional," Ruppel-Shell says. "Researchers can't say they have to ask someone for permission in order to comment. They can't hide behind the hierarchy or institution. They have to have the courage of their convictions and be forthcoming, otherwise freedom of speech is gone."

Journalists point out that while you can ask a reporter to read back your quote, you appear naive if you ask a reporter to show you a copy of their story so that you can vet it before it goes to press. Reporters don't make deals like that. Indeed, they will expect you or your PR officer to do much of their legwork for them. In this area of health and medical research, reporters have grown accustomed—perhaps too accustomed—to being spoon-fed. They may want you to send them not only your new study, but all the studies you have done on the subject. They probably will want to talk to patients who have benefited from the research. They may want to shoot footage and interview people in your hospital. They may expect you to arrange it. They may want you to provide the names of other people they can talk to about the subject, including those who differ from you. They may want you to propose policy solutions or practical tips for patients that they can use in their story. You will have to decide how much time and energy to put into promotion. Assistance from PR staff can be essential.

Selecting Studies and Making Their Implications Clear

While nursing doesn't have the resources that medicine does, it can nevertheless pursue any number of venues to make nursing research more widely known.

Look for research articles that will interest a wide public. If you want to go to a mainstream media outlet, ask yourself if your study affects a broad swath of its audience. Studies on cancer pain, heart disease, or care of sick children, the elderly, and nursing homes obviously do. Research that affects a smaller segment of the population might be a story if it has good news values.

Explain that it will save lives, and how many; that it will save money, and how much; prevent suffering, and what kind; change the way care is given, and how.

When discussing a study on delays in getting treatment after a heart attack, talk about how many people this problem affects. Describe the kinds of health problems such delays create. Calculate the differences in the cost of treating someone early versus treating someone who has delayed getting help. Draw attention to the additional burden of care borne by family members for the patient who delays such treatment.

If you have written a book on an important topic, send a complimentary copy to key journalists. Try to alert journalists to the publication of the book well before its release date.

Using Meetings to Promote Nursing Research

Professional meetings provide wonderful promotional possibilities. Nursing groups hold meetings in every large city in the US and Canada. These cities are home to local, and perhaps national, media outlets. Before arranging a national or regional meeting, organizers could take a tally of the researchers who will attend, get copies of their work and devise promotional strategies.

Here's the procedure. Send news releases to journalists who cover the areas that will be discussed. Call them to inform them of specific research findings that will be presented at the conference. Give them background information and encourage them to attend the sessions where pertinent research will be

Translate Your Research into Ordinary Language

At our request, Kathleen Dracup, an internationally known researcher in cardiac care, co-editor of the *American Journal of Critical Care* and dean of the University of California, San Francisco School of Nursing, presented a summary of her work—one in researchese and one that would be more attractive to the public or the media.

First summary

We conducted a research study to identify predictors of delay behavior in patients who experience an acute myocardial infarction. A logistic regression revealed the following factors to be important characteristics affecting time to seek treatment: advanced age, low income, low educational level, embarrassment about calling for help, fearing what might happen in the future, and worrying about troubling others. These predictors can be used to tailor appropriate patient education interventions.

Second summary

People who seek treatment immediately when they experience the symptoms of a heart attack are more likely to survive, have fewer complications, and have better outcomes than people who delay getting that treatment. Unfortunately, many people wait hours or even days after they first experience symptoms before they go to the hospital.

Nurse researchers who conducted studies in the US and Australia found that individuals are more likely to delay getting treatment if they are older, poor, and less educated. We also found that people who had a second heart attack delayed just as long the second time as the first.

Why do people delay getting help? Here are a few reasons. Some people felt embarrassed about calling for help. Some feared what might happen if they had to go to the hospital, or worried about troubling others.

"We're now testing an intervention to reduce the delay by encouraging patients to seek treatment immediately. This research can be life saving— particularly for people at high risk for having a heart attack and for those who may delay treatment if they do. The public needs to know about the benefits of immediate treatment. It's simple: If you want to save your life, minutes count!"[12,13]

presented. If they can't come to you, tell them you'll be glad to bring the researcher to them. If researchers will be attending but not presenting, arrange interviews with them. Ask a select group of researchers if they would be willing to meet with journalists. Request summaries of their research for distribution to the press.

Do not assume that because you post a release about your meeting on a Web site that anyone will see it or attend your meeting because of it. Make personal contacts and use the Web as a supplement to those contacts.

Be sure to give the names of any journalists you expect to attend to the people at the registration desk. Never ask a journalist to pay a registration fee. A journalist would attend as an observer, not a participant. Make sure there is a packet of conference materials waiting for the journalist. A PR representative or someone else knowledgeable about the proceedings should be available to greet the journalist and see if he or she has any questions. Be available to introduce him or her to speakers upon request, but don't hover or act like the reporter needs a keeper.

As we pointed out in chapter six, celebrity keynoters generally don't draw journalists into the tent, unless there is something special about who they are or what they will say. If a political candidate plans to deliver a major policy speech at the conference, the media probably will come. But they won't necessarily stay around to explore nursing issues unless it is clear to them that there is another story to cover or unless they think the reaction of the conference participants might be newsworthy. If a journalist is a guest speaker at the meeting, ask him or her to meet with a select group of nurse researchers who can talk about new developments.

It would be worthwhile for small groups of leading researchers to make annual visits to health care journalists at major newspapers, magazines and television outlets in such cities as New York, Washington, D.C., Los Angeles, Chicago, Toronto, Ottawa, Vancouver, and Montreal. A public relations specialist can help them to set up these "dog-and-pony shows" and prepare presentations on current research and its impact on health and illness.

Encourage Nursing Journals to Do More Outreach

If journals are too small to have full or part-time PR staff, perhaps a group of journal editors could start a cooperative project to promote articles from their journals. They could track who uses their releases and who doesn't and then call those outlets that have not used the research.

Nursing journal editors have told us that many publishers balk at spending money to promote nursing research. Some have told us that publishing companies that own and publish medical as well as nursing journals often have a double standard. They pay physician-editors a fee to edit the journals and provide administrative and promotional support for them. "We aren't paid a cent for our work," one editor of a nursing journal told us. "Plus, we have to pay for the postage to send out articles to peer reviewers."

Given the relevance of nursing and nursing research, these biased attitudes and practices should not be tolerated and nurses should be willing to make them public. Top researchers and nursing leaders should meet with publishers to discuss discriminatory patterns and insist on steps that would end them.

Look for On-going Opportunities to Promote Your Research

Certain subjects will reappear in the news. Researchers can take studies that are even a few years old to reporters if they illuminate a timely or hot issue in the news. It is not only timeliness, but the way research is packaged that influences coverage.

A good place to present your research is at conventions and meetings of associations of journalists who cover health care. You might approach conference organizers and suggest a presentation on why nursing research matters to the public.

Foundations, disease associations and international organizations sponsor conferences for journalists on specific health problems, social issues and health policy problems at which MDs and PhDs present overviews of recent research. Get into the network and convince the public relations people who plan these programs to highlight nursing as well as medical research.

There are a number of university-based journalism fellowship programs that give journalists an opportunity to study for a semester or year. These fellowship programs arrange presentations from experts in various fields. You may be invited just by virtue of being visible in the media in connection with a timely issue like health care legislation. This is another venue where presentations can be proposed.

Practically every school of nursing that conducts extensive research is situated in a university that has a communication or journalism school or department. Some journalism schools have science/health/medical writing courses and a few have graduate programs in this area. Public relations programs may also have a track for those students who want to go into health or science PR. Nursing researchers can go to these departments and ask to do class presentations on cutting-edge research.

Tell the Story in Various Ways

You can also promote your research in what you might consider to be unconventional ways. The *American Journal of Nursing* news release discussed at the beginning of this chapter grabbed attention through a dramatic story about a nurse's personal experience. Many journalists undoubtedly were drawn to the story of a nurse taking a risk to do what she considered the right thing for her patient and his or her family. This nurse would be an excellent subject for a general or woman's magazine profile.

Once papers pick up on a study like family presence, researchers, or members of the Emergency Nurses Association (which developed guidelines for the study), can keep the story alive by writing op-eds, letters to the editor, or other kinds of articles on their own experiences with families in treatment rooms. Debate over the issue would be equally compelling.

Women's and self-help magazines are an avenue for discussion of all sorts of human-interest subjects. Once the first wave of reporting on research has crested, it's time to expand the audience even further by producing articles that help patients and family members turn theory into practice. Some researchers may want to write these articles themselves. An organization concerned with these developments can find a nurse writer or pitch the story to an editor who will assign an article to a staff or freelance writer.

In the case of the study on delaying treatment after a heart attack, an excellent prospect would be a piece on how to deal with a loved one who may have suffered a heart attack. The title might be: Ten Things You Need to Do to Keep Your Husband Alive after He's Had a Heart Attack.

A similar spin-off on family presence could be Ten Things You Need to Know When Your Child (Spouse, Parent) Goes to the ER.

Using Research to Strengthen Advocacy

Research is an essential tool in any campaign or struggle waged by nurses for better working conditions, staffing, improvements in patient care and the institutional and societal resources needed to support quality care. All of the campaigns we described in chapter eight, for example, contained a research component. The media, policy makers and health care administrators all require documented research to demonstrate the importance of nursing care to patients and the conditions necessary to support nursing.

Any organization fighting for better patient care and better treatment of RNs will need research to underpin its arguments. "If you don't have the data, you will have trouble supporting your arguments," says Charlene Harrington. "To win, you need a combination of sound statistical research and anecdote." To be effective, Harrington says, there must be more contact between nursing researchers and nursing, patient and consumer groups working for improvements in clinical practice and health care policy.

The Canadian Federation of Nursing Unions (CFNU) initiated such a partnership to influence regional health authorities and hospital administrators that had been replacing RNs with LPNs and unlicensed assistive personnel.

"We wanted to convince them that RNs were the best buy for the money because we have a diversity of skills and knowledge allowing us to provide a better range of services," says Debra McPherson, acting president of the CFNU. "But of course, they weren't going to take our word for it. They felt that we were guarding our turf and our jobs."

Politicians and administrators, the CFNU leadership knew, would only be swayed if research documented the cost and care-effectiveness of registered nurses. The union approached Judith Shamian, then vice-president of Nursing at Mount Sinai Hospital in Toronto and a researcher involved in an international project on nursing workforce and outcomes, spearheaded by University of Pennsylvania researchers Linda Aiken and Julie Sochalski.

"We asked Judith Shamian and her colleague Donna Thomson to put together a review of all the literature on the cost-effectiveness of nurses," says McPherson. "We knew they had to be objective and report everything they found, even if it didn't support our arguments. We told them up front that we accepted that. We felt it would be useful to know what didn't support our argument because it would point to the gaps in research that we could address in future projects." Shamian and Thomson produced a 36-page study and accompanying slide presentation entitled, "The Effectiveness and Efficiency of Nursing Care—Cost and Quality."

"Nursing unions in this country are very effective because they have done two things," says Shamian. "While they represent the interests of nurses they are also strong advocates for a publicly funded health care system and equity for all Canadians. Secondly, there is agreement that nursing has to play a significant role in any discussion about the future of the health care system. This basic understanding has allowed us to look at where different groups agree and disagree and figure out how we can collaborate." By using research findings, professional associations and unions can present arguments that are based on evidence rather than emotional appeal, Shamian says.

In the United States, collaborations between researchers and advocates have also been effective. California governor Gray Davis was put under great pressure by a coalition of advocates— including the California Advocates for Nursing Home Reform, the Service Employees International Union (SEIU), American Association of Retired Persons (AARP), the California Nurses Association, and two nursing home industry associations—after he vetoed a 1999 bill passed by the legislature that would significantly increase nursing home staffs, salaries and benefits. Additionally, a television series on nursing home abuses highlighting the Davis veto resulted in a letter writing campaign to the governor. In his "state of the state" address in January 2000, Davis said he would propose new nursing home legislation and make it a high priority.

The arguments of all these groups, Charlene Harrington says, were grounded in sound data.

In the spring of 1999, New York University researcher Christine Kovner worked with the health care union 1199, which is part of the SEIU, to help nurses bring about improved quality of care. "Part of their contract with the League of Voluntary Hospitals in New York included setting up committees to establish safe staffing levels," Kovner explains. "I worked in an advisory role to teach staff more about how to measure quality and to work with management to set staffing levels."

Later the SEIU launched a national project to make the findings of nursing outcome studies more accessible and usable by activists by putting them into ordinary language. "We originally planned to assemble a bibliography of relevant nursing research and make it available to our members," says SEIU's Jamie Cohen. "But we quickly realized that nurses did not have the time to search for these articles. Nor would they be able to translate them into political arguments once they had read them. So we will help them do that."

Endnotes

1. NIH funding information is available on-line at www.nih.gov.

2. R. Rubin and D.H.L. Rogers, Jr., *Under the Microscope: The Relationship between Physicians and the News Media* (The Freedom Forum First Amendment Center at Vanderbilt University, 1993).

3. *Ibid.*

4. M.S. Wilkes and R.L. Kravitz, "Medical Researchers and the Media: Attitudes Toward Public Dissemination of Research," *Journal of the American Medical Association,* 268 no. 8 (26 August 1992): pp. 999–1003.

5. University of Pennsylvania Health System Invitational Conference for Nurse Executives, 11 June 1999, Philadelphia, Pennsylvania.

6. Rubin *et al., Under the Microscope.*

7. *Ibid.*

8. *Ibid.*

9. J. A. Fox and J. Levin, "How to Work with the Media," *Survival Skills for Scholars,* M. Allen, Ed. (Newbury Park: Sage Publications, 1993).

10. "Cutting through the Clutter: Increasing Media Coverage of Nurses and Nursing Research," conference sponsored by the National Institute of Nursing Research, Sigma Theta Tau International, American Association of Colleges of Nursing, and American Organization of Nurse Executives, 23 October 1998, Washington, D.C.

11. L. Rosa *et al.,* "A Close Look at Therapeutic Touch," *Journal of the American Medical Association,* 279 (1998): pp. 1005–1010.

12. K. Dracup, S.M. McKinley and D. Moser, "Australian Patients Delay in Response to Heart Attack Symptoms," *Medical Journal of Australia*, 166 (1997): pp. 233–236.

13. K. Dracup and D.K. Moser, "Beyond Sociodemographics: Factors Influencing the Decision to Seek Treatment for Symptoms of Acute Myocardial Infarction," *Heart & Lung*, 26 (1997): pp. 253–262.

Chapter 12
THE CONSTRUCTIVE
"COLLISION
OFPUBLICITY"

It's 9:45 on a Tuesday night. The theater house lights have just come on after the final astonishing scene of Wit, *the Pulitzer prize-winning, off-Broadway hit play about a terminally ill English professor and her experience as a patient in a cancer treatment program. The audience is heading for the doors. But Tuesday nights are different from other nights at the Union Square Theatre in New York.*

Wit raises such important questions about the care of the dying and the mission of health care that once a week the cast remains after the show for a post-performance discussion of the play led by a guest moderator. A sonorous male voice interrupts the exodus to invite playgoers to stay and participate in a "talk back."

Tonight's moderator is Peter Halperin, a psychiatrist who directs the division of behavioral medicine at the School of Medicine, State University of New York at Stony Brook on Long Island. Halperin explains that he has brought several medical students and colleagues—one of them an oncologist—along with him. He begins by reflecting on the painfully realistic scene in which Professor Vivian Bearing, the lead character, is informed in almost unintelligible medicalese by her oncologist that she has advanced ovarian cancer.

The play's oncologist not only fails to deal with his patient's shock and feelings of terror, he leads Bearing into a course of treatment almost as devastating to her body, soul and self-esteem as the disease itself. Soon she finds herself in the hands of her physician's young research associate, an oncology fellow far more interested in cancer cells than in the human beings who have them. How, Halperin wonders, can doctors relate more humanely than this to their patients?

The cast, now dressed in street clothes, joins Halperin on stage. Kathleen Chalfant, who plays Bearing, sits to his left. The actor who portrays the senior oncologist takes his seat as well. Finally, Paula Pizzi enters. She plays Bearing's nurse, Susie Monahan, BSN.

In the unfolding of the play, Monahan's knowledge is the knowledge that counts. It is the nurse who stops the male oncology fellow from degrading the patient during a pelvic exam. It is the nurse who protests that the doctors are far too aggressive with the highly toxic chemotherapy that is robbing the patient of any peace. (The doctors persist, nevertheless, in following the course they have charted for Bearing.)

It is the nurse who diagnoses the patient's pain and recommends the kind of treatment that would maintain this intellectual's most prized possession, her mental acuity. (The doctors dismiss the suggestion.) When it is clear that the experimental chemotherapy is failing, it is the nurse who has the courage to talk to her patient about her code status. Because of this conversation, the patient chooses to forego futile treatment that will only prolong her death. To get the eager, young oncology fellow to respect his patient's last wishes, the nurse must literally throw herself between the doctor and his dead patient.

The play's poignancy depends on the nurse's ability to penetrate Bearing's intellectual defenses so she can comfort the terrified woman hiding underneath. If the nurse did not reach through the patient's fortress of intellectualism, the audience would never glimpse her humanity. Her redemption would not be possible. Without that, the play would be an exercise in despair rather than the uplifting theatrical event that drew audiences night after night in New York and later in Boston, Washington, D.C., and other cities.

In this play doctors have only critical intelligence. The nurse has critical intelligence informed by emotional intelligence that allows her to understand her patient's needs. As a result, Pizzi has just received the second largest round of applause after that bestowed on Chalfant for her unforgettable depiction of the patient.

As the discussion resumes, Halperin's colleague, the oncologist, and several cancer patients in the audience recount their experiences with the impersonal world of high-tech medicine. For the next ten minutes, the subject of doctors and how they practice medicine holds center stage.

Finally, a physician in the audience challenges those on stage and in the audience to look at playwright Margaret Edson's work in a different way. "It seems to me this play is about the failure of abstract, critical intelligence," he says. "The only character who 'gets it' is the one who's supposedly not that sharp, and that's the nurse. Why are we focusing exclusively on the doctor-patient relationship when we should be looking at the nurse-patient relationship and what doctors can learn from nurses?"

As he speaks the audience erupts in spontaneous applause. More hands flash up. Behind him, an elderly woman, who turns out to be the widely known children's writer, Madeleine L'Engle, adds her emphatic agreement.

"The only healer in this drama is the nurse," she says. Others relate stories about the role nurses played when they or a loved one was seriously ill. Thanks to this exchange, the doctors begin to talk about what they can learn from caregiving and nursing.

Wit is a remarkable play. Margaret Edson, its author, is a public school kindergarten teacher in Atlanta, Georgia. The play, her first theatrical venture, was written after she left a job as a unit clerk in a research hospital.

"They were doing the first clinical trials of AZT for Kaposi's sarcoma. They were also working on a couple of different protocols for ovarian cancer and for non-Hodgkin's lymphoma," Edson tells us in an interview. "People came from all over the country to participate in these clinical trials. I thought the nurses were wonderful. They were so good at what they were doing. I admired the way they were able to express their compassion through skilled action. Like Susie, the nurse in the play, they were always doing something. Everyone in the audience is so moved that the nurse puts lotion on the dying patient's hands. But that's a typical nursing intervention."

What is also remarkable about this play is the way it captures the central dilemma of modern nursing: that nurses are given the awesome responsibility of caring for the sickest, most vulnerable human beings in our society without being given the commensurate authority and resources necessary to fulfill their mission. To cope with this untenable situation, the nurse in the play, like nurses in real life, is a kaleidoscope of strength and deference, courage and self-deprecation. She both manifests and conceals her intelligence and power. She is, like many real nurses, "afraid to speak up in routine situations but able to do so forcefully and courageously when they're really mad," Anne Schott of the New York State Nurses Association says after seeing the play.

In *Wit* the nurse finally gets really mad, and demonstrates real courage. But along the way, countless opportunities for self-assertion and agency are lost.

The health care problems prevalent in our society—aging, chronic illness, increased disability—are not those that medicine alone can remedy. They require the kind of intelligence the nurse in *Wit* displayed, the kind of intelligence nurses throughout North America and the world display everyday. But that kind of nursing care can only exist if we are willing to acknowledge that nursing intelligence is an *intelligence*, that nursing knowledge is *knowledge*, and that we must give nurses the authority and resources, both financial and emotional, that they need to do their work. Most of us won't do that unless nurses illuminate the knowledge and intelligence embedded in what can appear to be the most trivial, routine and basic nursing care.

We feel, as we conclude this book, that we have come full circle. We began our relationship with nurses during the nursing shortage of the late 1980s, when two visions of how to promote nursing competed for dominance. Many

RNs wanted to make visible the challenges and complexity of caring for the sick—the work that most nurses have done and always will do. They wanted to build a basic understanding and respect for hands-on nursing. Appreciation for nurses who do other work such as research, teaching, primary care, and management would depend on this foundation. They wanted to use mass communication to challenge conventional understandings of caregiving/women's work to improve significantly the conditions of that work. Then the best and the brightest would not flee the bedside or nursing.

Others favored a different approach. They wanted to downplay the traditional work of nurses as hands-on caregivers in order to highlight the work of those who appear to be more detached from the care of the body. Some nursing leaders tried to appeal to potential nursing students by emphasizing all the avenues that would lead nurses away from the care of the sick. We were told that the nursing degree could be a launching pad to a career as a nurse anthropologist, nurse historian, nurse attorney, or nurse entrepreneur. The message of this sales pitch is clear: Borrow the social legitimacy of another profession or occupation to hide the lack of status of nursing. In this approach, nursing is a career path not a career.

Today, nurses are again being driven from the profession, and many are discouraging others from entering it. This is because of deplorable work conditions stemming from underfunding of nursing in particular and health care in general. Once again, there is a question of approach. Is this an "image" or political problem? Does it require a short-term public relations campaign or a long-term, political and social struggle?

We don't think you can trick people into becoming nurses, or into valuing nurses. If our society does not understand what the core member of the profession does in her or his work in hospitals, clinics, nursing homes, schools, homes, and hospices, it cannot really value nursing, however "elevated" or "advanced." If we don't want to pay for the care of the sick and vulnerable, the aging and the dying, anyone with the word nurse in his or her professional title will ultimately be diminished by their connection to the sick, dependent and vulnerable.

Selling the nurse as anything but a nurse also sells the public short. In more than a decade of writing about nursing, we have been struck by how receptive people are to stories and presentations about the work of nurses. Like the audience at *Wit*, or the editor at the *Boston Globe* who remembered his teenage experience in a hospital, most people who have benefited from good nursing are supportive of nurses. When they learn about the things nurses put up with they are stunned. Even people who are deprived of a nurse's attention are often sympathetic to the burdens nurses bear when RNs explain the conditions imposed on their work. As political campaigns in Canada and the US have amply demonstrated, the public will fight for nurses and the resources to support quality patient care when nurses ask the public for help.

In this way, moving from silence to voice helps nurses and their patients, as Florence Nightingale herself concluded:

"If we were perfect, no doubt an absolute hierarchy would be the best kind of government for all institutions. But, in our imperfect state of conscience and enlightenment, publicity, and the collision resulting from publicity are the best guardians of the interests of the sick."[1]

Endnote

1. Lucy Ridgly Seymer, Ed., *Selected Writings of Florence Nightingale* (New York, Macmillan Publishing Co. Inc., 1954), pp. 222–223.

AFTERWORD

The media's portrayal of nurses is at the top of my mind as I reflect on the wisdom expressed by Suzanne Gordon and Bernice Buresh in *From Silence to Voice*. As I write this, in April 2000, I am struck by the strong contradictions we continue to witness in media reports about nursing and the public understanding of the profession. Yesterday, a friend called to congratulate me on my participation in a national radio interview. At a conference of the Canadian Association of Nurses in AIDS Care, where I was a speaker, my remarks on the reasons for, and impacts of, the current nursing shortage were reported as a national news story. I sensed that the media were finally beginning to recognize the negative impact on patient care that the Canadian Nurses Association has been trying to convey for the past two years. Here was good coverage of the role that nurses play in the health care system.

This positive coverage, however, appeared in stark contrast to a recent column in our national weekly news magazine, *Maclean's*. In her often-controversial column, writer Barbara Amiel referred to nurses as "increasingly loutish and indifferent" and stated: "In societies like ours, where people can find more congenial occupations (than nursing) pretty easily, intelligent and higher-quality people naturally choose less strenuous work—unless they are saintly." Amiel neglected to point out that it is not nursing work that is uncongenial. Rather our societal failure to appreciate and support that work is what makes it so difficult for good nurses to do good nursing.

Thankfully Barbara Amiel's column resulted in what the magazine's editors called an "email flood ... followed quickly by a torrent of faxes and mailed letters." Many of the quick responses were from nurses (including the CNA), and several appeared in the magazine the following week. But what was also needed were more letters from members of the public defending nursing and criticizing this failure of the media to correctly inform the public about nursing's important work.

CNA takes seriously the responsibility to present an accurate and compelling view of nursing to the public. We know that the image of the profession will only change with a concerted effort by all nurses, not just those who are active in associations and unions. While it is the unfortunate circumstance of an emerging shortage and recent labour unrest that has resulted in unprecedented media interest in nursing, we must take advantage of all opportunities to exercise our "voice of agency" and to keep exercising it.

CNA understands that the problems nurses confront are global, not just local, which is also why this book is important. It is a truly international look at the challenges nurses face when they try to communicate their work to the public. These challenges will only escalate as societies around the world deal with aging populations with an even greater burden of chronic illness. If we want to make sure that high quality, knowledgeable nursing care is adequately funded, and that nurses receive the reward, recognition and respect they deserve, communication with the public—not only with patients and families—has to be viewed as part of the nursing process.

The communication skills Buresh and Gordon give us in *From Silence To Voice* need to be taught to nurses from their first days in nursing education programs and then must be reinforced by health care institutions, professional organizations and unions throughout nurses' careers. We also have to be alert to the ways in which we ourselves may inadvertently acquiesce to or reinforce negative societal stereotypes. It isn't always comfortable to read about behaviours that Buresh and Gordon suggest contribute to our invisibility in the press and in the public debate about health care. Not always comfortable, but a very important exercise!

If we can confront our own cultural biases against visibility and voice we can learn to apply the practical tools that *From Silence to Voice* give us. This will allow us to more comfortably take our places on the public stage. Simplifying the often-daunting process of writing a press release or a letter to the editor, or telling us how to present ourselves before the television camera, this book is an excellent communication guide. Although I have spent many years doing media interviews, I picked up some excellent ideas from this book.

To make sure our health care systems stay healthy, nurses around the world have a responsibility to speak out. Bernice and Suzanne help to show us how.

Mary Ellen Jeans, RN, PhD
Executive Director, Canadian Nurses Association

INDEX